Cell Culture in the Neurosciences

CURRENT TOPICS IN NEUROBIOLOGY

Series Editor

Samuel H. Barondes
Professor of Psychiatry
School of Medicine
University of California, San Diego
La Jolla, California

Tissue Culture of the Nervous System
Edited by Gordon Sato

Neuronal Recognition
Edited by Samuel H. Barondes

Peptides in Neurobiology
Edited by Harold Gainer

Neuronal Development
Edited by Nicholas C. Spitzer

Neuroimmunology
Edited by Jeremy Brockes

Cell Culture in the Neurosciences
Edited by Jane E. Bottenstein and Gordon Sato

A continuation Order Plan is available for this series. A continuation order will bring delivery of each new volume immediatedly upon publication. Volumes are billed only upon actual shipment. For further information please contact the publisher.

Cell Culture
in the
Neurosciences

Edited by

JANE E. BOTTENSTEIN

The Marine Biomedical Institute and
Department of Human Biological Chemistry and Genetics
The University of Texas Medical Branch at Galveston
Galveston, Texas

and

GORDON SATO

W. Alton Jones Cell Science Center, Inc.
Lake Placid, New York

Plenum Press • New York and London

Library of Congress Cataloging in Publication Data

Main entry under title:

Cell culture in the neurosciences.

  (Current topics in neurobiology)
  Includes bibliographies and index.
  1. Neurons. 2. Cell culture. I. Bottenstein, Jane E. II. Sato, Gordon. III. Series. [DNLM: 1.
Cells, Cultured. 2. Electrophysiology. 3. Neurons—cytology. 4. Neurons—physiology.
WL 102.5 C3924]
QP356.C45   1985   599'.0188   85-3435
ISBN 0-306-41942-4

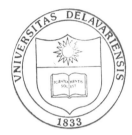

©1985 Plenum Press, New York
A Division of Plenum Publishing Corporation
233 Spring Street, New York, N.Y. 10013

Printed in the United States of America

Contributors

JEFFERY L. BARKER   Laboratory of Neurophysiology
National Institute of Neurological and
     Communicative Disorders and Stroke
National Institutes of Health
Bethesda, Maryland

JANE E. BOTTENSTEIN   Marine Biomedical Institute and
Department of Human Biological
     Chemistry and Genetics
University of Texas Medical Branch
Galveston, Texas

DOUGLAS E. BRENNEMAN   Laboratory of Developmental
     Neurobiology
National Institutes of Health
Bethesda, Maryland

MICHEL DARMON   Unité de Génétique Cellulaire
Institut Pasteur
Paris, France
     and
Département de Biologie Cellulaire
Centre International de Recherches
     Dermatologiques Sophia Antipolis
Valbonne, France

JEAN DE VELLIS   Departments of Anatomy and Psychiatry
                         UCLA School of Medicine and
                         Mental Retardation Research Center
                         Laboratory of Biomedical and
                             Environmental Sciences
                         University of California
                         Los Angeles, California

BERNARD EDDÉ   Unité de Génétique Cellulaire
                         Institut Pasteur
                         Paris, France
                                     and
                         Laboratoire de Biochimie Cellulaire
                         Collège de France
                         Paris, France

KAY FIELDS   Departments of Neurology and
                             Neuroscience
                         Albert Einstein College of Medicine
                         Bronx, New York

GORDON GUROFF   Section on Growth Factors
                         National Institute of Child Health and
                             Human Development
                         National Institutes of Health
                         Bethesda, Maryland

PAUL HONEGGER   Institute of Physiology
                         University of Lausanne
                         Lausanne, Switzerland

LI-YEN MAE HUANG   Marine Biomedical Institute and
                         Department of Physiology and Biophysics
                         University of Texas Medical Branch
                         Galveston, Texas

STORY C. LANDIS   Department of Neurobiology
                         Harvard Medical School
                         Boston, Massachusetts

PHILLIP G. NELSON   Laboratory of Developmental
                             Neurobiology
                         National Institutes of Health
                         Bethesda, Maryland

J. Regino Perez-Polo — Department of Human Biological Chemistry and Genetics, University of Texas Medical Branch, Galveston, Texas

Russell P. Saneto — Departments of Anatomy and Psychiatry, UCLA School of Medicine and Mental Retardation Research Center, Laboratory of Biomedical and Environmental Sciences, University of California, Los Angeles, California

Fritz Sieber — Department of Medicine, The Johns Hopkins University School of Medicine, Baltimore, Maryland

Maya Sieber-Blum — Department of Cell Biology and Anatomy, The Johns Hopkins University School of Medicine, Baltimore, Maryland

Thomas G. Smith, Jr. — Laboratory of Neurophysiology, National Institute of Neurological and Communicative Disorders and Stroke, National Institutes of Health, Bethesda, Maryland

Preface

A fundamental problem in neuroscience is the elucidation of the cellular and molecular mechanisms underlying the development and function of the nervous system. The complexity of organization, the heterogeneity of cell types and their interactions, and the difficulty of controlling experimental variables in intact organisms make this a formidable task. Because of the ability that it affords to analyze smaller components of the nervous system (even single cells in some cases) and to better control experimental variables, cell culture has become an increasingly valuable tool for neuroscientists. Many aspects of neural development, such as proliferation, differentiation, synaptogenesis, and myelination, occur in culture with time courses remarkably similar to those *in vivo*. Thus, *in vitro* methods often provide excellent model systems for investigating neurobiological questions.

Ross Harrison described the first culture of neural tissue in 1907 and used morphological methods to analyze the cultures. Since that time the technique has been progressively modified and used to address an ever widening range of developmental questions. In recent years a convergence of new or improved cell culture, biochemical, electrophysiological, and immunological methods has occurred and been brought to bear on neurobiological questions. This volume is intended not to be comprehensive but rather to highlight some of the latest findings, with a review of previous important work as well, in which combinations of these methods are used. The chapters cover a broad range of topics, but they can be divided into two major sections: (1) morphological and biochemical studies and (2) electrophysiological studies. All of the authors have made significant contributions in their respective areas of research.

The section on morphological and biochemical studies comprises nine chapters. The chapter by Bottenstein briefly describes the different types of culture preparations, the major components of a culture system, and, in more detail, the study of the molecular requirements for growth of cultured neurons and glial cells using serum-free methods. The importance of soluble and extracellular matrix factors and the cell type-specificity of these requirements are described. Fields reviews the antigenic markers presently available that have proven so useful for unambiguously identifying the different neural cell types *in vitro*. She describes neural cell surface antigens, including a discussion of their use in perturbing cellular function and in cell separation. Both polyclonal and the newer monoclonal antibodies are described, some of which discriminate between subpopulations of neurons and glial cells. Perez-Polo describes the discovery of nerve growth factor and other more recent neuronotrophic factors and their importance in neuronal survival, differentiation, and possibly regeneration. He discusses the benefits of using clonal cell lines for studying the responses to neuronotrophic factors. The chapter by Saneto and de Vellis covers the area of hormonal regulation of the proliferation and differentiation of primary CNS glial cells. They emphasize the advantages of using isolated populations of cells for studying these phenomena. Landis describes the classic experiments which first demonstrated the plasticity of the neurotransmitter phenotype in superior cervical ganglion cells in response to epigenetic regulation. Analysis at the single-cell level provides evidence for a transition from noradrenergic to cholinergic function, with an intermediate dual-function stage, as a result of interaction with target cells. The ability to distinguish induction from selection for already committed cells is only possible using *in vitro* methods. She also correlates the *in vitro* results with *in vivo* data, including electron microscopic analysis. Sieber-Blum and Sieber discuss the influence of soluble factors and the extracellular matrix on the migration and differentiation of neural crest cells. Clonal cultures of neural crest cells indicate that differentiation into melanocytes and adrenergic neurons can occur in the absence of noncrest cells, contrary to a widely accepted belief. Honegger's biochemical studies of reaggregate cultures of fetal rat brain, containing a mixture of cell types, illustrate the influence of several growth factors and hormones on both neuronal and glial differentiation. The effects on cholinergic neurons are described in the greatest detail. Serum-free culture methods provide a significant improvement for analyzing these phenomena. Guroff compares the properties of the PC12 clonal cell line with adrenal chromaffin cells and sympathetic neurons. He concludes that PC12 cells are an excellent model system for studying the mechanism of action of nerve growth factor and some aspects of neuronal differentiation, e.g., neurite extension and synapse formation. The chapter by Eddé and Darmon reviews the work of several groups investigating neuronal differentiation in embryonal carcinoma cells, which are multipotential stem cells able to give rise to derivatives of all three germ layers. When these cells differentiate, they are no longer tumorigenic and thus provide a unique model system. The authors describe several inducers of neuronal differentiation.

The section on electrophysiological studies comprises three chapters. The role of electrical activity in modulating neuronal survival and cholinergic differentiation in fetal mouse spinal cord neurons is discussed by Brenneman and Nelson. Blockade of electrical activity results in decreased survival and expression of cholinergic function. They also defined the critical period and suggested that electrical activity releases trophic factors that mediate the effects seen. Smith and Barker give a general introduction to classical electrophysiological techniques, i.e., intracellular stimulation and recording. They describe the underlying ionic mechanisms of neurotransmitter-mediated inhibitory and excitatory postsynaptic potentials in embryonic spinal cord and hippocampal neurons in culture. Quantitative analyses, including the use of voltage-clamping, can be made with cultured neurons that are difficult if not impossible to apply to CNS neurons *in vivo*. The more recent development of the patch-clamp method is discussed by Huang. Further biophysical analysis of single ion channels and their regulation, including aggregation of channels, is now possible using cultured neurons. Conventional neurotransmitter-activated and voltage-sensitive channels are described, as is the discovery of several new species of channels.

The authors have used a variety of preparations and asked many different questions. They have described the advantages and the limitations of their respective preparations and have given us a preview of future directions. Many of the experiments described here illustrate the individuality of growth and differentiation requirements of different neural cell types and their enormous plasticity during development in response to environmental influences. While cell culture is not the only or necessarily the best method to study a particular neurobiological question, this volume contains some of the best examples of when cell culture can be most profitably employed in neuroscience.

Jane E. Bottenstein
Gordon Sato

Galveston, Texas
Lake Placid, New York

Contents

3. Neuronotrophic Factors
J. REGINO PEREZ-POLO

6. *In Vitro* Analysis of Quail Neural Crest Cell Differentiation
   MAYA SIEBER-BLUM AND FRITZ SIEBER

7. Biochemical Differentiation in Serum-Free Aggregating
   Brain Cell Cultures
   PAUL HONEGGER

8. PC12 Cells as a Model of Neuronal Differentiation
GORDON GUROFF

9. Neural Differentiation of Pluripotent Embryonal Carcinoma Cells
   BERNARD EDDÉ AND MICHEL DARMON

II. Electrophysiology

10. Neuronal Development in Culture: Role of Electrical Activity
    DOUGLAS E. BRENNEMAN AND PHILLIP G. NELSON

I
Morphology and Biochemistry

1

Growth and Differentiation of Neural Cells in Defined Media

JANE E. BOTTENSTEIN

1. INTRODUCTION

The anatomical, physiological, and biochemical complexity of mammalian nervous systems is greater than that in other tissues and presents a formidable barrier to elucidating the cellular and molecular mechanisms involved in the development of these systems. Not only are there an abundance of complex cellular phenotypes, but the interactions of neural cells are exceedingly complex. One approach to this problem is to use culture methods in an attempt to simplify and control experimental variables.

There are two basic types of cell culture: (1) primary culture in which tissue is removed from an organism, placed in a culture vessel in an appropriate fluid medium, and has a finite lifetime (up to many months); and (2) continuous cell lines which proliferate and can thus be subcultured, i.e., passaged repeatedly into new culture vessels. The latter cells can also be stored for long periods of time in the frozen state in the vapor phase of liquid nitrogen when a cryopreservative is present, e.g., 10% dimethylsulfoxide or glycerol. In primary culture, small portions of a nervous system can be analyzed in isolation and systemic influences

JANE E. BOTTENSTEIN • Marine Biomedical Institute and Department of Human Biological Chemistry and Genetics, University of Texas Medical Branch, Galveston, Texas 77550.

are eliminated. Three-dimensional fragments or explants of neural tissue, restricted to 1 mm^3 or less because of diffusion limitations, are used to study discrete areas of the peripheral or central nervous system. Cytoarchitectural integrity, and thus the original cell–cell interactions, is best preserved with explant cultures. On the other hand, two-dimensional dissociated cell cultures permit visualization of individual cells which facilitates morphological and electrophysiological studies. The latter cultures contain a mixed population of cell types. It is often desirable to study the different cell types in isolation from each other; and it is possible to obtain populations of cells enriched for specific cell types, i.e., neurons, astrocytes, Schwann cells, or oligodendrocytes, by a variety of methods (Wood, 1976; Varon, 1977; Dvorak *et al.*, 1978; Schengrund and Repman, 1979; Bhat *et al.*, 1981; Meier *et al.*, 1982; Abney *et al.*, 1983). It is useful to obtain neuron-enriched cultures, for neurons rarely divide in culture whereas nonneurons (which may include glial cells, macrophages, endothelial cells, meningeal cells, and fibroblasts) may proliferate extensively and overgrow the cultures. Mitotic inhibitors, e.g., cytosine arabinoside or fluorodeoxyuridine, have been used to suppress nonneuronal proliferation. The investigation of cell–cell interactions is facilitated by comparing cultures of an isolated or enriched cell type with recombined cultures of different cell types. Alternatively, dissociated primary cells can be grown in suspension cultures, in which gentle agitation prevents their adhering to the culture vessel surface and promotes the formation of three-dimensional cellular reaggregates. This is followed by sorting out of the cells within the aggregates, reconstruction of their histotypic cellular organization, and normal expression of many biochemical and physiological neural properties (Seeds, 1983). Overgrowth by nonneuronal cells does not occur in reaggregate cultures as it can in monolayer cultures of primary cells. Continuous cell lines derived from normal or tumorigenic tissue (i.e., neuroblastoma, glioma, or pheochromocytoma) have the additional benefit of the ability to generate large numbers of cells in a short period of time for biochemical analyses. Cells that divide can often be cloned and are also useful for selecting mutants and variants. Some of these continuous cell lines are diploid and genetically stable, while others are not. Somatic cell hybrids, formed from the fusion of two different cells, have created a number of interesting cell lines, some of which have differentiated properties not found in either parent (Bottenstein, 1981b). Thus, each type of preparation has its advantages and also its particular limitations.

All of these preparations, however, have the common advantage of the ability to limit and control extrinsic factors that may influence cellular survival, growth, proliferation, and/or differentiation. Manipulations of the culture medium, substratum, gaseous environment, and other parameters are easily varied *in vitro*. These methods are useful in the cellular and molecular analyses of a wide spectrum of neurobiological questions, e.g., regulation of neurogenesis and gliogenesis, cell–cell interactions, trophic factors, neuronal and glial membrane properties, formation of synapses, determination of neurotransmitter phenotype, and regulation of myelination. Clearly, the microenvironment of neural cells (neurons and glial cells) plays a key role in the expression and modulation of these properties. In particular, culture methods are useful for studying early stages of neural development, since the embryonic mammalian nervous system is not readily accessible to experimental modification.

Ross Harrison (1907, 1910) first demonstrated the feasibility of culturing neural cells. He was able to maintain frog neural tube explants in frog lymph. Conventional culture techniques now involve plating explants, dissociated cells, or continuous cell lines into tissue culture vessels containing a basal synthetic medium supplemented with undefined biological fluids derived from a variety of species and developmental stages, e.g., serum, plasma, embryo extract, or combinations thereof. Modification of culture surfaces with collagen or polylysine coating is often employed for neural cultures. The variability, complexity, and undefined nature of these biological fluids are well-recognized problems, but only recently have serum-free defined culture conditions been described for neural cells (Bottenstein, 1983a,b). It has become increasingly apparent that more defined conditions and further refinements in culture methodology are necessary to enhance the yield of information derived from *in vitro* studies of the nervous system. Recognition of cell type- and developmental stage-specific requirements for maintaining neural cells in culture and the development of a broader range of culture conditions are required. In order to accomplish this, we need to (1) identify additional molecules that influence survival, cell division, differentiation, and both homotypic and heterotypic cell–cell interactions and to (2) further characterize some molecules already identified to have these influences. These regulatory molecules may be integral to plasma membranes, of extracellular matrix origin, or soluble in nature. In addition, some of the difficulties in culturing and sustaining dividing neuroblasts, oligodendrocytes, or adult neural tissue in primary cultures, for example, may be due in part to deficiencies in the culture methods. This has been shown for other cell types, e.g., thyroid cells (Ambesi-Impiombato *et al.*, 1980) and adult hepatocytes (Enat *et al.*, 1984).

This chapter will briefly review the major components of a culture system and in more detail our investigation of the molecular growth requirements of cultured neurons (Bottenstein and Sato, 1979, 1980; Bottenstein *et al.*, 1980; Darmon *et al.*, 1981; Bottenstein, 1984a) and glial cells (Michler-Stuke and Bottenstein, 1982a,b; Michler-Stuke *et al.*, 1984) using serum-free methods. The elimination of undefined substances, such as serum, from the culture system removes their possible inhibitory or interfering action, and it both simplifies the interpretation of experimental results and improves their reproducibility. The importance of developing optimal culture methods to better approximate *in vivo* conditions, where cells do not normally encounter the biological fluids used in conventional culture techniques, is emphasized. The strategy employed in defining the growth requirements for neural cells *in vitro* was to first analyze the requirements for growth of continuous neural cell lines (neuroblastomas, gliomas, or somatic cell hybrids). It was hypothesized that their growth requirements would reflect those of their cellular origin, and that the normal cell counterparts might well have additional requirements, since tumor cells often produce growth factors (Todaro, 1982) that are autostimulatory.

2. COMPONENTS OF THE CULTURE SYSTEM

2.1. Synthetic Medium and Supplements

A number of synthetic basal media are commercially available. They differ in their content of amino acids, vitamins, inorganic salts, buffering agents, and energy source (Bottenstein, 1983a). The pH of the medium markedly affects growth rates, neurite formation, and enzyme activities in neural cultures, with optimal expression attained within a narrow range of pH values (Bear and Schneider, 1976; Olson and Holtzman, 1981; Bottenstein, 1983a). Neural cultures are generally maintained at pH 7.2–7.6 and must also have the appropriate osmolarity. Most of the basal media were designed to support the continued proliferation of nonneural continuous cell lines, and are thus not optimized for neural cells and may be least suitable for postmitotic neurons. A higher requirement for glucose appears to be necessary for both neuron survival and optimal myelination (Bottenstein, 1983a). Basal media differ in their survival- or growth- and differentiation-promoting abilities. For example, dissociated fetal rat brain cells proliferate better in Dulbecco's modified Eagle's medium (DME) but have higher choline acetyltransferase (CAT) activity in Ham's F12 medium (Shapiro and Schrier, 1973); a human glial (Michler-Stuke and Bottenstein, 1982a) and a rat pheochromocytoma cell line (Bottenstein, 1984a) both exhibit markedly better proliferation in DME than in F12 medium; and fetal mouse brain reaggregation and subsequent biochemical differentiation depend greatly on the basal medium used for culture (Seeds, 1983).

Most neural cells will not survive for long in a viable condition or divide in synthetic medium alone and require further supplementation to permit long-term culture. Nerve growth factor (NGF) is required for embryonic dorsal root and sympathetic ganglionic neurons in culture, but thus far no NGF requirement has been demonstrated for CNS-derived neurons *in vitro* (Coyle *et al.*, 1973; Shoemaker *et al.*, 1979; Dreyfus *et al.*, 1980). Conventional culture methods generally supplement medium with biological fluids, such as serum, plasma, or embryo extract. These largely undefined fluids contain variable amounts of hormones, growth factors, transport proteins, substratum-modifying factors, vitamins, trace elements, and other unknown factors. Thyroid hormone, growth hormone, steroid hormones, and insulin are known to be present in biological fluids and have significant effects on the development of the nervous system, as shown in studies *in vivo* and *in vitro* (Lissack, 1971; MacLusky and Clark, 1980). The survival- or growth-promoting properties of these biological fluids vary between batches, and factors inhibitory to growth or differentiation may also be present. Experimental reproducibility can be significantly affected by the variability of these fluids, and their complexity and largely undefined nature complicate the analysis of the results obtained. Ideally, we need to establish culture conditions that more closely approximate the *in vivo* environment of neural cells, which do not normally come in contact with these fluids.

2.2. Substratum

In addition to interactions with soluble factors, most cells in vertebrate organisms are in contact with an extracellular matrix (ECM), a complex arrangement of interactive protein and polysaccharide molecules which are secreted locally and assemble into an intricate network in the spaces between cells. Hydrogen bonds, disulfide linkages, and other covalent bonds are important in maintaining the organization of the ECM. The major classes of ECM molecules are collagens, glycosaminoglycans (GAG), proteoglycans, and glycoproteins (e.g., fibronectin, laminin, entactin, and hyaluronectin). Laminin is the first ECM protein to appear during embryogenesis (Timpl *et al.*, 1983); it is present as early as the eight-cell stage (Wu *et al.*, 1983). Collagen type IV (Leivo *et al.*, 1980) and entactin (Wu *et al.*, 1983) appear several days after laminin in the mouse blastocyst. Fibronectin is also detected early in embryogenesis (Duband and Thiery, 1982); and cells in all three germ layers synthesize it (Hynes and Yamada, 1982). Hyaluronectin binds specifically to hyaluronic acid *in vitro* and first appears in the mesenchyme bordering the neural tube and somites in 10-day-old rat embryos (Delpech and Delpech, 1984). In the mature nervous system it is found at the nodes of Ranvier in PNS and CNS tissue and surrounding about 10% of neurons (Delpech *et al.*, 1982). Oligodendrocytes of newborn rat brains, but not astrocytes, stain with antihyaluronectin (Asou *et al.*, 1983). The ectodermal ECM of early neural-fold rat embryos contains the GAGs hyaluronic acid and chondroitin sulfates primarily (Morriss and Solursh, 1978). A common pattern of GAGs exists in the brains of a variety of vertebrate species, including rat and man (Singh *et al.*, 1969). Hyaluronic acid comprises 63% of the total GAGs in spinal cord and peripheral nerve and 41% in brain. The next most abundant GAG in the nervous system is chondroitin-4-sulfate, followed by heparan sulfate. Both heparan sulfate and chondroitin-6-sulfate levels are lower in spinal cord and peripheral nerve than in brain. *In vitro*, collagen is synthesized by embryonic chick spinal cord epithelium (Trelstad *et al.*, 1973), and laminin is produced by both mouse neuroblastoma (Alitalo *et al.*, 1980, 1982) and Schwann cells (Cornbrooks *et al.*, 1983). Although embryonic rat astrocytes produce laminin *in vitro* (Liesi *et al.*, 1983), this glycoprotein is not found in the adult CNS (Wan *et al.*, 1984). Fibronectin appears to be produced by brain fibroblasts but not neurons or glial cells (Schachner *et al.*, 1978; Raff *et al.*, 1979). It is now generally accepted that ECMs play a dynamic role in the regulation of cellular adhesion, proliferation, migration, cytodifferentiation, and morphogenesis. More recently, studies of the involvement of ECM in neural development have appeared (Toole, 1976; Sanes, 1983).

Neural cells in culture adhere to a substratum which corresponds to the ECM *in vivo*. Most *in vitro* studies use enzymatic treatment to dissociate cells in primary tissue or to remove cells from the culture surface during a subculture, and this procedure alters or removes the ECM. Thus, subcultured cells must be provided an exogenous matrix or be able to readily reconstruct a functional one. The original use of glass culture vessels was superseded in about 1965 by polystyrene vessels chemically treated to favor cell attachment (Curtis *et al.*, 1983). In addition, vessel surfaces are often coated with collagen (Bornstein, 1958; Iversen *et al.*, 1981) or polylysine (Yavin and Yavin, 1974; Sensenbrenner *et al.*, 1978; Bottenstein and Sato, 1980; Michler-Stuke and Bottenstein, 1982a,b; Michler-Stuke *et al.*, 1984). More recently, fibronectin has been used to modify the culture surface (Bottenstein and Sato, 1980; Michler-Stuke and Bottenstein, 1982a,b; Michler-Stuke *et al.*, 1984). Adsorption of fibronectin to the culture surface is necessary to acquire its affinity for cell surface receptors (Pearlstein, 1978). It may be added to culture medium before the cell inoculum instead of precoating dishes. Undefined medium supplements, such as serum or embryo extract, also contribute molecules, including fibronectin, which adhere to the culture surface. Fibronectin enhances the growth of neuroblastoma cells (Bottenstein, 1983a), established glial cell lines (Michler-Stuke and Bottenstein, 1982a), astrocytes (Michler-Stuke *et al.*, 1984), and Schwann cells (Baron-Van Evercooren *et al.*, 1982a). Fibronectin also influences the neurotransmitter phenotype of neural crest cells *in vitro* (see Chapter 6) and their migration (Rovasio *et al.*, 1983). Both fibronectin and polylysine influence neurite formation and orientation (Akers *et al.*, 1981). Laminin enhances the growth of processes of human fetal sensory neurons *in vitro* more than does fibronectin or collagen, and antibodies directed against laminin suppress all neurite growth (Baron-Van Evercooren *et al.*, 1982b). Neurite elongation is also enhanced by laminin—compared to fetal calf serum-coated substrata in cultures of fetal hypothalamic neurons maintained in a defined medium (Faivre-Bauman *et al.*, 1984).

Cells *in vitro* are able to synthesize ECM molecules and secrete them to form an insoluble matrix on the culture vessel surface. Cell-derived ECMs can be prepared by removing cells with detergents or a calcium chelator, and homotypic or heterotypic cells may then be plated on such surfaces (Gospodarowicz *et al.*, 1980; Michler-Stuke and Bottenstein, 1981). An exogenous ECM provided to cultured cells may modulate the expression of ECM molecules produced by the cells themselves (Tseng *et al.*, 1983). Several soluble factors also influence the synthesis of ECM molecules. Ascorbate, for example, is required for optimal collagen production (Murad *et al.*, 1981) but has no effect on laminin synthesis (Prehm *et al.*, 1982). Other soluble factors that affect the expression of ECM molecules in a variety of cell types include insulin (Stevens *et al.*, 1981; Foley *et al.*, 1982; Risteli *et al.*, 1982), somatomedins (Stevens *et al.*, 1981; Nevo, 1982), glucocorticoids (Heifetz and Snyder, 1981; Baumann and Eldredge, 1982), epidermal growth factor (EGF) (Lembach, 1976; Chen *et al.*, 1977), retinoids (Shapiro and Mott, 1981), GAGs (Meier and Hay, 1974), and fibroblast growth factor (FGF) (Tseng *et al.*, 1982). In addition, the type of basal medium (Nathanson, 1983) and the pH (Lie *et al.*, 1972; Nigra *et al.*, 1973) influence the ECM profile.

In the last few years our knowledge of the chemical composition of different ECMs has increased, although the mechanism of their assembly into functional matrices is not known. It is difficult to interpret studies that purport to modify or interfere with one component of the ECM, since it is probably the three-dimensional structure, created by the interaction of the various matrix molecules, that confers its bioactivity. Furthermore, multiple interactions occur between the ECM and the cell surface. For example, fibronectin appears to interact with microfilament bundles across the plasma membrane (Hynes, 1981). The cell–substratum interaction influences the shape of cells, which has been shown to be tightly coupled to DNA synthesis and proliferation of endothelial cells (Folkman and Moscona, 1978). The substratum has also been shown to modulate the responses of cells to hormones and growth factors (Bottenstein and Sato, 1980; Michler-Stuke and Bottenstein, 1981; Salomon *et al.*, 1981; Gospodarowicz, 1983; Gatmaitan *et al.*, 1983; Michler-Stuke *et al.*, 1984).

2.3. Gaseous Environment

Cultured cells are usually maintained in a carbon dioxide/air mixture or air alone, depending on the buffering system. The former is more widely used, since carbon dioxide/bicarbonate is the natural buffering system in the blood. Cells are usually equilibrated with 5% carbon dioxide/95% air with the appropriate amount of sodium bicarbonate in the culture medium. Nonvolatile organic buffers (Good *et al.*, 1966), such as HEPES, or basic amino acid and phosphate buffers (Leibowitz, 1963) do not require equilibration with carbon dioxide. Neural cells have a high oxygen requirement relative to other cell types (Hudspeth *et al.*, 1950). Oxygen is an essential metabolic requirement, and the amount dissolved in the culture medium must be sufficient for normal cellular function. Air contains approximately 18% O_2. Dissociated cells are more sensitive to high oxygen levels than explant cultures. Mouse neuroblastoma cells markedly increase their oxygen uptake at the onset of differentiation (Nissen *et al.*, 1973). A systematic study of the influence of various gases on neural cell growth and differentiation has not been undertaken. However, studies with mammalian fibroblasts indicate that clonal or sparse growth is increased when oxygen concentrations are lowered to 1–3%; and this is the result of increased proliferation rather than more efficient attachment or survival (Taylor *et al.*, 1978).

3. SERUM-FREE DEFINED MEDIA FOR NEURONAL CELLS

3.1. Neuronal Cell Lines

We have demonstrated that undefined biological fluids can be replaced by defined supplements for many neuronal cell lines (Bottenstein, 1983a, 1984a). Our strategy has been to replace biological fluids with purified molecules, which include hormones, growth factors, trans-

Table I. Defined Medium Supplements for Neuronal Cells[a]

Supplement	N1	N2	N3
Insulin	5 µg/ml	5 µg/ml	5 µg/ml
Transferrin	5 µg/ml	100 µg/ml	50 µg/ml
Progesterone	20 nM	20 nM	20 nM
Putrescine	100 µM	100 µM	100 µM
Selenium	30 nM	30 nM	30 nM

[a] Supplements are added to basal medium in concentrated form. Values shown are the final concentrations.

port proteins, trace elements, vitamins, and substratum-modifying factors. We began these studies with the B104 rat CNS neuroblastoma. After a long series of experiments we found that serum could be replaced by adding these soluble factors to a 1:1 mixture of Ham's F12 (F12) and DME: human transferrin, bovine insulin, sodium selenite, progesterone, and putrescine (Bottenstein and Sato, 1979). Initially, cells were plated into serum-containing medium, and after 18 hr and extensive washing of the cells it was replaced with medium containing the defined supplements (N2 medium; Table I). Only two of the defined supplements had any effect by themselves, transferrin and insulin, whereas the combination of five supplements had a highly synergistic growth-stimulating effect (Table II). Deletion of any single supplement results in markedly diminished growth (Bottenstein, 1980). A typical growth curve for B104 cells is shown in Fig. 1. The cells fare poorly in basal medium without supplementation and eventually die. The population doubling time in serum-containing medium is about 75% of that in N2 medium, and final cell densities are equivalent. B104 cells show enhanced morphological

Table II. Response of B104 Cells to Individual Growth Stimulants[a]

Treatment	Cells/60-mm dish $\times$ 10^{-5}	Relative increase
No addition	0.64 ± 0.02	1.0
Insulin, 5 µg/ml	1.34 ± 0.04	2.1
Transferrin, 100 µg/ml	1.90 ± 0.05	3.0
Progesterone, 20 nM	0.65 ± 0.02	1.0
Selenium, 30 nM	0.62 ± 0.06	1.0
Putrescine, 100 µM	0.76 ± 0.04	1.2
All (N2)	16.36 ± 0.09	25.6

[a] Additions were made to serum-free Ham's F12 and Dulbecco's modified Eagle's medium (1:1); cells were counted on day 5. Values are expressed as the mean ± S.D. of triplicate cultures.

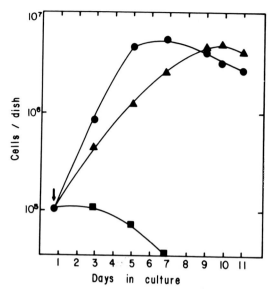

Figure 1. Growth curve for B104 rat neuroblastoma cells. ■, basal medium alone; ▲, N2 medium; ●, basal medium and 10% fetal calf serum. Arrow indicates end of serum preincubation period. (From Bottenstein and Sato, 1979.)

differentiation in N2 medium, and express action potentials and CAT activity comparable to their serum-grown counterparts. We were later able to eliminate the necessity for serum when plating the cells by precoating the culture dishes with poly-D-lysine and adding fibronectin to the culture medium (Bottenstein and Sato, 1980). It is not necessary to precoat the dishes with fibronectin, since fibronectin rapidly adheres to the culture surface and is added prior to the inoculum of cells. Both polylysine precoating and fibronectin are required to obtain proliferation of B104 cells in defined medium. Each has an effect by itself, but a synergistic effect is obtained with simultaneous treatment (Table III). There is no response to the soluble defined supplements unless the substratum is modified. Figure 2 shows the morphology of B104 cells in serum-containing medium and in N2 medium (after more than 50 population doublings and 6 subcultures in the absence of serum). N2 medium is more favorable for the expression of neurites, which are longer, contain varicosities, and exhibit growth cones. Clonal growth, i.e., low density, is supported by N2 medium as well as serial subculturing, and B104 cells can also be viably stored in liquid nitrogen vapor for extended periods of time in N2 medium containing 10% dimethylsulfoxide or glycerol (cryoprotective agents).

Table III. Effect of Substratum Modification on Growth of Trypsin-Detached B104 Cells in Serum-Free Medium[a]

Substratum modification	Medium	Relative increase
None (control)	Basal	1.0
None	N2	1.4
Fibronectin, 10 μg/ml	N2	2.8
Fibronectin precoat	N2	2.5
Polylysine, 25 ng/ml	N2	1.3
Polylysine precoat	N2	2.9
Fibronectin precoat + polylysine	N2	2.4
Fibronectin precoat followed by polylysine precoat	N2	8.6
Polylysine + fibronectin	N2	3.4
Polylysine precoat + fibronectin	N2	10.4

[a] Inoculum was 20,000 cells/35-mm dish. Data from duplicate cultures were averaged and are expressed as the relative increase in cell number over the mean of control cultures after 4 days. Control cell number was 15,100. (Adapted from Bottenstein and Sato, 1980.)

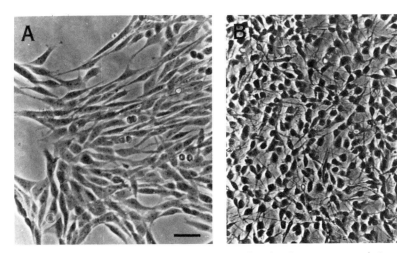

Figure 2. Phase-contrast micrographs of B104 cells after long-term growth in various media. (A) Stock culture maintained in serum-containing medium; (B) cells maintained on a polylysine-precoated dish with 10 μg/ml fibronectin added to N2 medium. Medium was changed every 5 days without readdition of fibronectin. Bar = 50 μm. (From Bottenstein and Sato, 1980.)

Table IV. Defined Medium for Growth of Neuronal Cell Lines[a]

Cell line	Origin	Basal medium	Supplement	Reference[b]
B104	Rat CNS neuroblastoma	DME/F12	N2	1–3
N1E-115	Mouse PNS neuroblastoma	DME/F12	N1	2, 4
NS20	Mouse PNS neuroblastoma	DME/F12	N1	2
LA-N-1	Human PNS neuroblastoma	DME/F12	N3	5
CHP 134	Human PNS neuroblastoma	DME/F12	N2	6
PC12	Rat pheochromocytoma	DME	N1	2
NX31	Mouse sympathetic ganglionic neuron × mouse PNS neuroblastoma	DME/F12	N1	7

[a] N1, N2, and N3 supplements and final concentrations are shown in Table I. All of these cell lines can be grown in defined medium on a polylysine- and fibronectin-modified substratum. Abbreviations: DME, Dulbecco's modified Eagle's medium; F12, Ham's F12 medium; DME/F12, 1:1 mixture of DME and F12. (From Bottenstein, 1984a.)

[b] 1, Bottenstein and Sato (1979); 2, Bottenstein *et al.* (1979); 3, Bottenstein and Sato (1980); 4, Bottenstein (1981b); 5, Bottenstein (1980); 6, Bottenstein (1981a); 7, Bottenstein (1983a).

A variety of other neuronal cell lines from the PNS of several different species and a pheochromocytoma cell line that can express neuronal properties are all able to proliferate in N1,N2, or N3 medium (Table IV). Some will grow in defined media with lower concentrations of transferrin (N1 or N3 medium; Bottenstein, 1983a, 1984a) than are required by B104 cells. One cell line (PC12) prefers DME medium to the 1:1 mixture of F12 and DME medium. Figure 3 shows phase-contrast micrographs of several of these cell lines growing in N2 medium. In all cases neurite extension is enhanced compared to their serum-grown counterparts. In the case of PC12 cells, when grown in serum they require NGF to extend neurites, whereas in N2 medium it is not required. Thus, N2 medium does not appear to have species-specificity, although the optimal concentrations of transferrin required do differ, and it satisfies the growth requirements of neuronal cell lines derived from both the CNS and the PNS. However, N2 medium does appear to be cell type-specific, since it does not support the continuous division of the glial, fibroblast, and skeletal muscle cell lines tested (Bottenstein, 1983a).

3.2. Primary Neurons

In addition to supplying the growth requirements of neuronal cell lines, the same defined supplements support the survival of a variety of postmitotic neurons in both PNS and CNS cultures (Bottenstein, 1983a,b). We first tested N1 supplements in DME medium on 19-day

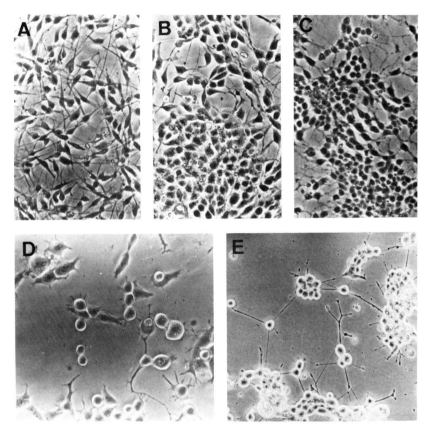

Figure 3. Morphology of neuronal cell lines grown in N2 medium. (A) B104 rat CNS neuroblastoma cells 7 days after plating on a polylysine- and fibronectin-modified substratum; (B) LA-N-1 human PNS neuroblastoma cells 6 days after plating on a polylysine- and fibronectin-modified substratum; (C) CHP 134 human PNS neuroblastoma cells 5 days after plating on a polylysine- and fibronectin-modified substratum; (D) N1E-115 mouse PNS neuroblastoma cells 3 days after switching from serum-containing medium (18 hr); (E) PC12 rat pheochromocytoma cells 14 days after plating on a fibronectin-modified substratum. Basal medium was a 1 : 1 mixture of Dulbecco's modified Eagle's (DME) and Ham's F12 medium, except for PC12 cells which was DME only. (From Bottenstein, 1984a.)

fetal rat brain explants of locus coeruleus, substantia nigra, cerebellum, caudate nucleus, and hypothalamus (Shoemaker *et al.*, 1979, 1985). Explants are plated on collagen-coated dishes in serum-supplemented medium with 0.4% Methocel and without NGF. After the explants are well attached to the substratum, the plating medium is removed, the explants are carefully washed, and N1 medium is added (Table I). Neuronal processes extend from the explants, but migration of cells does not occur as it does in serum-supplemented medium. Figure 4 is a fluorescence micrograph of sister substantia nigra explants after 21 days in serum-containing medium (Fig. 4A) and N1 medium (Fig. 4B). The accumulation of catecholamines is prominent under both conditions. Note the radial outgrowth of fibers in the former and the fasciculation of fibers in the latter, suggesting that perhaps N-CAM [cell adhesion molecule (Edelman, 1983)] may be differentially expressed in the two culture conditions. The absence of cellular outgrowth from the explants as well as a lack of increase in explant size suggested that nonneuronal cell proliferation might be impaired in N1 medium. This hypothesis was tested by measuring the DNA content and incorporation of [^{3}H]thymidine of locus coeruleus and substantia nigra explants. DNA content is reduced when cultures are in N1 medium, and the incorporation of [^{3}H]thymidine is markedly reduced compared to serum-grown cultures. Immunostaining for tetanus toxin receptors, glial fibrillary acidic protein, and galactocerebroside supports the conclusion that the number of neurons are similar whereas the nonneurons are reduced in N1 medium versus serum-supplemented medium. Both substantia nigra and locus coeruleus explants continue to synthesize and accumulate catecholamines after 21 days in N1 medium. Caudate nucleus and hypothalamus explants synthesize enkephalins and β-endorphin, respectively, in N1 medium. The substratum requirements for optimal culture of these CNS neurons have not been defined as yet. Fibronectin does not substitute satisfactorily for serum preincubation.

N1 supplements in Eagle's basal medium, with the addition of NGF, also support the selective survival *in vitro* of postmitotic sensory neurons from 8-day chick embryos (Bottenstein *et al.*, 1980). A collagen substratum is required, and fibronectin and polylysine cannot substitute for the initial plating in serum-containing medium for 48 hr, suggesting a possible requirement for additional or different ECM components. Dorsal root ganglionic neurons, Schwann cells, and fibroblasts can be identified morphologically in these dissociated cultures: neurons are phase-bright and neurite-bearing; Schwann cells are phase-dark and are closely associated with the neurons; and fibroblasts are flat, amorphous-shaped cells that show no particular affinity for neurons or Schwann cells at this cell density. Figure 5 illustrates the fate of the nonneurons in N1 medium. Although both Schwann cells and fibroblasts proliferate vigorously in serum-supplemented medium, they die in N1 medium after a few days. On the other hand, the neurons survive as well or better than their serum-grown counterparts. Figure 6A shows an initial culture at 48 hr just before switching to experimental medium. Four days after

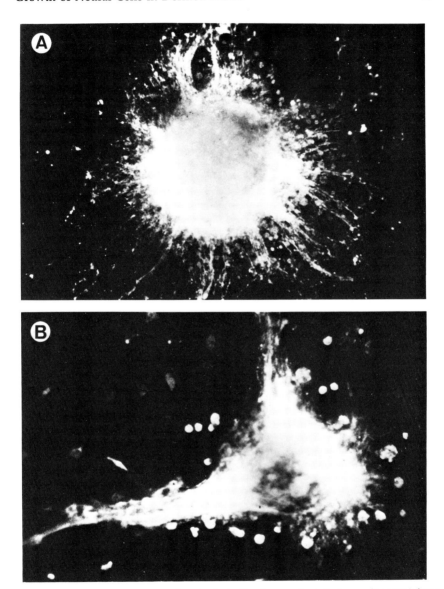

Figure 4. Fluorescence micrographs of substantia nigra explants (~1-mm diameter) from 19-day fetal rat brains. Explants were plated on a collagen substratum in Dulbecco's modified Eagle's medium supplemented with serum and Methocel. Five days later, the plating medium was removed and replaced with (A) serum-containing medium or (B) N1 medium. Sister cultures are shown 21 days after this procedure. Whole mount preparations were treated with formaldehyde vapor to visualize catecholamines. Some autofluorescence is apparent adajacent to the explants.

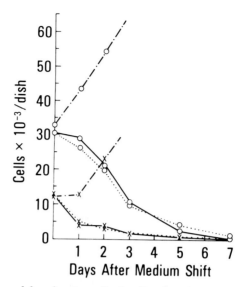

Figure 5. Nonneuronal dorsal root ganglionic cells cultured in serum-containing or serum-free supplemented medium. Collagen-coated 35-mm tissue culture dishes were seeded with 2×10^5 cells in 2 ml of basal medium containing 10% fetal calf serum (FCS) and 10 BU/ml nerve growth factor (NGF). After 48 hr, the cell monolayers were washed with three 1.5 ml aliquots of basal medium (each wash 20 min at 37°C). Cultures then received 2 ml of basal medium containing: 10% FCS and 10 BU/ml NGF (– · –); N1 supplements and 10 BU/ml NGF (——); N1 supplements only (·····). ○, Schwann cells; X, fibroblasts. Cell numbers were determined under phase-contrast microscopy and were plotted against the time after the washes and medium shift. Each point represents the average of two cultures. The extended lines represent the expected continued proliferation of the respective nonneuronal cell types. (Adapted from Bottenstein et al., 1980.)

replacing the serum-supplemented plating medium with identical fresh medium, the Schwann cells have divided and the fibroblasts have expanded in numbers to form a layer under the neural cells (Fig. 6B). In contrast, after 2 days in N1 medium, Schwann cells are still visible but disappearing and fibroblasts are almost gone (Figs. 6C, D). After 4 days in N1 medium, the cultures consist almost entirely of neurons (> 95%); and extensive neurite lengthening and arborization are apparent in some areas of the culture (Figs. 6E, F), a phenomenon not observed in the serum-containing cultures.

More recently, we have found that dissociated 11-day embryonic mouse dorsal root ganglion (DRG) or spinal cord cultures can be maintained for long periods (up to 4 months) in N2 medium (Table I) after initial plating in serum-supplemented medium on collagen-coated

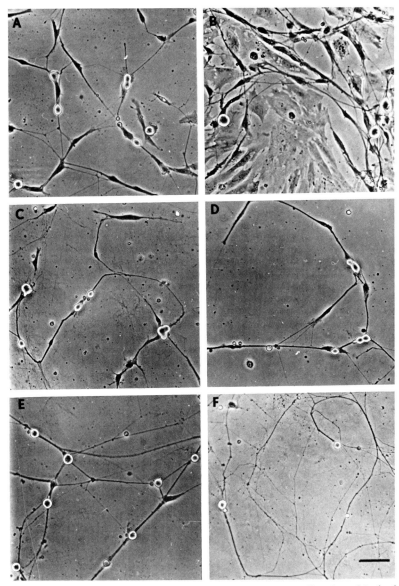

Figure 6. Phase-contrast micrographs of dorsal root ganglionic cells cultured in fetal calf serum (FCS)-containing medium or N1 medium. Cells were seeded in FCS-containing medium on collagen, washed with serum-free medium after 48 hr, and returned to FCS-containing medium or N1 medium. All cultures contained 10 BU/ml nerve growth factor. (A) 48 hr after seeding in FCS-containing medium; (B) 4 days after shift to fresh FCS-containing medium; (C, D) 2 days after shift to N1 medium; (E, F) 4 days after shift to N1 medium. Bar = 50 μm. (From Bottenstein *et al.*, 1980.)

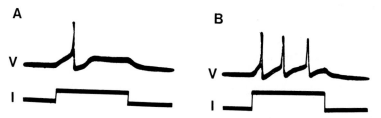

Figure 7. Intracellular recordings of an embryonic mouse spinal cord neuron grown in N2 medium. Membrane voltage (V) responses to intracellularly applied current (I) via a Wheatstone bridge are shown. (A) 1 nA current evokes a single action potential; (B) 1.5 nA current evokes multiple spikes. (From Bottenstein *et al.*, 1985.)

dishes (Bottenstein *et al.*, 1985). Intracellular recordings indicate that constant-current stimulation of spinal cord neurons evokes an action potential (Fig. 7A), and further depolarization results in multiple spikes (Fig. 7B). Similar results occur with DRG neurons in N2 medium. Figure 8 shows that similar I–V (current–voltage) curves are generated for DRG

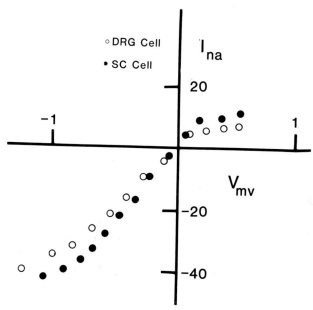

Figure 8. Current–voltage (I–V) curves of embryonic mouse spinal cord (SC) and dorsal root ganglion (DRG) cells grown in N2 medium from data similar to those shown in Fig. 7. (From Bottenstein *et al.*, 1985.)

and spinal cord neurons in N2 medium; and most cells exhibit delayed rectification with depolarization. Spontaneous activity is recorded in spinal cord neurons when extracellular magnesium is removed, including excitatory postsynaptic potentials, action potentials, and some inhibitory postsynaptic potentials. These neurons also have the appropriate responses to pressure ejection of GABA, glutamate, or glycine. Resting potentials and electrical responses are comparable to their serum-grown counterparts for both spinal cord and DRG neurons. Biochemical assays indicate that spinal cord cultures in N2 medium contain twice as much glutamic acid decarboxylase (GAD) activity as do serum-grown cultures; and immunoreactive GAD is present in 10–15% of the neurons. Also, CAT and acetylcholinesterase activities are detectable in these cultures, and the neurons specifically bind both radiolabeled benzodiazepines and opiates.

Thus, we have demonstrated that our defined medium designed for neurons supports both survival and the expression of many physiological and biochemical properties characteristic of differentiated neurons derived from the CNS and PNS. Many other investigators have also successfully used N1 or N2 medium, with little or no modification, to culture primary neural cells of several different species (Bottenstein, 1983a,b). Marked suppression of fibroblast proliferation occurs in all cases, while the magnitude of decreases in glial cell division differs depending on the species. In most cases differentiated properties of neurons are retained or even enhanced in defined medium. A remaining problem, however, is the need to define the substratum requirements for neurons, as most of the preparations still require a serum preincubation before changing the medium to a defined one. Fibronectin, laminin, and/or poly-D-lysine have all been tried with partial success but do not give optimal results.

4. SERUM-FREE DEFINED MEDIA FOR GLIAL CELLS

4.1. Glial Cell Lines

Following our success with defined medium for neurons, we attempted to define the culture conditions optimal for serum-free growth of glial cells. We followed the same strategy useful for the neuronal medium, i.e., to define the growth requirements of continuous cell lines first and subsequently to test the medium on their primary counterparts. We found that the sets of requirements for growth of glial cell lines are different from those for neuronal cell lines. I first reported a defined

Table V. Defined Medium Supplements for Glial Cells[a]

Supplement	G2	G3	G4	G5
Transferrin	50 µg/ml	50 µg/ml	50 µg/ml	50 µg/ml
Hydrocortisone	10 nM	—	10 nM	10 nM
Fibroblast growth factor	5 ng/ml	—	5 ng/ml	5 ng/ml
Biotin	10 ng/ml	10 ng/ml	10 ng/ml	10 ng/ml
Selenium	30 nM	30 nM	30 nM	30 nM
Insulin	—	—	5 µg/ml	5 µg/ml
Epidermal growth factor	—	—	—	10 ng/ml

[a] Supplements are added to Dulbecco's modified Eagle's medium in concentrated form on various substrata. Values shown are the final concentrations.

medium for growth of C6-2B cells in 1979 (Bottenstein, 1981a), and a further refinement of this medium (G2 medium; Table V) supports the proliferation of both C6-2BD and U-251 MGsp cells, which both express glial fibrillary acidic protein (GFA), a marker characteristic of mature astrocytes (Michler-Stuke and Bottenstein, 1982a,b). This medium consists of DME medium supplemented with human transferrin, bovine pituitary fibroblast growth factor, hydrocortisone, sodium selenite, and biotin; the substratum is modified with poly-D-lysine precoating and the addition of human fibronectin to the medium prior to the cells. Serum is not even required in the initial stage of these cultures. In the absence of our substratum modification, however, there is no growth response to the purified soluble supplements. The type of basal medium used has a profound effect on the stimulation of growth. Table VI shows the influence of the ratio of DME to F12 medium on growth of U-251 MGsp

Table VI. Influence of Different Ratios of DME:F12 Medium on Growth of U-251 Cells[a]

Basal medium DME:F12	Serum supplement (cpm/dish)	G2 supplement (cpm/dish)
1:0	49,200 ± 1,000	21,200 ± 278
3:1	36,200 ± 1,320	12,300 ± 504
1:1	26,700 ± 2,420	2,890 ± 208
1:3	16,600 ± 627	2,170 ± 26
0:1	11,700 ± 610	2,340 ± 225

[a] Cells (40,000/35-mm dish) were plated either in basal medium supplemented with 5% calf serum and 5% horse serum or in G2 medium on poly-D-lysine-coated dishes. Cells were labeled 24 hr before harvesting with [^{3}H]thymidine (specific activity 0.25 µCi/ml) and trichloroacetic acid-precipitable counts were determined on day 4. Values are expressed as the mean ± S.D. of triplicate cultures. (From Michler-Stuke and Bottenstein, 1982a.)

cells. Although a 1:1 mixture of these two media is optimal for neuronal cells, this is not the case for glial cells. Instead, there is a clear preference for DME medium alone, and this effect is more marked in defined medium than in serum-containing medium (a 10-fold versus 4-fold difference in the incorporation of [³H]thymidine). Biotin must be added when DME medium alone is used, since this important vitamin is missing from DME but not from F12 medium. If single supplements are deleted from G2 medium, there is a decrease in the number of U-251 MGsp or C6-2BD cells compared to the fully supplemented medium. Figure 9 shows growth curves for both of these cell lines in G2 medium. Figure 10 illustrates the different morphologies of C6-2BD cells in serum-containing versus G2 medium; more complex processes are evident in the defined medium (Bottenstein and Michler-Stuke, 1983). Similar effects of G2 medium on morphology are also observed with the U-251 MGsp and RN-22 cell lines (Michler-Stuke and Bottenstein, 1982a). The latter Schwannoma cell line does not require fibroblast growth factor or hydrocortisone and will grow in the simpler G3 medium (Table V). Process formation is enhanced in defined medium for all three glial cell lines. All of these glial cell lines have been maintained in defined medium for periods of several weeks to a month with several subcultures.

Unlike neuronal cells, U-251 MGsp, C6-2BD, and RN-22 cells do not require insulin for survival or proliferation. G2 medium does not support the continuous division of either human neuroblastoma or fibroblast cell lines. It is also not optimal for growth of a cell line expressing oligodendroglial properties, the CO-13-7 somatic cell hybrid (McMorris *et al.*, 1981). We are presently defining the growth requirements for this cell line derived from the fusion of a primary calf brain oligodendrocyte and a C6 rat glioma cell. Thus, it appears that glial cell lines derived from astrocytes, Schwann cells, and oligodendrocytes may differ in their sets of growth requirements, although there are some common elements.

4.2. Primary Glia

It is clear that N2 medium is not optimal for primary glial cell growth. Will G2 medium and the substratum modifications that support the proliferation of glial cell lines expressing astrocytic properties sustain the division of primary brain astrocytes? We tested these culture conditions on primary cultures of dissociated newborn rat brain cortical cells. The initial cultures contain a variety of cell types, including neurons, astrocytes, oligodendrocytes, fibroblasts, and others. We found that neuron- and fibroblast-like cells disappear from these cultures after

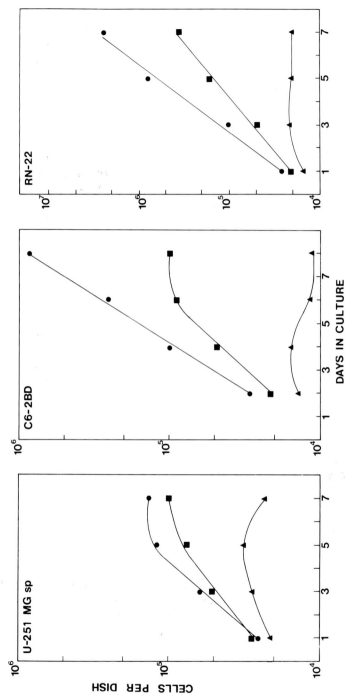

Figure 9. Growth curves for U-251 MGsp, C6-2BD, and RN-22 cells in defined media. Cells (25,000/35-mm dish) were plated in: Dulbecco's modified Eagle's medium (DME) with 5% calf serum and 5% horse serum (●); defined medium on poly-D-lysine- and fibronectin-modified dishes (■); or in serum-free DME alone (▲). Defined media: G2 medium for U-251 MGsp or C6-2BD cells; G3 medium for RN-22 cells. On day 5 cells were fed by replacing half the medium with fresh medium. Values are expressed as the mean of triplicate cultures and did not vary more than 10% from the mean. (From Michler-Stuke and Bottenstein, 1982a.)

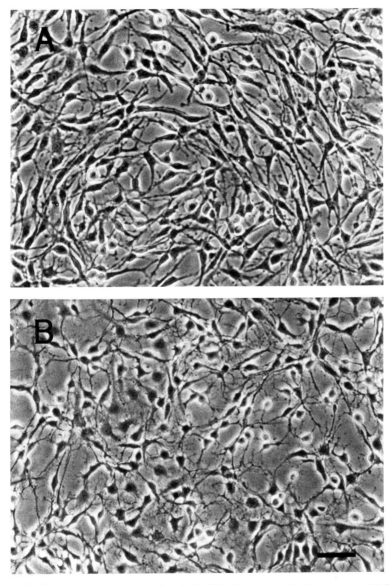

Figure 10. Phase-contrast micrographs of C6-2BD cells on day 6 after passage. (A) Dulbecco's modified Eagle's medium supplemented with 5% fetal calf serum and 5% horse serum; (B) G2 medium with a substratum modified with fibronectin and poly-D-lysine. Bar = 50 μm. (From Bottenstein and Michler-Stuke, 1983.)

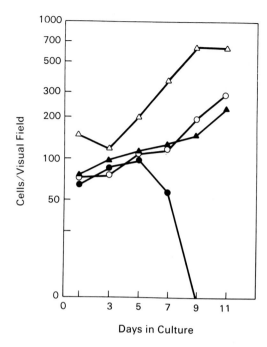

Figure 11. Growth curve for neonatal rat astrocytes in primary cultures. Cells were plated at 10^6 cells/35-mm dish in: Dulbecco's modified Eagle's medium supplemented with 10% fetal calf serum (○); G2 medium (●); G4 medium (▲); or G5 medium (△). Culture surfaces were modified with fibronectin and poly-D-lysine when using defined media (G2, G4, or G5). The cells were fed 4 days after plating and every 3–4 days thereafter. The S.E.M. of quadruplicate cultures was less than 10%. (Adapted from Michler-Stuke et al., 1984.)

a few weeks in G2 medium, but the remaining cells appear to undergo limited cell division initially (Michler-Stuke and Bottenstein, 1982b). These preliminary results were verified and extended in a later study (Michler-Stuke et al., 1984). Immunostaining for GFA indicated that the cultures are composed primarily of mature astrocytes. We then added additional supplements to improve G2 medium, since the astrocytes proliferate initially but begin to degenerate thereafter. The addition of bovine insulin to G2 medium increases the longevity of these cultures (G4 medium; Table V), whereas mouse EGF greatly enhances their growth rate. Figure 11 shows the increase in cell number observed with G2, G4, or G5 medium relative to serum-supplemented medium. Changes in the morphology of rat brain astrocytes occur in all of these defined media compared to serum-supplemented medium (Michler-Stuke et al., 1984). Figure 12 shows that GFA-stained astrocytes grown in serum-containing medium are morphologically undifferentiated, whereas in G5 medium they have long processes and more closely resemble the morphology of fibrous astrocytes in vivo. If defined medium is replaced with serum-supplemented medium, the astrocytes revert to the more undifferentiated morphology. Cultures in G5 medium have

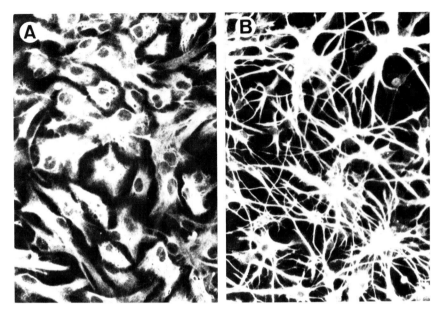

Figure 12. Fluorescence micrographs of cultured neonatal rat astrocytes after 7 days. Cells were plated at 10^6 cells/35-mm dish in: (A) Dulbecco's modified Eagle's medium supplemented with 10% fetal calf serum; (B) G5 medium on culture surfaces modified with fibronectin and poly-D-lysine. Cells were immunostained for glial fibrillary acidic protein.

been subcultured as many as 4 times and after more than 2 months the cells still appear healthy. Almost pure (>98%) astrocyte cultures result after the first subculture. Various substratum modifications indicate that poly-L-ornithine precoating can substitute for poly-D-lysine and that collagen is an inferior substratum. Furthermore, fibronectin is required with G4 medium, but not with G5 medium. The addition of hyaluronic acid or chondroitin sulfate A (chondroitin-4-sulfate) further enhances the growth of astrocytes on fibronectin-modified surfaces in G4 medium, but has no effect in G5 medium; and each of these GAGs can substitute for fibronectin modification when G4 medium is employed. Chondroitin sulfate C (chondroitin-6-sulfate) has no growth-stimulating effect. These results suggest that EGF may stimulate the endogenous production of ECM components by the astrocytes so that an exogenous supply is not required. This is consistent with results in human fibroblasts that EGF stimulates fibronectin synthesis (Chen *et al.*, 1977) and enhances the synthesis and deposition of hyaluronic acid (Lembach, 1976).

We have demonstrated that the defined medium (G2 medium) designed for glial cell lines which express GFA has to be further supplemented to sustain continued proliferation of primary astrocytes *in vitro*. In addition, we have provided evidence that not only the defined medium supplements but also the substratum requirements of primary neurons and astrocytes differ substantially. Whether any of these defined media are optimal for primary Schwann cell proliferation is not known yet; presumably, G3 medium would be the best presently available candidate. Even though it has been reported that embryonic Schwann cells derived from rodents, but not chicks, will proliferate moderately in N2 medium, optimal growth of these cells has not yet been achieved in a defined medium. After optimization of the medium and substratum for the CO-13-7 cell line, which expresses a variety of oligodendroglial markers, we will determine whether these conditions are also capable of sustaining the survival and/or proliferation of primary oligodendrocytes. Our initial immunocytochemical data indicate a marked increase in galactocerebroside-positive rat brain cells maintained in our present defined medium for CO-13-7 cells compared to sister cultures in serum-supplemented medium (Bottenstein, 1984b).

5. SERUM-FREE DEFINED MEDIA FOR NEURAL PRECURSOR CELLS

We know that the neuronal and glial media defined above are relatively cell type-specific without apparent species-specificity. What would be the result of culturing stem cells in such media? We investigated this question with a multipotential embryonal carcinoma cell line—the 1003 subclone of the C17-S1 mouse embryonal carcinoma (EC) cell line. These cells are capable *in vivo* of generating derivatives of all three germ layers, thus corresponding to the blastocyst stage. This and other EC cell lines are unique model systems for investigating various aspects of development, since their malignant nature can be reversed when they are induced to differentiate. N2 medium (Table I) with a fibronectin-modified substratum is able to induce selective neurogenesis of 1003 EC cells. Further study indicated that progesterone and putrescine are not required for this effect (Darmon *et al.*, 1981). Chapter 9 gives more details about the neuronal characteristics of these differentiated cells. The 1003 cells remain undifferentiated when maintained at subconfluent levels in serum-containing medium (Fig. 13A), but begin to differentiate 1 day after exposure to defined medium (Fig. 13B) and subsequently form interconnected clusters of neurite-bearing neurons (Fig. 13C). Figure 14 shows at higher magnification the extensive radial outgrowth in defined medium of neurites from a cluster of these neurons

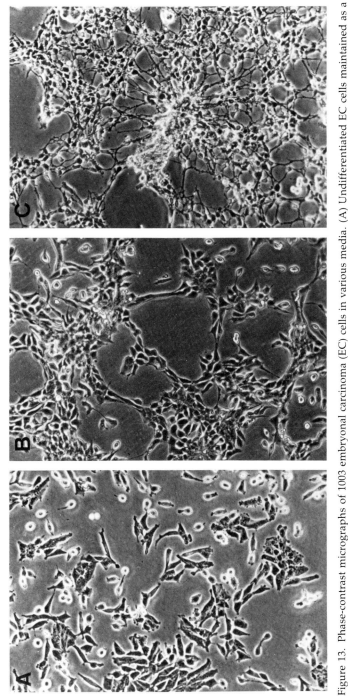

Figure 13. Phase-contrast micrographs of 1003 embryonal carcinoma (EC) cells in various media. (A) Undifferentiated EC cells maintained as a stock cell line in a 1:1 mixture of Ham's F12 and Dulbecco's modified Eagle's medium (DME) supplemented with 8% fetal calf serum; (B) after 1 day in T2 medium on a fibronectin-modified substratum; (C) after 27 days in T2 medium on a fibronectin-modified substratum. T2 medium consists of DME supplemented with 5 μg/ml insulin, 100 μg/ml transferrin, and 30 nM sodium selenite.

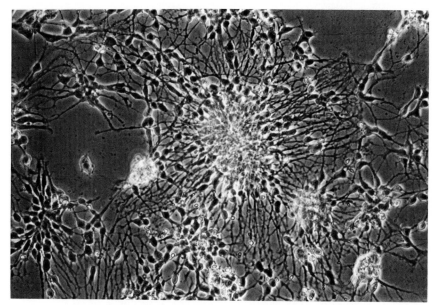

Figure 14. Phase-contrast micrograph of cultured aggregates of 1003 embryonal carcinoma cells. Initially, 200,000 cells were plated in a 100-mm dish in T2 medium (see Fig. 13) with an unmodified culture surface. Cells formed aggregates and were subcultured 6 days later in T2 medium on a fibronectin-modified surface. Cells were again subcultured without dissociation 15 days later and are shown 4 days after this second subculture in T2 medium on a fibronectin-modified surface. The cells have been exposed to T2 medium for a total of 25 days. More extensive process formation is observed using this procedure than the one in Fig. 13C.

and the interconnections with nearby neurons. We have recently measured the activities of CAT, tyrosine hydroxylase (TH), and GAD in the differentiated cultures of 1003 cells. We found that there is no detectable TH or GAD activity; and by high-performance liquid chromatography no serotonin is detected. However, in our preliminary results there is very high CAT activity—817 pmoles/min per mg protein. After 11 days in defined medium, 1003 cells exhibit both regenerative responses and delayed rectification in response to anode-break stimulation (J. Bottenstein and A. Ritchie, unpublished results). Thus, 1003 cells can be induced to become primarily neurons with cholinergic properties and excitable membranes. We are now interested in using this model system to address a variety of developmental questions. For example, we are interested in (1) establishing a continuous neuroepithelial cell line, (2) defining the molecular requirements for continued growth and/or arrest of differentiation of the neuroepithelial precursor cells, (3) investigating the hormonal, growth factor, trace element, and other molecular influences on neurotransmitter phenotype (other than cholinergic) in the neurons we are able to generate, and (4) determining the conditions for inducing glial differentiation of 1003 cells. The effect of our neuronal and glial defined media and substrata on primary neural precursor cells remains to be investigated, and we also intend to pursue this line of research.

Another group of investigators has recently found that a slight modification of N2 medium can induce extensive neuronal differentiation of a human retinoblastoma cell line, including neurite-bearing cells that are neuron-specific enolase-positive (Kyritsis *et al.*, 1984). Dibutyryl cAMP treatment causes an increase in GFA-positive glial cells. In contrast, in serum-containing medium the cell line retains a small round cell morphology, lacks processes, and expresses neuronal but not glial antigens. The histogenesis of this tumor cell line is controversial, but their results suggest that it may originate from a neuroepithelial stem cell.

6. CONCLUSION

6.1. In Vivo vs. in Vitro Growth and Differentiation Requirements

The following data and correlations suggest that the growth and differentiation requirements we have defined for neural cells *in vitro* may be important during normal development of the nervous system. Deficiencies in the availability of these factors or of their receptors might then be expected to result in various neuropathological conditions.

We find that the glycoprotein transferrin, a β_1-globulin with iron-transporting ability, is required by all neural cells tested thus far. While most mammalian cells have cell surface transferrin receptors, their density is greatly increased during proliferative stages (Larrick and Cresswell, 1979; Omary *et al.*, 1980; Shindelman *et al.*, 1981). The actual mechanism of iron transport across the plasma membrane is unknown, but it is generally agreed that specific binding of diferric transferrin to receptors is an obligatory step in the uptake of iron by cells (Lamb *et al.*, 1983). Neither metal-free apotransferrin nor transferrin complexed with chromium, manganese, copper, cadmium, cobalt, zinc, or nickel improves survival or growth of a variety of cell types *in vitro*, including chick embryo spinal cord cells (Saito *et al.*, 1982). Neurons in these latter cultures survive well in 50 μM ferrous or ferric ion or 1 μM iron-bound transferrin, but do poorly in their absence.

In addition to its anabolic effects on postnatal target tissue, the polypeptide hormone insulin is thought to act as a growth factor during fetal development (Straus, 1981; Persson, 1981). Our studies suggest that while insulin is required for survival of neurons *in vitro*, astrocytes do not exhibit such a requirement although their proliferation is enhanced by inclusion of insulin within the culture medium. Supraphysiological concentrations of insulin are required for survival of neurons or enhanced proliferation of astrocytes *in vitro* in defined medium. Extremely high levels of insulin in the presence of serum also enhance neuron survival in dissociated fetal rodent cell cultures (Sotelo *et al.*, 1980). Since insulin binds with low affinity to somatomedin receptors, which are prevalent in mammalian brain (Sara and Hall, 1979), it may be that somatomedins are the relevant physiological ligand in some cases. Somatomedins are elevated in fetal relative to adult human brain tissue (Sara *et al.*, 1981a), there is a significant correlation between fetal growth *in vivo* and serum somatomedin levels (Sara and Hall, 1980), and somatomedins have a direct growth-stimulating effect on human fetal brain cells in culture (Sara *et al.*, 1981b). Furthermore, somatomedins are synthesized *in vitro* by many different cell types derived from the mouse fetus, including brain cells (D'Ercole *et al.*, 1980). Growth hormone stimulates the production of somatomedins and insulin-like growth factors (Kaufmann *et al.*, 1978), and a deficiency *in vivo* of this hormone decreases brain cell number, size, and myelination (Pelton *et al.*, 1977). Specific insulin receptors, however, are also present in both mammalian (Posner *et al.*, 1974; Landau *et al.*, 1976; Havrankova *et al.*, 1981) and invertebrate CNS (Schot *et al.*, 1981), immunoreactive insulin is found in extracts of mammalian and invertebrate brains (Baskin *et al.*, 1983), and insulin is detectable immunocytochemically in mammalian CNS neurons (Havrankova *et al.*, 1978; Dorn *et al.*, 1981, 1982; Weyhenmeyer and Fellows, 1983). Rat astrocytes bind insulin with a specificity and affinity similar to that in cerebral homogenates (Albrecht *et al.*, 1982). Insulin concentrations in whole brain extracts are about 25 times greater than in plasma and between 10 and 100 times greater in discrete brain areas, e.g., hypothalamus, olfactory bulb, cerebral hemispheres, and brain stem (Havrankova *et al.*, 1978). Both insulin receptors and the concentration of insulin in rodent brains are independent of peripheral insulin levels, suggesting that local synthesis or sequestration of insulin occurs within the CNS (Havrankova *et al.*, 1979). Raizada (1983) recently reported that insulin-like immunoreactivity was restricted to neuronal cells and presented evidence suggesting that fetal rat brain neurons may synthesize this material.

The diamine putrescine is the precursor of the polyamines, spermidine and spermine, which are found in higher levels in proliferating cells (Tabor and Tabor, 1976; Pegg and McCann, 1982) and also at early stages of development (Heby, 1981). Putrescine is also a precursor of the neurotransmitter GABA (Seiler et al., 1979). The activity of ornithine decarboxylase, which synthesizes putrescine, is correlated with neuronal proliferation and growth in the developing rat brain (Anderson and Schanberg, 1972); and putrescine levels are correlated with neurogenesis in mouse brain (Jasper et al., 1982). The development of sympathetic neurons is markedly impaired if polyamine synthesis is inhibited in neonatal rats (Slotkin et al., 1983). In addition, polyamine synthesis appears to be required for the survival of sympathetic neurons after axonal injury (Gilad and Gilad, 1983). Lower levels of ornithine decarboxylase activity and of polyamines are found in differentiated mouse neuroblastoma cells than in undifferentiated ones (Chen et al., 1982), and putrescine transport is also decreased in the differentiated cells (Chen and Rinehart, 1981). Depletion of polyamines in vitro results in major chromosomal aberrations and multinucleated cells, leading to disturbances in mitosis and cytokinesis (Sunkara et al., 1979; Knuutila and Pohjanpelto, 1983). Proliferation inhibited by treatment with difluoromethylornithine can be reversed by adding polyamines to the culture medium (Stoscheck et al., 1982). Furthermore, micromolar exogenous putrescine stimulates human fibroblast proliferation in a concentration-dependent manner in low-density or low-serum cultures (Pohjanpelto, 1973) and also stimulates the growth of hamster fibroblast cells (Ham, 1964). This suggests that under certain culture conditions cells are unable to synthesize sufficient putrescine or are losing it into the culture medium. Thus, our data are consistent with the hypothesis that astrocytes and gliomas do not have a polyamine deficiency in our defined media, whereas some neurons and neuroblastomas do.

There are high-affinity cytoplasmic progesterone receptors in several rat brain regions, and specific saturable nuclear uptake also occurs (MacLusky and Clark, 1980). Estrogen-independent progesterone receptors are more abundant during early neural development. We find that embryonic neurons and tumor cells derived from them have a requirement for progesterone, whereas glial cells or their tumor derivatives do not. However, glucocorticoids do stimulate the growth of astrocytes and tumor cells derived from them, although Schwannoma cells do not have a growth response to these hormones. Glucocorticoid receptors are present in both cytoplasmic and nuclear compartments in rodent brain (MacLusky and Clark, 1980). Whereas corticosterone is concentrated preferentially by neurons, the synthetic glucocorticoid dexamethasone is taken up by a variety of cell types, including neurons and glia. Glucocorticoid cytosol binding sites have been described for rat glial cells in the optic nerve (Meyer and McEwen, 1982). These investigators did not, however, distinguish whether a subclass or all classes of glial cells contain these receptors. Thus, neurons and glia appear to have different responses to these steroid hormones.

The mitogenic and survival-promoting effects of NGF are well known and amply reviewed elsewhere (Greene and Shooter, 1980; see Chapter 3). It is essential for the survival of embryonic sensory and sympathetic neurons, but not CNS neurons, in the presence of serum or in our defined medium. EGF receptors are found predominantly on astrocytes in mouse (Leutz and Schachner, 1982) and rat brain cultures (Simpson *et al.*, 1982). Fibroblast growth factor (FGF) is present in both the brain and the pituitary gland (Gospodarowicz and Mescher, 1980); however, receptors for FGF have not yet been identified on any cell type. Neonatal rat astrocytes are stimulated to divide by FGF in serum-containing cultures (Pruss *et al.*, 1982). We find that in our defined medium FGF is required by all cells of astrocytic lineage and EGF by primary astrocytes only.

Several trace elements are known to be required *in vivo* and also *in vitro* (Underwood, 1977; Ham, 1981). Iron is an essential requirement for all vertebrate cells in culture and plays an important role in energy metabolism (see the discussion about transferrin above). Requirements for zinc and selenium are also well established. During embryogenesis, maternal zinc deficiency causes congenital CNS malformations (Dvergsten *et al.*, 1983). Selenium is a cofactor for the seleno-enzyme glutathione peroxidase, which protects cellular membranes from lipid peroxide damage (Stadtman, 1974, 1980). Because of their contaminating presence in basal media, it has been more difficult to demonstrate a requirement *in vitro* for copper, manganese, chromium, vanadium, nickel, silicon, tin, or molybdenum. The interaction of several of these essential trace elements is probably important during prenatal and postnatal development of the nervous system. We find that selenium is an absolute requirement for both neurons and glia after 3–4 days in serum-free medium.

6.2. Future Directions

The mechanisms of action of hormones, growth factors, neurotransmitters, and neuromodulators can be more easily investigated using rigorously defined culture conditions. In addition, the potential for identifying new regulatory factors is increased when undefined substances are absent from the culture environment. Further clarification of the role of endogenous factors and heterotypic cell–cell interactions is possible when isolated populations of particular cell types and their recombinations are used in conjunction with defined culture conditions. However, the requirements for coculture of different neural cell types will need to be optimized for the mixed cell type cultures. Developmental, locus-specific, and subclass-specific requirements will be defined where and if they exist. It may also be possible in the future to maintain neural cells *in vitro* which are difficult or impossible at the present time, e.g., proliferating neuroblasts or oligodendroblasts and many adult neural cells. As our knowledge of the molecular requirements for the survival, proliferation, and differentiation of neurons and glia increases, our understanding of normal and pathological development of the nervous system will expand correspondingly.

ACKNOWLEDGMENTS

I would like to thank Drs. Gordon Sato, William Shoemaker, Silvio Varon, and Angelika Michler-Stuke for their collaboration in different aspects of the work reviewed and Ms. Terry Klassen for assistance in preparing the manuscript. Portions of my research have been supported by grants from the National Institutes of Health, Concern Foundation, California Institute for Cancer Research, UCLA Cancer Research Coordinating Committee, California Department of Health Services, and National Science Foundation.

REFERENCES

Abney, E., Williams, B., and Raff, M., 1983, Tracing the development of oligodendrocytes from precursor cells using monoclonal antibodies, fluorescence-activated cell sorting, and cell culture, *Develop. Biol.* **100**:166–171.
Akers, R., Mosher, D., and Lilien, J., 1981, Promotion of retinal neurite outgrowth by substratum-bound fibronectin, *Develop. Biol.* **86**:179–188.
Albrecht, J., Wroblewska, B., and Mossakowski, M., 1982, The binding of insulin to cerebral capillaries and astrocytes of the rat, *Neurochem. Res.* **7**:489–494.
Alitalo, K., Kurkinen, M., Vaheri, A., Virtanen, I., Rohde, H., and Timpl, R., 1980, Basal lamina glycoproteins are produced by neuroblastoma cells, *Nature* **287**:465–466.
Alitalo, K., Kurkinen, M., Virtanen, I., Mellström, K., and Vaheri, A., 1982, Deposition of basement membrane proteins in attachment and neurite formation of cultured murine C-1300 neuroblastoma cells, *J. Cell. Biochem.* **18**:25–36.
Ambesi-Impiombato, F., Parks, L., and Coon, H., 1980, Culture of hormone-dependent functional epithelial cells from rat thyroids, *Proc. Natl. Acad. Sci. USA* **77**:3455–3459.
Anderson, T., and Schanberg, S., 1972, Ornithine decarboxylase activity in developing rat brain, *J. Neurochem.* **19**:1471–1481.

Asou, H., Brunngraber, E., and Delpech, B., 1983, Localization of hyaluronectin in oligodendroglial cells, *J. Neurochem.* **40**:589–591.

Baron-Van Evercooren, A., Kleinman, H., Seppa, H., Rentier, B., and Dubois-Dalcq, M., 1982a, Fibronectin promotes rat Schwann cell growth and motility, *J. Cell Biol.* **93**:211–216.

Baron-Van Evercooren, A., Kelinman, H., Ohno, S., Marangos, P., Schwartz, J., and Dubois-Dalcq, M., 1982b, Nerve growth factor, laminin, and fibronectin promote neurite growth in human fetal sensory ganglia cultures, *J. Neurosci. Res.* **8**:179–193.

Baskin, D., Porte, D., Guest, K., and Dorsa, D., 1983, Regional concentrations of insulin in the rat brain, *Endocrinology* **112**:898–903.

Baumann, H., and Eldredge, D., 1982, Dexamethasone increases the synthesis and secretion of a partially active fibronectin in rat hepatoma cells, *J. Cell Biol.* **95**:29–40.

Bear, M., and Schneider, F., 1976, The effect of medium pH on rate of growth, neurite formation and acetylcholinesterase activity in mouse neuroblastoma cells in culture, *J. Cell. Physiol.* **91**:63–68.

Bhat, S., Barbarese, E., and Pfeiffer, S., 1981, Requirement for nonoligodendrocyte cell signals for enhanced myelinogenic gene expression in long-term cultures of purified rat oligodendrocytes, *Proc. Natl. Acad. Sci. USA* **78**:1283–1287.

Bornstein, M., 1958, Reconstituted rat-tail collagen as substrate for tissue cultures on coverslips in Maximow slides and in roller tubes, *Lab. Invest.* **7**:134–137.

Bottenstein, J., 1980, Serum-free culture of neuroblastoma cells, in: *Advances in Neuroblastoma Research* (A. Evans, ed.), Raven Press, New York, pp.161–170.

Bottenstein, J., 1981a, Proliferation of glioma cells in serum-free defined medium, *Cancer Treat. Rep.* **65**(Suppl. 2):67–70.

Bottenstein, J., 1981b, Differentiated properties of neuronal cell lines, in: *Functionally Differentiated Cell Lines* (G. Sato, ed.), Liss, New York, pp. 155–184.

Bottenstein, J., 1983a, Growth requirements of neural cells in vitro, in: *Advances in Cellular Neurobiology*, Volume 4 (S. Fedoroff and L. Hertz, eds.), Academic Press, New York, pp. 333–379.

Bottenstein, J., 1983b, Defined media for dissociated neural cultures, in: *Current Methods in Cellular Neurobiology*, Volume 4 (J. Barker and J. McKelvy, eds.), Wiley, New York, pp. 107–130.

Bottenstein, J., 1984a, Culture methods for growth of neuronal cell lines in defined media, in: *Cell Culture Methods for Molecular and Cell Biology*, Vol. 4 (D. Barnes, D. Sirbasku, and G. Sato, eds.), Liss, New York, pp. 3–13.

Bottenstein, J., 1984b, Growth of primary neural cells in chemically defined media, in: *Growth and Differentiation of Cells in Defined Environment* (H. Murakami, I. Yamane, D. Barnes, J. Mather, I. Hayashi, and G. Sato, eds.) Springer-Verlag, Berlin, in press.

Bottenstein, J., and Michler-Stuke, A., 1983, Proliferation of glial-derived cell lines in serum-free defined medium, in: *Developing and Regenerating Vertebrate Nervous Systems* (P. Coates, R. Markwald, and A. Kenny, eds.), Liss, New York, pp. 185–189.

Bottenstein, J., and Sato, G., 1979, Growth of a rat neuroblastoma cell line in serum-free supplemented media, *Proc. Natl. Acad. Sci. USA* **76**:514–517.

Bottenstein, J., and Sato, G., 1980, Fibronectin and polylysine requirement for proliferation of neuroblastoma cells in defined medium, *Exp. Cell Res.* **129**:361–366.

Bottenstein, J., Mather, J., and Sato, G., 1979, Growth of neuroepithelial-derived cell lines in serum-free hormone-supplemented media, *CSH Conf. Cell Prolif.* **6**:531–544.

Bottenstein, J., Skaper, S., Varon, S., and Sato, G., 1980, Selective survival of neurons in chick sensory ganglionic cultures utilizing serum-free supplemented medium, *Exp. Cell Res.* **125**:183–190.

Bottenstein, J., Mazzetta, J., Caserta, M., Kapatos, G., Neale, J., Plishka, R., and Smith, T., 1985, Differentiated properties of mouse embryonic spinal cord neurons in defined medium, in preparation.

Chen, K., and Rinehart, C., 1981, Difference in putrescine transport in undifferentiated versus differentiated mouse NB-15 neuroblastoma cells, *Biochem. Biophys. Res. Commun.* **101**:243–249.

Chen, K., Presepe, V., Parken, V., and Liu, A., 1982, Changes of ornithine decarboxylase activity and polyamine content upon differentiation of mouse NB-15 neuroblastoma cells, *J. Cell. Physiol.* **110**:285–290.

Chen, L., Gudor, R., Sun, T., Chen, A., and Mosesson, M., 1977, Control of a cell surface major glycoprotein by epidermal growth factor, *Science* **197**:776–778.

Cornbrooks, C., Carey, D., McDonald, J., Timpl, R., and Bunge, R., 1983, In vivo and in vitro observations on laminin production by Schwann cells, *Proc. Natl. Acad. Sci. USA* **80**:3850–3854.

Coyle, J., Jacobowitz, D., Klein, D., and Axelrod, J., 1973, Dopaminergic neurons in explants of substantia nigra in culture, *J. Neurobiol.* **4**:461–470.

Curtis, A., Forrester, J., McInnes, C., and Lawrie, F., 1983, Adhesion of cells to polystyrene surfaces, *J. Cell Biol.* **97**:1500–1506.

Darmon, M., Bottenstein, J., and Sato, G., 1981, Neural differentiation following culture of embryonal carcinoma cells in a serum-free defined medium, *Develop. Biol.* **85**:463–473.

Delpech, A., and Delpech, B., 1984, Expression of hyaluronic acid-binding glycoprotein, hyaluronectin, in the developing rat embryo, *Develop. Biol.* **101**:391–400.

Delpech, A., Girard, N., and Delpech, B., 1982, Localization of hyaluronectin in the nervous system, *Brain Res.* **245**:251–257.

D'Ercole, A., Applewhite, G., and Underwood, L., 1980, Evidence that somatomedin is synthesized by multiple tissues in the fetus, *Develop. Biol.* **75**:315–328.

Dorn, A., Bernstein, H., Hahn, H., Ziegler, M., and Rummelfönger, H., 1981, Insulin immunohistochemistry of rodent CNS: Apparent species differences but good correlation with radioimmunological data, *Histochemistry* **71**:609–616.

Dorn, A., Bernstein, H., Rinne, A., Hahn, H., and Ziegler, M., 1982, Insulin-like immunoreactivity in the human brain: A preliminary report, *Histochemistry* **74**:293–300.

Dreyfus, C., Peterson, E., and Crain, S., 1980, Failure of nerve growth factor to affect fetal mouse brain stem catecholaminergic neurons in culture, *Brain Res.* **194**:540–547.

Duband, J., and Thiery, J., 1982, Appearance and distribution of fibronectin during chick embryo gastrulation and neurulation, *Develop. Biol.* **94**:337–350.

Dvergsten, C., Fosmire, G., Ollerich, D., and Sandstead, H., 1983, Alterations in the postnatal development of the cerebellar cortex due to zinc deficiency. I. Impaired acquisition of granule cells, *Brain Res.* **271**:217–226.

Dvorak, D., Gipps, E., and Kidson, C., 1978, Isolation of specific neurones by affinity methods, *Nature* **271**:564–566.

Edelman, G., 1983, Cell adhesion molecules, *Science* **219**:450–457.

Enat, R., Jefferson, D., Ruiz-Opazo, N., Gatmaitan, Z., Leinwand, L., and Reid, L., 1984, Hepatocyte proliferation in vitro: Its dependence on the use of serum-free hormonally defined medium and substrata of extracellular matrix, *Proc. Natl. Acad. Sci. USA* **81**:1411–1415.

Faivre-Bauman, A., Puymirat, J., Loudes, C., Barret, A., and Tixier-Vidal, A., 1984, Laminin promotes attachment and neurite elongation of fetal hypothalamic neurons grown in serum-free medium, *Neurosci. Lett.* **44**:83–89.

Foley, T., Nissley, S., Stevens, R., King, G., Hascall, V., Humbel, R., Short, P., and Rechler, M., 1982, Demonstration of receptors for insulin and insulin-like growth factors on Swarm rat chondrosarcoma chondrocytes, *J. Biol. Chem.* **257**:663–669.

Folkman, J., and Moscona, A., 1978, Role of cell shape in growth control, *Nature* **273**:345–349.

Gatmaitan, Z., Jefferson, D., Ruiz-Opazo, N., Biempica, L., Arias, I., Dudas, G., Leinwand, L., and Reid, L., 1983, Regulation of growth and differentiation of a rat hepatoma cell line by the synergistic interactions of hormones and collagenous substrata, *J. Cell Biol.* **97**:1179–1190.

Gilad, G., and Gilad, V., 1983, Polyamine biosynthesis is required for survival of sympathetic neurons after axonal injury, *Brain Res.* **273**:191–194.

Good, N., Winget, G., Winter, W., Connolly, T., Izawa, F., and Singh, R., 1966, Hydrogen ion buffers for biological research, *Biochemistry* **5**:467–477.

Gospodarowicz, D., 1983, The control of mammalian cell proliferation by growth factors, basement lamina, and lipoproteins, *J. Invest. Dermatol.* **81**:40s–50s.

Gospodarowicz, D., and Mescher, A., 1980, Fibroblast growth factor and the control of vertebrate regeneration and repair, *Ann. N.Y. Acad. Sci.* **339**:151–174.

Gospodarowicz, D., Delgado, D., and Vlodavsky, I., 1980, Permissive effect of the extracellular matrix on cell proliferation in vitro, *Proc. Natl. Acad. Sci. USA* **77**:4094–4098.

Greene, L., and Shooter, E., 1980, The nerve growth factor: Biochemistry, synthesis, and mechanism, *Annu. Rev. Neurosci.* **3**:353–402.

Ham, R., 1964, Putrescine and related amines as growth factors for a mammalian cell line, *Biochem. Biophys. Res. Commun.* **14**:34–38.

Ham, R., 1981, Survival and growth requirements of nontransformed cells, in: *Tissue Growth Factors* (R. Baserga, ed.), Springer-Verlag, Berlin, pp. 13–88.

Harrison, R., 1907, Observations on the living developing nerve fiber, *Anat. Rec.* **1**:116–118.

Harrison, R., 1910, The outgrowth of the nerve fiber as a mode of protoplasmic movement, *J. Exp. Zool.* **9**:787–846.

Havrankova, J., Schmechel, D., Roth, J., and Brownstein, M., 1978, Identification of insulin in rat brain, *Proc. Natl. Acad. Sci. USA* **75**:5737–5741.

Havrankova, J., Roth, J., and Brownstein, M., 1979, Concentrations of insulin and insulin receptors in the brain are independent of peripheral insulin levels, *J. Clin. Invest.* **64**:636–642.

Havrankova, J., Brownstein, M., and Roth, J., 1981, Insulin and insulin receptors in rodent brain, *Diabetologia* **20**:268–273.

Heby, O., 1981, Role of polyamines in the control of cell proliferation and differentiation, *Differentiation* **19**:1–20.

Heifetz, A., and Snyder, J., 1981, The effects of hydrocortisone on the biosynthesis of sulfated glycoconjugates by human fetal lung, *J. Biol. Chem.* **256**:4957–4967.

Hudspeth, E., Swann, H., and Pomerat, C., 1950, Preliminary observations on the effect of various concentrations of oxygen on the in vitro growth of spinal cord from embryonic chicks, *Tex. Rep. Biol. Med.* **8**:341–349.

Hynes, R., 1981, Fibronectin and its relation to cellular structure and behavior, in: *Cell Biology of the Extracellular Matrix* (E. Hay, ed.), Plenum Press, New York, pp. 295–334.

Hynes, R., and Yamada, K., 1982, Fibronectins: Multifunctional modular glycoproteins, *J. Cell Biol.* **95**:369–377.

Iversen, P., Partlow, L., Stensaas, L., and Moatamed, F., 1981, Characterization of a variety of standard collagen substrates: Ultrastructure, uniformity, and capacity to bind and promote growth of neurons, *In Vitro* **17**:541–552.

Jasper, T., Luttge, W., Benton, T., and Garnica, A., 1982, Polyamines in the developing mouse brain, *Develop. Neurosci.* **5**:233–242.

Kaufmann, U., Zapf, J., and Froesch, E., 1978, Growth-hormone dependence of non-suppressible insulin-like activity (NSILA) and of NSILA-carrier protein in rats, *Acta Endocrinol. (Copenhagen)* **87**:716–727.

Knuutila, S., and Pohjanpelto, P., 1983, Polyamine starvation causes parallel increase in nuclear and chromosomal aberrations in a polyamine-dependent strain of CHO, *Exp. Cell Res.* **145**:222–226.

Kyritsis, A., Tsokos, M., Triche, T., and Chader, G., 1984, Retinoblastoma—origin from a primitive neuroectodermal cell?, *Nature* **307**:471–473.

Lamb, J., Ray, F., Ward, J., Kushner, J., and Kaplan, J., 1983, Internalization and subcellular localization of transferrin and transferrin receptors in HeLa cells, *J. Biol. Chem.* **258**:8751–8758.

Landau, B., Abrams, M., White, J., Takaoka, Y., Taslitz, N., Austin, P., Austin, J., and Chernicky, C., 1976, Insulin action on the primate hypothalamus, *Diabetes* **25**(Suppl. 1):322.

Larrick, J., and Cresswell, P., 1979, Modulation of cell surface iron transferrin receptors by cellular density and state of activation, *J. Supramol. Struct.* **11**:579–586.

Leibowitz, A., 1963, The growth and maintenance of tissue-cell cultures in free gas exchange with the atmosphere, *Am. J. Hyg.* **78**:173–180.

Leivo, I., Vaheri, A., Timpl, R., and Wartiovaara, J., 1980, Appearance and distribution of collagens and laminin in the early mouse embryo, *Develop. Biol.* **76**:100–114.

Lembach, K., 1976, Enhanced synthesis and extracellular accumulation of hyaluronic acid during stimulation of quiescent human fibroblasts by mouse epidermal growth factor, *J. Cell. Physiol.* **89**:277–288.

Leutz, A., and Schachner, M., 1982, Cell type-specificity of epidermal growth factor (EGF) binding in primary cultures of early postnatal mouse cerebellum, *Neurosci. Lett.* **30**:179–182.

Lie, S., McKusick, V., and Neufeld, E., 1972, Simulation of genetic mucopolysaccharidoses in normal human fibroblasts by alteration of pH of the medium, *Proc. Natl. Acad. Sci. USA* **69**:2361–2363.

Liesi, P., Dahl, D., and Vaheri, A., 1983, Laminin is produced by early rat astrocytes in primary culture, *J. Cell Biol.* **96**:920–924.

Lissack, K., 1971, *Hormones and Brain Function*, Plenum Press, New York.

MacLusky, N., and Clark, C., 1980, Hormone receptors in the central nervous system, in: *Proteins of the Nervous System*, 2nd ed. (R. Bradshaw and D. Schneider, eds.), Raven Press, New York, pp. 331–383.

McMorris, F., Miller, S., Pleasure, D., and Abramsky, O., 1981, Expression of biochemical properties of oligodendrocytes in oligodendrocyte × glioma cell hybrids proliferating in vitro, *Exp. Cell Res.* **133**:395–404.

Meier, D., Lagenauer, C., and Schachner, M., 1982, Immunoselection of oligodendrocytes by magnetic beads. I. Determination of antibody coupling parameters and cell binding conditions, *J. Neurosci. Res.* **7**:119–134.

Meier, S., and Hay, E., 1974, Stimulation of extracellular matrix synthesis in the developing cornea by glycosaminoglycans, *Proc. Natl. Acad. Sci. USA* **71**:2310–2313.

Meyer, J., and McEwen, B., 1982, Evidence for glucocorticoid target cells in the rat optic nerve: Physicochemical characterization of cytosol binding sites, *J. Neurochem.* **39**:435–442.

Michler-Stuke, A., and Bottenstein, J., 1981, Homotypic extracellular matrices enhance the proliferation of human neuroblastoma cells, *Soc. Neurosci. Abstr.* **7**:149.

Michler-Stuke, A., and Bottenstein, J., 1982a, Proliferation of glial-derived cells in defined media, *J. Neurosci. Res.* **7**:215–228.

Michler-Stuke, A., and Bottenstein, J., 1982b, Defined media for the growth of human and rat glial-derived cells, *CSH Conf. Cell Prolif.* **9**:959–971.

Michler-Stuke, A., Wolff, J., and Bottenstein, J., 1984, Factors influencing astrocyte growth and development in defined media, *Int. J. Develop. Neurosci.* **2(6)**:575–584.

Morriss, G., and Solursh, M., 1978, Regional differences in mesenchymal cell morphology and glycosaminoglycans in early neural-fold stage rat embryos, *J. Embryol. Exp. Morphol.* **46**:37–52.

Murad, S., Grove, D., Lindberg, K., Reynolds, G., Sivarajah, A., and Pinnell, S., 1981, Regulation of collagen synthesis by ascorbic acid, *Proc. Natl. Acad. Sci. USA* **78**:2879–2882.

Nathanson, M., 1983, Analysis of cartilage differentiation from skeletal muscle grown on bone matrix. III. Environmental regulation of glycosaminoglycan and proteoglycan synthesis, *Develop. Biol.* **96**:46–62.

Nevo, Z., 1982, Somatomedins as regulators of proteoglycan synthesis, *Connect. Tissue Res.* **10**:109–113.

Nigra, T., Martin, G., and Eagle, H., 1973, The effect of environmental pH on collagen synthesis by cultured cells, *Biochem. Biophys. Res. Commun.* **53**:272–281.

Nissen, C., Ciesielski-Treska, J., Hertz, L., and Mandel, P., 1973, Regulation of oxygen consumption in neuroblastoma cells: Effect of differentiation and potassium, *J. Neurochem.* **20**:1029–1035.

Olson, J., and Holtzman, D., 1981, Factors influencing the growth and respiration of rat cerebral astrocytes in primary culture, *Neurochem. Res.* **6**:1337–1343.

Omary, M., Trowbridge, I., and Minowada, J., 1980, Human cell-surface glycoprotein with unusual properties, *Nature* **286**:888–891.

Pearlstein, E., 1978, Substrate activation of cell adhesion factor as a prerequisite for cell attachment, *Int. J. Cancer* **22**:32–35.

Pegg, A., and McCann, P., 1982, Polyamine metabolism and function, *Am. J. Physiol.* **243**(Cell Physiol. 12):C212–C221.

Pelton, E., Grindeland, R., Young, E., and Bass, N., 1977, Effects of immunologically induced growth hormone deficiency on myelinogenesis in developing rat cerebrum, *Neurology* **27**:282–288.

Persson, B., 1981, Insulin as a growth factor in the fetus, in: *The Biology of Normal Human Growth* (M. Ritzen, ed.), Raven Press, New York, pp. 213–221.

Pohjanpelto, P., 1973, Relationship between putrescine and the proliferation of human fibroblasts in vitro, *Exp. Cell Res.* **80**:137–142.

Posner, B., Kelly, P., Shiu, R., and Friesen, H., 1974, Studies of insulin, growth hormone and prolactin binding: Tissue distribution, species variation and characterization, *Endocrinology* **95**:521–531.

Prehm, P., Dessau, W., and Timpl, R., 1982, Rates of synthesis of basement membrane proteins by differentiating teratocarcinoma stem cells and their modulation by hormones, *Connect. Tissue Res.* **10**:275–285.

Pruss, R., Bartlett, P., Gavrilovic, J., Lisak, R., and Rattray, S., 1982. Mitogens for glial cells: A comparison of the response of cultured astrocytes, oligodendrocytes and Schwann cells, *Develop. Brain Res.* **2**:19–35.

Raff, M., Fields, K., Hakomori, S., Mirsky, R., Pruss, R., and Winter, J., 1979, Cell-type specific markers for distinguishing and studying neurons and the major classes of glial cells in culture, *Brain Res.* **174**:283–308.

Raizada, M., 1983, Localization of insulin-like immunoreactivity in the neurons from primary cultures of rat brain, *Exp. Cell Res.* **143**:351–357.

Risteli, J., Draeger, K., Regitz, G., and Neubauer, H., 1982, Increase in circulating base-ment membrane antigens in diabetic rats and effects of insulin treatment, *Diabetologia* **23**:266–269.

Rovasio, R., Delouvee, A., Yamada, K., Timpl, R., and Thiery, J., 1983, Neural crest cell migration: Requirements for exogenous fibronectin and high cell density, *J. Cell Biol.* **96**:462–473.

Saito, K., Hagiwara, Y., Hasegawa, T., and Ozawa, E., 1982, Indispensibility of iron for the growth of cultured chick cells, *Develop. Growth Differ.* **24**:571–580.

Salomon, D., Liotta, L., and Kidwell, W., 1981, Differential response to growth factor by rat mammary epithelium plated on different collagen substrata in serum-free medium, *Proc. Natl. Acad. Sci. USA* **78**:382–386.

Sanes, J., 1983, Roles of extracellular matrix in neural development, *Annu. Rev. Physiol.* **45**:581–600.

Sara, V., and Hall, K., 1979, Growth hormone, growth factors, and the brain, *Trends Neurosci.* **2**:263–265.

Sara, V., and Hall, K., 1980, Somatomedins and the fetus, *Clin. Obstet. Gynecol.* **23**:765–778.

Sara, V., Hall, K., Rodeck, C., and Wetterberg, L., 1981a, Human embryonic somatomedin, *Proc. Natl. Acad. Sci. USA* **78**:3175–3179.

Sara, V., Hall, K., and Wetterberg, L., 1981b, Growth hormone dependent polypeptides and the brain, in: *The Brain as an Endocrine Target Organ in Health and Disease* (D. de Wied and A. van Keep, eds.), MTP Press, London, pp. 63–72.

Schachner, M., Schoonmaker, G., and Hynes, R., 1978, Cellular and subcellular locali-zation of LETS protein in the nervous system, *Brain Res.* **158**:149–158.

Schengrund, C., and Repman, M., 1979, Differential enrichment of cells from embryonic rat cerebra by centrifugal elutriation, *J. Neurochem.* **33**:283–289.

Schot, L., Boer, H., Swabb, D., and Van Noorden, S., 1981, Immunocytochemical dem-onstration of peptidergic neurons in the central nervous system of the pond snail *Lymnaea stagnalis* with antisera raised to biologically active peptides of vertebrates, *Cell Tissue Res.* **216**:273–291.

Seeds, N., 1983, Neuronal differentiation in reaggregated cell cultures, in: *Advances in Cellular Neurobiology*, Volume 4 (S. Fedoroff and L. Hertz, eds.), Academic Press, New York, pp. 57–79.

Seiler, N., Schmidt-Glenewinkel, T., and Sarhan, S., 1979, On the formation of gamma-aminobutyric acid from putrescine in brain, *J. Biochem.* **86**:277–278.

Sensenbrenner, M., Maderspach, K., Latzkowitz, L., and Jaros, G., 1978, Neuronal cells from chick embryo cerebral hemispheres cultivated on polylysine-coated surfaces, *Develop. Neurosci.* **1**:90–101.

Shapiro, D., and Schrier, B., 1973, Cell cultures of fetal rat brain: Growth and marker enzyme development, *Exp. Cell Res.* **77**:239–247.

Shapiro, S., and Mott, M., 1981, Modulation of glycosaminoglycan biosynthesis by reti-noids, *Ann. N.Y. Acad. Sci.* **359**:306–321.

Shindelman, J., Ortmeyer, A., and Sussman, H., 1981, Demonstration of the transferrin receptor in human breast cancer tissue: Potential marker for identifying dividing cells, *Int. J. Cancer* **27**:329–334.

Shoemaker, W., Bottenstein, J., Milner, R., Clark, B., and Bloom, F., 1979, Serum-free culture medium maintains differentiated properties of neurons in fetal rat brain ex-plants, *Soc. Neurosci. Abstr.* **5**:758.

Shoemaker, W., Bottenstein, J., Schlumpf, M., Milner, R., and Bloom, F., 1985, Explant cultures of locus ceruleus: Lack of requirement for NGF, in preparation.

Simpson, D., Morrison, R., de Vellis, J., and Herschman, H., 1982, Epidermal growth factor binding and mitogenic activity on purified populations of cells from the central nervous system, *J. Neurosci. Res.* **8**:453–462.

Singh, M., Chandrasekaran, E., Cherian, R., and Bachhawat, B., 1969, Isolation and characterization of glycosaminoglycans in brain of different species, *J. Neurochem.* **16**:1157–1162.

Slotkin, T., Whitmore, W., Lerea, L., Slepetis, R., Weigel, S., Trepanier, P., and Seidler, F., 1983, Role of ornithine decarboxylase and the polyamines in nervous system development: Short-term postnatal administration of alpha-difluoromethylornithine, an irreversible inhibitor of ornithine decarboxylase, *Int. J. Develop. Neurosci.* **1**:7–16.

Sotelo, J., Gibbs, C., Gajdusek, D., Toh, B., and Wurth, M., 1980, Method for preparing cultures of central neurons: Cytochemical and immunochemical studies, *Proc. Natl. Acad. Sci. USA* **77**:653–657.

Stadtman, T., 1974, Selenium biochemistry, *Science* **183**:915–922.

Stadtman, T., 1980, Selenium-dependent enzymes, *Annu. Rev. Biochem.* **49**:93–110.

Stevens, R., Nissley, S., Kimura, J., Rechler, M., Caplan, A., and Hascall, V., 1981, Effects of insulin and multiplication-stimulating activity on proteoglycan biosynthesis in chondrocytes from the Swarm rat chondrosarcoma, *J. Biol. Chem.* **256**:2045–2052.

Stoscheck, C., Erwin, B., Florini, J., Richman, R., and Pegg, A., 1982, Effects of inhibitors of ornithine and S-adenosylmethionine decarboxylases on L6 myoblast proliferation, *J. Cell. Physiol.* **110**:161–168.

Straus, D., 1981, Minireview: Effect of insulin on cellular growth and proliferation, *Life Sci.* **29**:2131–2139.

Sunkara, P., Rao, P., Nishioka, K., and Brinkley, B., 1979, Role of polyamines in cytokinesis of mammalian cells, *Exp. Cell Res.* **119**:63–68.

Tabor, C., and Tabor, H., 1976, 1,4-Diaminobutane (putrescine), spermidine, and spermine, *Annu. Rev. Biochem.* **45**:285–306.

Taylor, W., Camalier, R., and Sanford, K., 1978, Density-dependent effects of oxygen on the growth of mammalian fibroblasts in culture, *J. Cell. Physiol.* **95**:33–40.

Timpl, R., Engel, J., and Martin, G., 1983, Laminin—A multifunctional protein of basement membranes, *Trends Biochem. Sci.* **8**:207–209.

Todaro, G., 1982, Autocrine secretion of peptide growth factors by tumor cells, *Natl. Cancer Inst. Monogr.* **60**:139–147.

Toole, B., 1976, Morphogenetic role of glycosaminoglycans (acid mucopolysaccharides) in brain and other tissues, in: *Neuronal Recognition* (S. Barondes, ed.), Plenum Press, New York, pp. 275–329.

Trelstad, R., Kang, A., Cohen, A., and Hay, E., 1973, Collagen synthesis in vitro by embryonic spinal cord epithelium, *Science* **179**:295–297.

Tseng, S., Savion, N., Stern, R., and Gospodarowicz, D., 1982, Fibroblast growth factor modulates synthesis of collagen in cultured vascular endothelial cells, *Eur. J. Biochem.* **122**:355–360.

Tseng, S., Savion, N., Gospodarowicz, D., and Stern, R., 1983, Modulation of collagen synthesis by a growth factor and by the extracellular matrix: Comparison of cellular response to two different stimuli, *J. Cell Biol.* **97**:803–809.

Underwood, E., 1977, *Trace Elements in Human and Animal Nutrition*, 4th ed., Academic Press, New York.

Varon, S., 1977, Neural cell isolation and identification, in: *Cell, Tissue, and Organ Cultures in Neurobiology* (S. Fedoroff and L. Hertz, eds.), Academic Press, New York, pp. 237–261.

Wan, Y., Wu, T., Chung, A., and Damjanov, I., 1984, Monoclonal antibodies to laminin reveal the heterogeneity of basement membranes in the developing and adult mouse tissues, *J. Cell Biol.* **98:**971–979.

Weyhenmeyer, J., and Fellows, R., 1983, Presence of immunoreactive insulin in neurons cultured from fetal rat brain, *Cell. Mol. Neurobiol.* **3:**81–86.

Wood, P., 1976, Separation of functional Schwann cells and neurons from normal peripheral nerve tissue, *Brain Res.* **115:**361–374.

Wu, T., Wan, Y., Chung, A., and Damjanov, I., 1983, Immunohistochemical localization of entactin and laminin in mouse embryos and fetuses, *Develop. Biol.* **100:**495–505.

Yavin, Z., and Yavin, E., 1974, Attachment and culture of dissociated cells from rat embryo cerebral hemispheres on polylysine-coated surface, *J. Cell Biol.* **62:**540–546.

2

Neuronal and Glial Surface Antigens on Cells in Culture

KAY FIELDS

1. INTRODUCTION

1.1. Scope

This review will emphasize cell surface antigenic markers and practically ignore work with most of the described cytoplasmic antigens, simply because this field is growing so fast that it is impractical to try to cover all the new antigens. The emphasis here is on antigens that have been used with success in cultures of the nervous system.

It is often quite difficult to recognize the different cell types in neural cultures. In this situation cell type-specific antigens are very useful, and more and more effort is being made to identify antigens that distinguish between subpopulations of neurons or glia. Both cytoplasmic and surface markers can help in the evaluation of mixed cultures or in judging the success of procedures designed to separate and grow single cell types; surface antigens can also be used to select, separate, or kill off cell populations. Antigens can also provide information about the level of differentiation of cells in the nervous system. Two examples are the expression of myelin-specific proteins and lipids by glia or the synthesis of the glycoprotein surface antigen Thy-1 by neurons.

KAY FIELDS • Departments of Neurology and Neuroscience, Albert Einstein College of Medicine, Bronx, New York 10461.

Table I. Positive Antigenic Markers for Most Neurons in Culture[a]

Marker	Qualification or comment	Section
Tetanus toxin receptors	Very good specificity	1.2
Cholera toxin receptors	Shared with other cell types	1.2
A2B5	Erratic specificity	3.5
A4	CNS only	1.3
T61	Chicken CNS neurons	5
38/D7	PNS only; rat only	1.3
UC45	Also on macrophages	1.3
NILE-GP	Also on Schwann cells	2.1
N-CAM, D2, NS-4, BSP-2	CNS and PNS neurons in culture	2.2
CG-5	All chicken neurons	4.3
N10	SCG neurons and in brain	4.4
C4/12	Also on some astrocytes	4.2
GM_1 ganglioside	Shared with other cell types	3.3
GT_{1b} and/or GD_{1b} gangliosides	—	3.4
GQ ganglioside(s)	See A2B5	3.5

[a] See text at indicated section for references and full description. Not all exceptions are noted here.

Surface proteins and complex lipids are likely to play roles in cell–cell interactions or to have other functions at the cell surface, such as combination with soluble or matrix-bound ligands. Most antigens have unknown functions, but in this review I have tried to point out what tests for function have been made. There is also considerable detail here about the gangliosides and glycoprotein antigens involved in adhesion, since antisera to these molecules affect neurite outgrowth, although in quite different ways.

Rather than focus on work done only in one laboratory, I have tried to bring together and compare the work of many groups, especially those working on the adhesion glycoproteins. In other areas, the emphasis is on work done in the last few years, since there was a volume devoted to neuroimmunology (Brockes, 1982) that contains excellent reviews by many of the leading groups working on surface antigens. Another broad review (Morris, 1982) contains an extensive bibliography and a discussion of techniques, which have not been stressed here at all.

1.2. Toxins as Neuronal Markers

The most successful application so far for some of the defined surface and cytoplasmic antigens is for cell identification in a variety of tissue culture systems (Table I). Tetanus toxin was one of the first neuron-specific surface markers, and its binding continues to be exceedingly useful whenever morphology is not sufficient for neuronal identification (Fields *et al.*, 1982). Originally, the toxin was labeled with ^{125}I and its binding to neuronal cell bodies and processes was detected by counting and visualized by autoradiography (Dimpfel *et al.*, 1975, 1977). Soon thereafter it was detected by immunological methods using rabbit or mouse anti-tetanus toxoid and a fluorescein- or rhodamine-labeled anti-immunoglobulin (Mirsky *et al.*, 1978). By using two different fluorochromes, toxin binding can be used to establish the specificity of other antigens of neuronal or nonneuronal cell types.

Tetanus toxin is particularly useful for the positive identification of neurons. First, it has a broad species-specificity for chick, rodent, human, and amphibian neurons in culture (Mirsky, 1982). Second, antitoxoid antibodies are readily raised in a wide variety of species, allowing great flexibility for double-label experiments with antisera to other antigens. Third, toxin binding has been demonstrated in tissue sections (Beale *et al.*, 1982), so it can be used to compare the *in vivo* with the *in vitro* distribution of markers. Fourth, very young neurons have been examined, E10 in the mouse (Schnitzer and Schachner, 1981a; Koulakoff *et al.*, 1982) and late neurula stage embryos of an amphibian (Vulliamy and Messenger, 1981), and found to bind toxin. Most other neuronal markers are not expressed so early in development.

By combining immmunocytochemistry to detect tetanus toxin binding with [^{3}H]thymidine autoradiography, Koulakoff *et al.* (1983) showed that dividing cells had no toxin receptors, but cells in the CNS acquired toxin receptors within 7 hr after the last period of DNA synthesis, as they converted from dividing neuroblasts to postmitotic neurons. In contrast, at least some dorsal root ganglion (DRG) neurons apparently had toxin receptors before they ceased division. Quail neuroretina cells transformed by Rous sarcoma virus also have toxin receptors while dividing (Crisanti-Combes *et al.*, 1982). In contrast, PC12 pheochromocytoma cells fail to bind either tetanus or cholera toxin, but acquire both receptors when treated with nerve growth factor (NGF) (K. Fields, unpublished observations). Mouse neuroblastoma cells, on the other hand, synthesized no detectable di- or trisialogangliosides and had very few tetanus toxin-binding sites unless the cells were grown with exogenous gangliosides added to the medium (Dimpfel *et al.*, 1977).

The only exceptions to the generalization that all neurons, and only neurons, express tetanus toxin receptors are: (1) adrenal chromaffin cells from neonatal rats have few if any toxin receptors (K. Fields, unpublished observations), although NGF-treated rat adrenal medullary cells do become positive (Lietzke and Unsicker, 1983); (2) retinal photoreceptors do not bind toxin (Beale *et al.*, 1982); (3) thyroid tissue homogenates bind toxin (Kohn *et al.*, 1980); and (4) there is weak binding to some astrocytes and a glial precursor cell (Abney *et al.*, 1983; Raff *et al.*, 1979, 1983a,b).

The chemical identity of the toxin receptor is of some interest. Brain or thyroid homogenates bind toxin, as do ganglioside fractions purified from either source. When separated brain gangliosides were tested for toxin binding, the most active fractions were those containing GD_{1b} and GT_{1b} (van Heyningen, 1974). More recently, binding by gangliosides in the order $GQ_{1b} \cong GT_{1b} \cong GD_{1b} > GT_{1a} > GM_1 > GD_{1a} > GM_3$ was shown (Holmgren *et al.*, 1980). It is hard to establish that it is the major ganglioside in these fractions that does indeed adsorb the toxin, and it is also uncertain that the relatively abundant binding sites visualized by indirect immunofluorescence are chemically the same as the sites involved in the lethal effects of the toxin. Toxin receptors seen by immunofluorescence on neurons are insensitive to glutaraldehyde fixation but are destroyed by alcohol, as expected for glycolipids. There have been no published experiments testing the Pronase- or neuraminidase-sensitivity of the binding sites on the neuronal cell surface. However, in the absence of any evidence to the contrary, it is widely accepted that the tetanus toxin receptors seen are one or all of the complex gangliosides of the *b* series.

One of the more awkward aspects of using tetanus toxin is its extraordinary toxicity, second only to botulinum toxin. Immunization of all lab personnel and prompt inactivation of toxin solutions and washes during the staining procedure are our usual precautions. The nontoxic tetanus toxin fragment IIc substitutes nicely for the whole toxin and is detected by antitoxoid antibody (Koulakoff *et al.*, 1982). It is the preferred probe but is not yet as widely available as whole toxin.

To some extent cholera toxin can be employed instead of tetanus toxin in cultures and in tissue sections (Raff *et al*, 1979; Willinger and Schachner, 1980). Unfortunately, immature neurons may not bind cholera toxin (Willinger and Schachner, 1980) and other cells, in particular oligodendrocytes, bind this toxin in large amounts (Raff *et al.*, 1979). In CNS and PNS cultures, other nonneuronal cells bind lesser but variable amounts of cholera toxin (Raff *et al.*, 1979), which increases with longer times in culture (K. Fields, unpublished observations). Although it shows much less cell type-specificity than tetanus toxin, cholera toxin is commercially available, is quite a stable protein, and it appears to bind to many more sites per neuron than tetanus toxin. Its receptor is the ganglioside GM_1 (Fishman and Brady, 1976).

Willinger and Schachner (1980) have done the most interesting experiments with cholera toxin, measuring the appearance of toxin receptors on the granule cells of mouse cerebellum as they migrate and differentiate. From the distribution of toxin binding in tissue sections of mice of increasing age and from the binding *in vitro*, where cultured cells were labeled *in vivo* with [^{3}H]thymidine, they could measure the expression of this surface marker relative to cellular DNA synthesis. They concluded that there are many more cholera toxin receptors on postmitotic neurons than on dividing neuroblasts.

1.3. Monoclonal Antibodies That Bind to Neurons

The anti-retinal cell monoclonal antibody A2B5 (Eisenbarth *et al.*, 1979) has been reported to be a reagent useful for the positive identification of neurons (Walsh, 1980; Dickson *et al.*, 1982). However, in some species or culture systems not all neurons are positive and not all nonneurons are negative, so that this antibody must be used with discrimination in cell identification. The findings with A2B5 will be summarized at length in Section 3.5.

Two monoclonal antibodies discriminate between CNS and PNS neurons. A4 is specific for CNS neurons in rat (Cohen and Selvendran, 1981) and human cultures (Dickson *et al.*, 1982), whereas 38/D7 binds to the surface of PNS neurons (Vulliamy *et al.*, 1981). A4 appears to label immature cerebellar cells in the external granular layer more intensely than neurons of the internal granular layer (Cohen and Selvendran, 1981), and very early (E10) embryo brain has only 1% of adult levels of this antigen. Human, ovine, porcine, bovine, and rabbit brains had antigen levels similar to rat brain, whereas guinea pig, mouse, chicken, and frog brains had no detectable antigen. The antigen resisted protease or neuroaminidase digestion and was heat-sensitive and detergent-soluble (Cohen and Selvendran, 1981). More recently, A4 antigen was shown on glial precursor cells along with tetanus toxin receptors and A2B5 antigen (Abney *et al.*, 1983), as discussed in Section 3.5.

A counterpart of A4, the monoclonal 38/D7 binds to all PNS neurons, but in DRG cultures a few flat cells were also positive. Adrenal medullary cells, if treated with NGF, had antigen on chromaffin cells (Vulliamy *et al.*, 1981). The pheochromocytoma cell line PC12 was positive, whereas electrically active cell lines from CNS tumors were negative. Unlike A4, this antigen was trypsin-sensitive and rat-specific. Since many PNS neurons are obvious by their morphology, the use of 38/D7 may not become widespread. The low density and rat-specificity of this antigen may also reduce its utility.

A surface marker shared by macrophages and neurons is defined by monoclonal antibody UC45 (Hogg *et al.*, 1981). This antibody binds to needlelike projections formed by a variable proportion of adherent macrophages, but not to other hemopoietically derived cells. It also binds to processes of CNS and PNS neurons in culture, but not to non-neuronal cells. The antigen is found on rat, mouse, and human neurons. Interestingly, neither the macrophages in rat brain cultures nor process-bearing fibrous astrocytes were positive with UC45. The cell line PC12, which can express many neuronal properties (see Chapter 8) did not bind UC45.

1.4. Cross-Reactions of Monoclonal and Conventional Antibodies

The monoclonal antibody UC45 illustrates two interesting kinds of cross-reactions, both of which must be kept in mind by those using antibodies. The first is that antibodies that are functionally cell type-specific may bind to other cell types in a different region of the nervous system or in nonneural tissues. UC45, for example, binds to the surface of neurons and to a subset of nonneural macrophages. The antigens on the two types of cells are different although they share a common antigenic determinant. The monocyte surface antigen is the 66,000-dalton chain of fibrin, but the neuronal antigen is not, and its size is still unknown. In the second type of cross-reaction, which may be especially difficult with tissue sections, when neural cultures were fixed all cells were positive, since the antibody, in addition to its reaction with a neuronal surface antigen, reacts with a ubiquitous mitochondrial protein of 45,000 daltons (Hogg, 1983).

A reaction with both a surface antigen and a seemingly unrelated cytoplasmic antigen was also found with about 10% of all anti-Thy-1.1 monoclonal antibodies. They reacted with cytoplasmic intermediate filament structures in fibroblasts, independent of whether the cells were genetically Thy-1.1 or Thy-1.2 (Dulbecco *et al.*, 1981). It seems unlikely that two cross-reacting antigens, one associated with the cell surface and one with a cytoplasmic organelle, are closely related.

Rabbit antigalactocerebroside (GalC) sera were reported to react not only with the surface galactolipid but also with cytoplasmic elements of epithelial cells (Sakakibara *et al.*, 1981a). In a kidney epithelial cell line, the cytoplasmic antigen was found to be associated with colchicine-sensitive, microtubulelike structures inside the fixed cells, but the antigen was extracted by lipid solvents (Sakakibara *et al.*, 1981b). It was not clear whether cells with the cytoskeleton-associated antigen had surface galactospingolipids or not.

Staining by monoclonal A2B5 of fibrous cytoskeletal elements inside cells that are negative for A2B5 surface antigen has been reported by Sommer and Schachner (1981). They noted similar staining by O1, O2, and O3 monoclonal antibodies of fixed astrocytes *in vitro* that did not have the O-antigens on their surface. Since the staining was abolished by chloroform–methanol treatment, it was probably due to glycolipids at both sites. Monoclonal antibodies O2 and O3 also reacted with Bergmann glial fibers in tissue sections, showing that some astrocytes *in vivo* also have the cytoplasmic O2 and O3 antigens.

Thus, there are already numerous examples of the cross-reaction of monoclonal antibodies with surface components and seemingly unrelated cytoplasmic antigens. Staining of cell surface antigens in tissue sections is particularly hard to obtain for all but the most plentiful of plasma membrane components, and it is not always easy to distinguish between surface and cytoplasmic labeling at the light microscopic level, especially if the cells are small and have only a thin rim of cytoplasm. In cell culture, if reagents that have been shown to be cell type-specific by experiments using live cells are applied to fixed cells, it may again be difficult to tell cytoplasmic from surface labeling. Fixation is a particular temptation with neural cells, for it is often difficult to avoid washing away neurons or oligodendrocytes during the staining procedures. In cultures without an astrocyte monolayer beneath the round cells, the problem is especially frustrating. Very careful fixation with aldehydes can give unbroken membranes, with little penetration of antibody inside the cell, but the more common situation is that numerous breaks occur, and both surface and cytoplasmic constituents are accessible to antibody. Staining patterns that are largely cytoplasmic, revealed by a clearly outlined nucleus and a lack of bright membrane-associated labeling, are all too often presented as evidence of cell identification using reagents for surface markers. Hopefully, those who do this have proof that the procedure is valid, in the face of the counterexamples given above.

2. LARGE GLYCOPROTEINS OF THE NEURONAL SURFACE

2.1. NILE Glycoproteins

Another neuronal marker is the NGF-inducible large, external glycoprotein (NILE-GP), originally identified on the PC12 cell line by comparing the surface glycoproteins of cells with and without added NGF (McGuire *et al.*, 1978). A rabbit antiserum raised to purified NILE-GP cut from SDS gels was found to react with a 230,000-dalton glycoprotein from PC12 solubilized membranes and to be adsorbed by PC12 cells or brain, but not by nonneural tissue (Salton et al., 1983a). Unlike earlier guinea pig antisera raised against whole PC12 cells or sympathetic neurons that had recognized multiple glycoprotein bands (Lee et al., 1981), the rabbit antiserum to NILE-GP, since it reacted only with the 230,000-dalton protein, was a more appropriate reagent for study of the NILE-GP. In CNS cell cultures, binding, assayed by indirect immunofluorescence, was only to neurons, whereas in PNS cultures, neurons and Schwann cells were both positive, although Schwann cells had less antigen. The antigen on CNS neurons had a molecular weight on gels of 200,000–210,000, smaller than the PNS or PC12 glycoprotein (Salton et al., 1983a,b). A monoclonal antibody that reacts with the NILE-GP, isolated by L. L. Y. Chun, and the rabbit antiserum of Salton et al. (1983a) were used by Sweadner (1983) to show that the surface glycoprotein B2 that she characterized on sympathetic neurons in culture was identical to the NILE-GP.

Stallcup et al. (1983) used conventional antisera to PC12 cells to show antibody binding to CNS and PNS neurons, adrenal chromaffin cells, and Schwann cells, all of which could be absorbed by brain tissue. Immunoprecipitates of ^{125}I-labeled PC12 proteins showed multiple bands on gels similar to those of Lee et al. (1981). Stallcup et al. (1983) concluded that a protein of about 200,000 daltons was shared by PC12, neurons, and Schwann cells. Again, their large glycoproteins had slightly different molecular weights from each source (215,000 to 235,000). They may have been examining the same protein as the PC12 NILE-GP and the "band 1" surface protein on mouse neuroblastoma cell line N18 described by Akeson and Hsu (1978).

Curiously, the only monoclonal antibody developed from mice immunized with PC12 cells failed to react with PC12 cells after selection and cloning, and instead it detected an antigen (G5) shared by brain and lymphoid cells with a molecular weight of 95,000–105,000 (Rodman and Akeson, 1981).

2.2. A Quartet of Related Glycoproteins: N-CAM, D2, NS-4, and BSP-2

One of the most important examples of a set of surface glycoproteins with developmental functions, or at least developmentally regulated synthesis, are the neural cell adhesion molecules (N-CAMs) studied by Edelman and his collaborators (Edelman, 1983). In addition to these adhesion molecules, rodent glycoproteins that antigenically and biochemically are closely related to them were independently characterized. They are the synaptosomal protein D2 (Jørgensen and Bock, 1974;

Jørgensen and Møller, 1980) and several cerebellar cell surface glyco-proteins, especially the NS-4 (Schachner *et al.*, 1975; Goridis *et al.*, 1978) and the BSP-2 antigens (Hirn *et al.*, 1981).

An interesting aspect of the work on N-CAM is the imaginative use of immunological methods in assays for the molecules mediating cell adhesion (Brackenbury *et al.*, 1977). The first antibody was a polyclonal rabbit antiserum against young chick embryo retinal cells that had been cultured briefly. Whole immunoglobulin from this serum agglutinated retinal cells, while monovalent immunoglobulin fragments (Fab') inhibited cell aggregation. The media from suspension cultures of retinal cells neutralized this Fab' activity. Three inhibitory polypeptides of 140,000, 120,000, and 65,000 daltons were purified from spent media, and a new antiserum, one giant step closer to being specific, was raised to a pool of the inhibitory fractions. This antiserum also inhibited adhesion. The major polypeptide of detergent-solubilized membranes to react with this antiserum had a molecular weight of 140,000 (Thiery *et al.*, 1977). It comigrated on gels with the surface protein previously named CAM, which was thought to be important in adhesion since it too was precipitated by an antiserum that inhibited cell adhesion (Rutishauser *et al.*, 1976).

Antibody to the 140,000-, 120,000-, 65,000-dalton pool of shed antigens ("specific anti-CAM") reacted with the surfaces of aggregated, fixed retinal cells and stained frozen sections of retina, other CNS regions, and PNS ganglia. Fourteen-day-old embryonic (E14) retina showed intense staining of the plexiform layers and little staining of the nuclear layers, perhaps reflecting the different density of surface membrane around the cell bodies compared to the layers of packed processes or perhaps indicating a preferential location of the antigen on membranes of processes rather than membranes around cell bodies (Rutishauser *et al.*, 1978a).

The biochemical characterization of N-CAM has been helped by the advent of monoclonal antibodies. These were raised to partially purified chick N-CAM, and hybridoma clones were sought that produced immunoglobulins that bound to N-CAM and inhibited retinal cell aggregation. From partially purified N-CAM preparations the resulting monoclonal antibodies precipitated proteins that ran on gels as a smear in the range of about 200,000–250,000 daltons. For the first time large amounts of chick N-CAM could be readily purified 100-fold in high yield from detergent extracts of whole embryonic chick brains by immunoaffinity chromatography using this monoclonal antibody (Hoffman *et al.*, 1982).

One monoclonal antibody (15G8), raised to chick tectal cell membranes, allowed the comparison of chick and mouse N-CAM activities.

This antibody immunoprecipitated purified chick N-CAM and a high-molecular-weight (200,000–220,000) smear of proteins from extracts of iodinated embryonic mouse brain vesicles. Mouse brain extracts run over 15G8 immunoaffinity columns yielded 1% of the protein and resulted in a 70-fold enrichment of material active in a mouse brain cell adhesion assay. Since 15G8 appeared to react with the sialic acid component of chick and mouse N-CAMs, another round of rabbit sera and mouse monoclonal antibodies was isolated from animals immunized with the 15G8 affinity-purified proteins from mouse brain. Fab' fractions of the resulting rabbit antiserum inhibited aggregation of mouse brain cells, and proteins that reacted with 15G8 neutralized this effect. A different monoclonal antibody, 9E11, probably reacts with the protein moiety of mouse N-CAM (Chuong et al., 1982).

Chicken and mouse N-CAM glycoproteins have similar biochemical properties. They are heterogeneous in size on SDS gels and are converted by boiling to lower-molecular-weight bands around 140,000 (Hoffman et al., 1982; Chuong et al., 1982). The protease V8 peptide maps of 15G8 or 9E11 affinity-purified mouse N-CAMs are the same, but they differ from chicken N-CAM. Both monoclonal antibodies stain neurons but not glial cells in rat brain cultures (Chuong et al., 1982), and in tissue sections antigen is found in both the CNS and the PNS. All these antigens have an unusually high sialic acid content. Chick N-CAM has 13.2 moles of sialic acid and 6.3 moles of other hexoses per 100 moles of amino acid. Overall, N-CAM contains 26% carbohydrate and 58% protein (Hoffman et al., 1982).

Thus, various chick, mouse, and rat brain N-CAMs are related molecules, with cross-reacting, highly unusual carbohydrate portions and, in some cases, cross-reactive protein structures. However, various chick N-CAMs are not identical. For example, N-CAM from the chick retina is smaller than N-CAM from chick brain, although both are reduced to 140,000-dalton bands by neuraminidase treatment (Hoffman et al., 1982). Embryonic and adult chick N-CAMs also differ: the antigen from adult brain has more protein at distinct bands of molecular weight 150,000 and 180,000, much less in the higher-molecular-weight regions of SDS gels, and the sialic acid content of the adult form is only 10% compared to 30% in embryonic N-CAM. Antigens from brains of both ages run as a doublet at 140,000 daltons after neuraminidase treatment, and the protein portions appear to be identical by various criteria (Rothbard et al., 1982).

There is a change during development of mouse N-CAM similar to that found in the chick (Edelman and Chuong, 1982). Multiple bands are reduced to a doublet at 120,000 daltons by neuraminidase. The 15G8 monoclonal antibody against the unique carbohydrate antigen reacts only with the very-high-molecular-weight forms, which were the major forms in embryonic brain and which disappeared by postnatal day 14. Other monoclonal antibodies detect antigenic differences between the N-CAM fractions from different brain regions.

There are neurological mouse mutants with well-characterized developmental defects. Edelman and Chuong (1982) showed that mice homozygous for the mutant allele at the staggerer locus (Sg/Sg) are different from wild-type mice or heterozygous littermates in their cerebellar N-CAM patterns. Sg/Sg mice had an abnormal persistence of embryonic N-CAM while other neurological mutants showed the normal conversion of high-molecular-weight N-CAM to the adult forms. They suggested that the defects in development in staggerer mice and the persistence of embryonic N-CAM might be due to defects in sialidation enzymes. Alternately, both could be secondary consequences of a different maturational defect. If staggerer mouse mutants contain a modified desialidation enzyme, for example, rather than low levels of the normal enzyme, this would be a strong argument for a direct connection of N-CAM to neuronal migration, survival, and synapse formation in the cerebellum. In fact, sialic acid-containing lipids, the gangliosides, are also abnormal in staggerer mice, with an abnormal persistence of the "immature" ganglioside GD_3 in the cerebellum of mutant compared to normal mice (Seyfried et al., 1982).

Reviews of the work of Edelman's group and the cell surface modulation theories which accompany it have recently been published (Edelman, 1983; Rutishauser, 1983). This immunological approach is also being applied to heterologous cell interactions, in particular the adhesion of neurons and glia (Grumet et al., 1984).

D2, one of three rat synaptosomal protein antigens defined by Bock and her colleagues (Bock, 1978), has been shown by direct experiments to cross-react with anti-N-CAM antibody (Jørgensen et al., 1980). Quantitative data on D2 were obtained using polyspecific rabbit antisynaptosome sera (Bock, 1978), including the determination of its molecular weight (139,000) (Jørgensen, 1979). However, immunohistochemical localization required a monospecific serum, and this was made by raising antisera to antigen–antibody complexes cut from immunoelectrophoretic separations of impure antigen preparations. When iterated, this resulted in successively more specific rabbit antisera (Jørgensen and Møller, 1980). With the final serum, the D2 antigen was shown to be present on the surface of CNS neurons in cultures (Bock et al., 1980), whereas in adult tissue the antigen was detected on presynaptic membranes but not on axonal or dendritic membranes (Jørgensen and Møller, 1980).

Like N-CAM, the D2 antigen changes its physical properties during the perinatal period. In a system responsive to net negative charge, the electrophoretic mobility of D2 from perinatal rats was 1.6-fold greater than that from adults. Neuraminidase converted the perinatal form into the adult form (Jørgensen and Møller, 1980). Later, neuraminidase was shown to act on chick N-CAM (Rothbard et al., 1982). Both anti-D2 and anti-N-CAM affect the fasciculation of neurites growing out of explants of PNS ganglia (Rutishauser et al., 1978b; Jørgensen et al., 1980). Anti-N-CAM was shown to inhibit the immunoprecipitation of D2 by anti-D2 antibody, evidence for a cross-reaction of rat D2 and chick N-CAM (Jørgensen et al., 1980).

A surface glycoprotein of the mouse that is probably closely related or identical to mouse N-CAM is the NS-4 antigen first described by Schachner et al. (1975). This antigen was defined by rabbit antisera to membranes of 4-day-old mouse cerebella, and it was present as two polypeptides of 145,000 and 200,000 daltons (Goridis et al., 1978). The same serum precipitated polypeptides of slightly different size from labeled retinal cells (Rohrer and Schachner, 1980). Goridis et al. (1978) found a developmental change in the size of the larger polypeptide of NS-4 antigen similar to the shifts of N-CAMs. This change was not found by Rohrer and Schachner (1980), whose peptide maps indicated that the 200,000- and 145,000-dalton polypeptides were unlikely to be "overtly structurally related." In dissociated cell cultures of the cerebellum the NS-4 antigen is seen by indirect immunofluorescence to be present predominantly, but not exclusively, on neuronal cells (Schnitzer and Schachner, 1981a). Like the N-CAM proteins, the NS-4 antigens are shed from cells in culture, and when new monoclonal antibodies to mouse N-CAM are available, a direct test of the relationship of NS-4 cerebellar and retinal antigens to mouse N-CAMs will be possible, as discussed by Rohrer and Schachner (1980).

While rabbit antisera defined the NS-4 antigen, the BSP-2 antigen is defined by a monoclonal antibody (BSP-2) isolated from rats immunized with short-term-cultured mouse cerebellar cells. BSP-2 antibody bound to the surface of cerebellar neurons in cultures, and from detergent extracts of the cultures it precipitated a triplet of glycoproteins with molecular weights on SDS gels of 180,000, 140,000, and 120,000 (Hirn et al., 1981). Adult brain regions had different amounts of these three antigens: cerebral cortex had bands of 140,000 and 120,000, spinal cord had only the 120,000, and DRG contained mainly the 180,000 component. A neuroblastoma cell line had a different form (150,000), and neonatal mouse tissue had antigen in the region of 180,000–250,000 on gels. Cleavage of the sugars resulted in a 90,000-dalton protein band, whether the starting material was neonatal 180,000- to 250,000-dalton proteins or the 180,000-, 140,000-, 120,000-dalton triplet of proteins. Tyrosine-containing tryptic peptides of neonatal and adult deglycosylated proteins showed no significant differences (Rougon et al., 1982). Developmental changes in the carbohydrate structures of BSP-2 consist mainly in modifications of the number and average length of $\alpha2\rightarrow8$-linked polysialosyl units (Finne et al., 1983). The sugar and amino acid compositions of BSP-2 antigens were nearly identical to those reported for mouse N-CAM by Chuong et al. (1982). All these data strongly support the interpretation that the various forms of BSP-2 antigen arise by posttranslational modification of a single protein (Rougon et al., 1982).

The BSP-2 antigen was present on the cell surface of neurons in culture, but early in postnatal cerebellar development it was found on Bergmann glia and astrocytes. Migrating neuronal granule cells appeared to acquire the antigen upon arrival at the internal granular layer at times when adult forms of the antigen were emerging. The data suggest that the diffuse 180,000- to 250,000-dalton band may only be on astrocytes and not on neurons. These authors showed by sequential immunoprecipitation experiments that BSP-2 and mouse D2 antigenic determinants are on the same proteins (Hirn et al., 1983). Surprisingly, I have not found a clear statement of whether the mouse antigens NS-4 and BSP-2 are now thought to be on the same molecule, but both NS-4 and D2 are found in the testis as well as brain (Schachner et al., 1975; Jørgensen and Møller, 1983).

Thus, between 1975 and the present, extensive work by several separate groups has come together. An adhesion protein, a synaptosomal protein, a brain antigen, and an antigenic glycoprotein on cultured cells all seem to be the same or at least closely related. Confirmation of this has been slowed by complications due to species differences and the unique carbohydrate portion of the glycoproteins and its processing.

Why should these proteins have such a bewildering variety of modified structures? Do the different forms have different adhesive properties? Using liposomes bearing adult or embryonic forms of BSP-2, Sadoul et al. (1983) showed that only the adult form can effectively mediate the adhesion of liposomes to neuroblastoma cells, and Hoffman and Edelman (1983) found that there is a fourfold difference in the aggregation activity of vesicles formed with embryonic versus adult N-CAM.

It is fairly clear that efforts in several laboratories will now concentrate on the relationship of N-CAM changes to the developmental events that this molecule may mediate. At the moment, however, the evidence

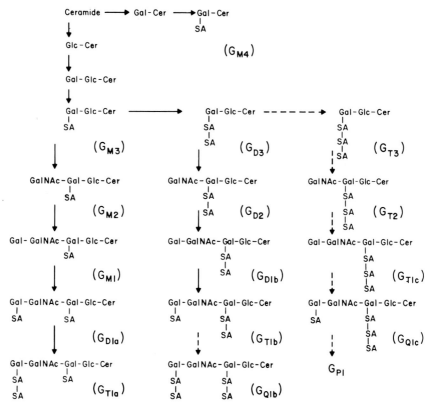

Figure 1. The proposed pathways for ganglioside synthesis. (From Yu and Ando, 1980.)

for a specific role in development is not yet very convincing. But it is increasingly clear that N-CAM and similar molecules are the strongest candidates for a surface component involved in cell–cell interactions.

3. GANGLIOSIDE ANTIGENS ON NEURONS AND GLIA

Gangliosides are complex, sialic acid-containing glycolipids that are present in low amounts in most cells of many animal species but are present in strikingly high concentrations in some neural cells. In Fig. 1 the structures of the major gangliosides and their proposed pathways of biosynthesis are summarized (Yu and Ando, 1980; Rapport, 1981a). The structures of the *a* and *b* series have long been established; the *c* series has been described more recently (Kasai and Yu, 1983).

While the biological functions of gangliosides in brain are still obscure, the consequence of abnormal ganglioside metabolism are devastating. Some inherited lipidoses primarily disrupt myelin; others apparently affect neurons (Brady, 1981). The role of gangliosides in neuronal differentiation, synaptogenesis, and regeneration is now a subject of intense interest (Rapport and Gorio, 1981; Ledeen et al., 1984), and cell culture models of the effects of ganglioside administration are being developed, starting from the observations of increased synapse formation (Obata et al., 1977) and neurite sprouting (Roisen et al., 1981).

It seems important to establish whether different gangliosides are on the cell surface of different cell types, since there are models in which gangliosides act as mediators of cell surface interactions. Surface labeling of live cells in culture with well-characterized antibodies is a very direct way of doing this. New monoclonal antibodies will help standardize this type of experiment and introduce an exquisite level of sensitivity and discrimination, especially when mixed populations of cells of different ganglioside compositions are present.

3.1. GM$_4$

Ceramide, a sphingolipid, is at a major branch point in ganglioside biosynthesis. There are two glycosyltransferases that act on ceramide—one adds a glucose residue, the other a galactose (Fig. 1). With slight exceptions, the latter enzyme appears to be restricted to oligodendrocytes and Schwann cells, and the product GalC is found only, or predominantly, in myelin or myelin-forming cells. The addition of a sialic acid residue to the galactose of GalC produces a monosialoganglioside, GM$_4$ (also called G$_7$ in another nomenclature), that is a major ganglioside species in purified myelin fractions of birds and some primates and is present to a variable extent in other species (Cochran et al., 1982). From its distribution, we might expect this ganglioside to be a specific glial marker (Ledeen et al., 1973), but antisera to GM$_4$ have not been used for immunochemistry. However, in most species little GalC is converted to the ganglioside and most of it remains in myelin membranes as GalC or its sulfated derivative, sulfatide (see Section 6.1).

3.2. GD$_3$

In most cells glucose, galactose, and a sialic acid residue are added to ceramide to form GM$_3$, a monosialoganglioside that is the branch point for the two major pathways of most species (Fig. 1). The ganglioside series a, b, and c differ in the number of sialic acid residues attached to the innermost galactosyl residue (Fig. 1). All the major gangliosides (except GM_4) of most mammalian brains have the same four-sugar backbone (Gal-GalNAc-Gal-Glc-Cer) and differ only in the number and location of sialic acid residues. Of their shorter-chain precursors (the "2" and "3" compounds in Fig. 1), only GD_3 is ever a major species in normal brain. In fact, GD_3 is the most abundant ganglioside early in development (Seyfried *et al.*, 1982), and it is the precursor of the complex gangliosides of the *b* and *c* series.

GD_3 was the only brain ganglioside to react with a monoclonal antibody, R24, raised against melanoma tumor cells (Pukel *et al.*, 1982). A minority of the neurons bound this antibody in cell cultures of rat cerebellum, brain stem, olfactory bulb, DRG, and superior cervical ganglion (SCG) (Fields, 1983b). The antigen was present on all somal, neurite, and growth cone surfaces of positive cells. The detected antigen was not neuron-specific for it was also expressed by small subpopulations of nonneural cells in all culture systems tested.

In vivo, GD_3 declines in amount as all the other gangliosides increase. It is possible that some of the neuroblast-specific lipid antigens that are being described, e.g., D1.1 (Stallcup *et al.*, 1983), are related to GD_3.

3.3. GM_1

The major gangliosides in adult brain are GM_1 and GD_{1a} from the *a* series, and GD_{1b} and GT_{1b} from the *b* series. GM_1 is weakly antigenic. Antisera to mixed ganglioside preparations contain some antibodies that react with GM_1 and with its desialylated derivative, asialo-GM_1 (Naiki *et al.*, 1974), but no monoclonal antibodies that react with GM_1 have been described. Such antibodies are actively being sought, so far without success (Hakomori, 1984). Perhaps mice do not make antibodies to this lipid because it is present on their lymphocytes (Revesz and Greaves, 1975). However, rabbits do respond; and affinity-purified antibodies have been used for antigen localization (deBaecque *et al.*, 1976), tests of neurite outgrowth (Schwartz and Spirman, 1982), and injection into brain (Rapport, 1981b). Many of these experimenters seem to assume that GM_1 antigenic sites are exposed on the surface of live cells. This would seem to be the location of the GM_1, for cholera toxin, usually assumed to bind only to GM_1 (Fishman and Brady, 1976), binds readily both to neurons and in lesser amounts to other live cells *in vitro*. However, with cells from the brain, where other complex gangliosides may well be on the cell surface that are not represented on nonneural cells, there may be other lipids that cholera toxin and anti-GM_1 antibodies bind to, for even antisera raised to purified GM_1 react with other gangliosides (Gregson and Hammer, 1980, 1982). It is difficult to know whether anti-GM_1 antibodies exert their effects by binding to GM_1 itself or to a related ganglioside, or even glycoprotein, in the membranes. Even blocking the effects with GM_1 does not show that the antibodies that can bind to GM_1 in solution were binding to GM_1 at the membrane.

Most cerebellar cells from rats can be lysed by complement and an antibody to gangliosides (Gregson *et al.*, 1977), but it was not determined which membrane gangliosides were the effective receptors. One study reported agreement of cholera toxin binding and anti-GM_1 binding (Raff *et al.*, 1979). It was also found that affinity-purified anti-GM_3 antibodies bound only to oligodendrocytes. Surprisingly, antigloboside antibodies bound to about 50% of DRG neurons in culture. What this glycolipid might be doing in DRG neurons is unclear since globoside is the major neutral glycolipid of red cells, has the same hexoses linked to ceramide as do the major gangliosides but has them linked in a different order, and has no sialic acid residues (Brady, 1981).

My attempts to show binding of anti-GM_1 antibodies to live cerebellar cells have not been successful (K. Fields, unpublished observations), even though I have tried antisera with high titers to GM_1 by other types of assays (Gregson and Hammer, 1980, 1982). Binding of cholera toxin to the neurons indicated that there were many GM_1 sites present and exposed on the live cells. The poor binding of most anti-GM_1 antibodies to the same cells suggests that most of the antibodies are not directed at the same part of GM_1 as cholera toxin binds to. Perhaps the antigenic sites are "buried" when the lipid is in the membrane of live cells. This explanation is currently being tested in an attempt to understand better whether some ganglioside antigens exist in "masked" conformations.

Several interesting questions about ganglioside localization were raised by Ganser *et al.* (1983) in a study of teased myelinated nerve fibers. Cholera toxin bound to fibers at the nodes of Ranvier, apparently to both axonal membranes and Schwann cell membranes near the node. Along the Schwann cell membrane between the nodes there was little binding, but if the nerve fibers were treated with neuraminidase, which converts higher gangliosides into GM_1, then there was binding all along the membrane around the myelin sheath. The authors concluded that the outer Schwann cell plasma membrane has polysialogangliosides, but little GM_1 except at the node itself. At what stage in development do Schwann cells, and perhaps oligodendroglia as well, start making more complex polysialogangliosides, and why do the GM_1 molecules persist only near the node? Is this GM_1 made by the neuron or the Schwann cell? Are there other inhomogeneities in ganglioside distribution; for example, are the closely packed inner myelin membranes the same as the outermost turn of membrane? Perhaps cell culture systems will provide appropriate material to study the synthesis and regional localization of gangliosides in myelin.

3.4. GD_{1b} and GT_{1b}

These gangliosides differ by one sialic acid and are both major ganglioside species in adult brain. An antiserum to purified GT_{1b} reacted with both species, as well as with other tested gangliosides (Gregson and Hammer, 1980, 1982). Unlike the anti-GM_1 antiserum, the binding of anti-GT_{1b} to live cells could be readily visualized by indirect immunofluorescence (Gregson, 1981).

Given the consistency of neuronal binding of tetanus and cholera toxins, it has been rather a shock to observe the relative variability of the ganglioside antigenic determinants (Fields, 1983b). However, for cell recognition and cell–cell interactions, molecules that can be modified by further glycosylation, surface modulation, or combination with other surface components may be important during normal development.

3.5. GQ

While the GQ ganglioside represents a minor portion (3%) of total ganglioside sialic acid, it is of interest here because the A2B5 monoclonal antibody was shown to bind to neurons in culture, to be cytotoxic for retinal cells, and to be adsorbed out by tetrasialoganglioside fractions. This monoclonal antibody has been made widely available by M. Nirenberg and his co-workers, and there are now published data for this antigen in chicken, rat, mouse, and human systems. In all of them, it is a fairly good marker for the neuronal cell surface, but it also binds to other cell types. No one has identified a functional activity blocked by A2B5; the formation, stability, and functioning of synapses appear unperturbed (Eisenbarth et al., 1979).

The A2B5 monoclonal antibody was raised by Eisenbarth et al., (1979) by immunization with glutaraldehyde-fixed retinal cells from chicken embryos. It bound to retinal cells and was one of a few antibodies that were cytotoxic. Ascites fluid containing A2B5 lysed retinal cells at a 1:300,000 dilution and could be used for immunofluorescence at 1:100. The hybridoma is available from the American Type Culture Collection, and the ascites fluid can be purchased (Accurate Scientific).

Immunofluorescent staining of fixed adult chicken retina tissue sections showed binding only to the cell bodies of retinal neurons and photoreceptor cells. The plexiform layers, which contain neuronal processes and synapses, were negative for A2B5 binding. The antigen was both surface and cytoplasmic, and antibody did not bind at all (or nearly as well) to Müller glial cell bodies or processes. In 24-hr cultures of retinal cells, A2B5 bound to more than 60% of the cell bodies, but not to the processes; however, chick DRG neurons had antigen on the entire cell surface (Eisenbarth et al., 1979). Schnitzer and Schachner (1982) confirmed this distribution on chicken retinal cells but observed that with mouse retinal cells and with neurons from other species and regions the antigen was present equally on cell bodies and processes.

Antigen in retina or brain tissue was extracted by chloroform–methanol, and when brain lipids were partitioned the antigen was in the ganglioside fraction. Consistent with it being a ganglioside, the antigen was heat-stable and neuraminidase-sensitive. Purified gangliosides absorbed the cytotoxic antibody, and after separation of the different gangliosides this activity was found only in the tetrasialoganglioside fraction (Eisenbarth et al., 1979). However, the complete structure of the antigenic ganglioside(s) is controversial. Kasai and Yu (1983) found binding of A2B5 to GQ_{1c} but not to GQ_{1b}, while Fredman et al. (1984) found a complex pattern of minor gangliosides bound the antibody. GQ_{1c} is present in large amounts in fish and chicken brains, but it is not known to be present to any great extent in the rat or mouse. The identity of the antigen on cells cultured from mammalian species is unclear.

Eisenbarth et al. (1981) showed that A2B5 antibody bound to pancreatic islets, but not to pancreatic acinar cells, and to some cells from the adrenal medulla. This was one of the first indications that it might not be a completely neuron-specific antigen. Brain and islet cells share this antigen, as they do another neuronal antigen, the cytoplasmic enzyme neuron-specific enolase (Marangos et al., 1982).

Schnitzer and Schachner (1982) analyzed the cell type-specificity of A2B5 in cell cultures. Most tetanus toxin-binding neurons from mouse cerebellum, retina, spinal cord, and DRG were found to be A2B5-positive; however, more than 10% of the astrocytes from mouse, chicken, and rabbit cerebellum or from chicken retina were also A2B5-positive. No rat cerebellar astrocytes or mouse retinal glial cells were positive. Less than 10% of immature oligodendrocytes were A2B5-positive, whereas none of the more mature oligodendrocytes with surface GalC bound A2B5 antibody. In all species, cells with tetanus toxin receptors (neurons) were all or nearly all positive for A2B5 antigen, and in no species were cells with extracellular fibronectin ever positive for surface

A2B5. However, every other marker tested [glial fibrillary acidic protein (GFA), vimentin, or O4] showed wide species variation. Even worse, *all* *cells* showed intracellular labeling with anti-A2B5 if treated with a permeabilizing fixative. Anyone contemplating the use of A2B5 should review in detail these results before expecting high specificity for certain cell types.

Berg and Schachner (1982) have studied the ultrastructure of the mouse cells in culture that bound antibody A2B5. Immature oligodendrocytes and immature astrocytes both had surface A2B5 antigen. Photoreceptor cells, identified by ribbon synapses, were A2B5-negative whereas other retinal neurons were positive. They did not observe A2B5-positive cells whose cell type could not be assigned using ultrastructural criteria.

A glial precursor cell that bore A2B5 antigen was identified by Abney *et al.* (1983). They found that GalC-positive oligodendrocytes did not develop in rat brain cultures exposed to either A2B5 or A4 antibody plus complement. The precursor cell itself apparently had the surface antigens; when cells were separated by a cell sorter into A2B5-positive and negative fractions, many GalC-bearing cells developed in cultures of antigen-positive fractions and none developed in those of negative fractions. In cell suspensions from newborn rat corpus callosum they found by immunofluorescence that 85% or more of the GalC-bearing cells had A4, A2B5, and tetanus toxin receptors. The idea that the cell with A4, A2B5, and tetanus toxin receptors is a precursor to both astrocytes (defined as GFA-positive cells) and oligodendrocytes (GalC-positive cells) was supported by experiments of Raff *et al.* (1983a), in which the A2B5-bearing cells from optic nerve were cultured in serum-containing or serum-free defined medium. In the presence of serum nearly all A2B5-positive cells became GFA-positive, but in defined medium they converted to A2B5-negative, GalC-positive cells.

We have also observed nonneuronal cells with intense surface staining for A2B5 in cultures of rat cerebellum, brain stem, SCG, and DRG (Fields, 1983b). The CNS cells either die or lose their A2B5 antigen after several days in culture. In the CNS cultures most positive cells were stellate and, in our hands, negative for tetanus and cholera toxin receptors, GalC, and Thy-1. They may have come from white matter, since they were much more abundant in cultures of brain stem than of cerebellum. Except that these cells were considered negative under our labeling conditions for tetanus toxin binding, they appear to be the same as the glial precursor cells described by others (Schnitzer and Schachner, 1982; Berg and Schachner, 1982; Raff *et al.*, 1983a,b). The flat A2B5-

bearing cells of the PNS cultures were not Schwann cells or astrocytes; their identity is still obscure.

All this work on immature glial cells means that we must modify the original picture of A2B5 as neuron-specific, for it is certainly untrue that all A2B5-positive cells are neurons; but are all neurons A2B5-positive? Walsh (1980) did not note any A2B5-negative neurons in rat cerebellar cultures, nor did he find any discrepancy in the distribution of A2B5 and other neuronal markers in cultures from human fetal brain or DRGs (Dickson *et al.*, 1982). Schnitzer and Schachner (1982) also found that most tetanus toxin-positive neurons were A2B5-positive. However, our own experience has been very different. In embryonic rat cerebellum and brain stem cultures tested between 2 and 40 days *in vitro*, nearly all neurons (tetanus toxin-binding cells bearing long, usually thin processes) were at first *negative* for A2B5-binding. With increasing time in culture, more and more of the neurons became positive, and eventually nearly all toxin-binding cells were strongly A2B5-positive (Fields, 1983b). Although there was some variation between experiments in the rate of "differentiation" of the neurons, the most striking variation was due to the age of the rat. Cerebellar and brain stem neurons from postnatal rats were nearly all A2B5-positive after 4–7 days *in vitro*, whereas embryonic rat neurons took much longer (20–30 days *in vitro*) to become positive. (Walsh (1980) tested cells from 5-day-old rats and found all cerebellar neurons A2B5-positive). Our results with DRG and SCG neurons were even more surprising. Perhaps because they are all Thy-1-positive, we expected them to be equally fully developed in their A2B5 expression. Instead, in our hands, A2B5 was a volatile surface marker. Dramatic differences in A2B5 expression were exhibited by adjacent PNS neurons. Antigen was often detected on less than 30% of all the neurons, and the pattern of expression found most often was a sharp decrease in the proportion of A2B5-positive DRG and SCG neurons during 1–2 weeks in culture. In all cases, a positive cell was high in antigen expression over its entire surface, including the tips of growing processes (Fields, 1983b).

At present it is rather difficult to claim a very deep understanding of ganglioside distribution, much less function, from the studies of antiganglioside sera binding. The observed patterns do not agree very well with the published findings of ganglioside content of neuronal and glial cell cultures from chick embryos (Dreyfus *et al.*, 1980). What is needed are monoclonal antibodies directed against nicely exposed and specific antigenic determinants and parallel studies of antibody binding and ganglioside labeling. Since antibodies to gangliosides may play a role in some diseases, such as Graves' disease, and may be present in patients with neurological disorders, including multiple sclerosis (see Ledeen *et al.*, 1984), we can expect to see much more work on these lipids in the future.

3.6. Thyrotropin Receptor

A monoclonal antibody to the thyrotropin receptor that behaved as if it were binding like thyrotropin itself has been described and named thyroid stimulator antibody. It reacted with a minor disialoganglioside component from the thyroid that was not present in brain (Lacetti *et al.*, 1984). Previously, it had been thought that thyrotropin bound to the same gangliosides as did tetanus toxin, but these antibodies seem to rule that notion out. Models have been suggested for the action of cholera and tetanus toxins, interferon, and thyrotropin that postulate interacting glycoprotein and glycolipid membrane components. The toxins and thyroid stimulator antibodies, either mouse monoclonal ones or autoimmune antibodies in patients with Graves' disease, apparently bypass the glycoprotein receptor component and stimulate adenylate cyclase directly after combining with the ganglioside (Lacetti *et al.*, 1984). Work on such models may clarify what roles gangliosides may have in brain development or function.

3.7. Chol-1, a Polysialoganglioside Antigen

An antiserum raised against synaptosomal membrane fractions from *Torpedo* electric organ, a densely and cholinergically innervated tissue, bound specifically to cholinergic nerve endings in several tissues as determined by immunohistochemistry (Jones *et al.*, 1981). The serum had a low titer of cytotoxic antibodies that released choline acetyltransferase from mammalian brain synaptosomes but did not release dopadecarboxylase or various smaller molecules (Richardson, 1983). There was antigen in ganglioside fractions from the electric organ and, to some extent, from mammalian brain. It was thought to be a polysialoganglioside, and its charge but not its antigenicity was decreased by neuraminidase treatment.

4. NEURONAL SUBSET-SPECIFIC MONOCLONAL ANTIBODIES

One of the most important questions that antibodies may help to answer is how neurons differ from one another. It is commonly held that neuronal synaptic specificity is established by mechanisms that discriminate between appropriate and inappropriate targets, in part by probing the surface of the potential synaptic partner. It is possible that neurotransmitter receptors play a role in this imagined probing and selecting, but attempts to demonstrate this at the neuromuscular junction have not been successful, and the mechanism by which the growing motor neuron discriminates between skeletal or smooth muscle, much less individual muscle fibers, is unknown.

However, there is continued optimism that antibodies, especially monoclonal reagents, because they can potentially detect any molecule, will become indispensible tools for understanding the molecular basis of neural development and function, especially if *in vitro* immunization allows us to circumvent some problems of tolerance in antibody generation. Some antibodies are directed at molecules specific to neurons and present on all of them; others recognize neuronal subsets. In this section, some of the best characterized antibodies that recognize some but not all neurons will be described. Again, the emphasis here is on antibodies that bind to cell surface antigens found on cultured cells (Table II). An important and rapidly expanding class of antigen, the neuropeptides and neurotransmitter-related enzymes, will not be reviewed, even though they clearly divide neurons into intelligible subpopulations, nor will antibodies to cytoskeletal proteins be assessed (Yen and Fields, 1981; Ostermann *et al.*, 1983; Huber and Matus, 1984).

4.1. Retinal Cell Subpopulations

One of the most thorough and successful studies using monoclonal antibodies concerns retinal antigens and has been the subject of two recent reviews (Barnstable, 1982; Barnstable *et al.*, 1983). Even though unfixed retinal membrane fractions were used for immunization, the hybridomas were screened on aldehyde-fixed retina homogenates and tissue sections, and two cell surface antigens could be localized at the electron microscopic level using glutaraldehyde-fixed tissue (Fekete and Barnstable, 1983). Their results showing antigen distribution on photoreceptors are very convincing, for the monoclonal antibodies analyzed react with the well-fixed and, therefore, well-preserved membranes.

Monoclonal antibodies that labeled the photoreceptors were of three classes: one (RET-P1) labeled the photoreceptor outer segments, inner segments, and cell bodies in the outer nuclear layer, but did not label photoreceptor cell processes in the outer plexiform layer. The second class (RET-P2) labeled only the outer segments of the photoreceptors, and the third (RET-P3) labeled only the photoreceptor cell bodies. More recently, monoclonal antibodies specific to other retinal neurons have

Table II. Positive Antigenic Markers for Neuronal Subsets in Culture[a]

Marker	Subset	Section
RET-P1,-P2,-P3	Retina photoreceptors	4.1
RET-B1	Bipolar cells in retina	4.1
HPC-1	Amacrine cells in retina	4.1
Thy-1	Retinal ganglion cells	4.1
	Other CNS and PNS populations	4.2
TOP	Toponymic distribution	4.1
GD$_3$ ganglioside	5–15% of cerebellar neurons	4.2
	A minority of other CNS or PNS neurons; a few nonneurons	3.2
D1.1	Neuroblasts	4.2
Globoside	50% of DRG neurons	3.3
Chol-1	Cholinergic neurons	3.7
NSP-4	Subsets of cerebellar and DRG neurons	4.2
NG2	Few cerebellar neurons and glia; extracellular matrix	4.2
CG-3	Chick ciliary ganglion neurons	4.3
CG-1, CG-4	Ciliary ganglion neurons and 5% of cranial neural crest cells	4.3
CG-2	Ciliary ganglion neurons and 12% of spinal cord neurons	4.3
180,000-dalton protein	*Torpedo* electric organ, mammalian motor neurons, SCG neurons	4.5

[a] See text at indicated section for references and full description. Not all exceptions are noted here.

been described. RET-B1 bound to bipolar cells; HPC-1, raised by immunization with hippocampal cells, bound to amacrine cells; and antibodies to intermediate filament proteins discriminated between subtypes of retinal neurons. Antineurofilament antibodies, in particular, bound to horizontal cells and ganglion cells. Parallel studies of antigen expression *in vivo* and in dissociated cell cultures were needed to identify neuron subsets in the cultures (Akagawa *et al.*, 1983; Barnstable *et al.*, 1983).

Müller cells, the radial glial cells of the retina, bound monoclonal antibodies RET-G1, G2, and G3. Each antibody reacted with different antigenic determinants, which differed in their expression during early development. Only RET-G1 was also present on membranes from cerebral cortex or cerebellum (Barnstable, 1980, 1982). Expression of the RET-G antigens in cultures has started to be examined (Akagawa *et al.*, 1983).

The ganglion cells, but no other retinal neurons, were stained *in vivo* by anti-Thy-1 antibody (Beale and Osborn, 1982). This antigen is an abundant glycoprotein of 25,000 daltons in brain and thymus (Williams *et al.*, 1977). Selective Thy-1 expression persists *in vitro*, and ganglion cells, after labeling by retrograde transport of a fluorescent dye, could be identified in cultures, where they survived only in cell aggregates (Akagawa *et al.*, 1983). Recently, the culture of retinal cells from neonatal rats was described, where the ganglion cells were labeled with dye and then purified 50- to 100-fold by gradient centrifugation. The ganglion cells in the initial cell suspension and in the cultures were shown to have the Thy-1 antigen, but they survived only for 48 hr (Sarthy *et al.*, 1983).

Studies of retinal antigens *in vivo* show beautifully the specialization of different parts of neurons, especially the photoreceptors. By electron microscopic localization, RET-P1 was shown to be on the plasma membrane, the ends of the disks, and at the inner face of the disks of broken rod outer segments (Fekete and Barnstable, 1983). Biochemical evidence suggests that RET-P2 antigen may not be present within the disks (Barnstable, 1982). The mechanism by which such regional variation in expression of surface components may be established is not known, but conceptually similar selective expression of specialized structures on different regions of plasma membranes occurs in many differentiated tissues. A discussion of the importance of regional membrane differences and neuronal function can be found in a review by Pfenninger (1978).

A2B5, as discussed earlier, is an antigen found only on the cell bodies, not on the processes, of neurons in the chick retina *in vivo* (Eisenbarth *et al.*, 1979). Curiously, Schnitzer and Schachner (1982) found this restriction to the cell body to apply only to chick retinal cells in culture, as cells from other regions of the chick CNS or from the retina of other species had an even distribution of antigen on cell bodies and neurites.

An important example of a molecule with a different kind of restricted distribution, in this case not according to cell type or membrane region but according to cell position within the retina, is the TOP ("toponymic") antigen discovered and defined by another monoclonal antibody (Trisler *et al.*, 1981). Developmental neurobiologists concerned with the formation of ordered synaptic connections and similar processes of neuronal recognition designed the experiments resulting in the isolation of this hybridoma. By immunizing mice with dorsal or ventral neural retina from chick embryos and then screening wells for antibody that bound better to cells from the immunizing sector than to the other sectors, Trisler *et al.* (1981) found one monoclonal antibody that showed preferential binding. There was 35-fold more antigen in dorsoposterior retina than in ventroanterior retina. This gradient persisted from early embryos through the adult stage. Molecules antigenically related to TOP were detected only in other birds, and the antigen was destroyed by boiling or trypsin treatment. A review is available that places this antigen in its context of the coding of positional information (Trisler, 1982).

Other monoclonal antibodies that bind to the chick retina have been described. One was not cell type-specific but regional-specific. It was present on the retina, not elsewhere in the brain or in the PNS, but was also present on liver and red blood cells. Other antigens were specific for retinal photoreceptors after day E14 and present on some cells in the optic tectum, whereas others had specificity for synaptic layers (Grunwald *et al.*, 1983). Clearly, the development of such specificity for the retina, its cell types, and local areas of membranes are topics that will be intensively studied with antibodies.

4.2. Cerebellar Neurons

Another part of the CNS that is particularly well suited for an analysis of neuronal subpopulations is the cerebellum. Here, as in the retina, there are a limited number of well characterized and distinctive neuronal cell classes. They are arranged in three layers, vary in size over the widest possible range, and are at least partially characterized with respect to their neurotransmitters. There have been extensive efforts to establish explant, microexplant, and dissociated cell culture systems for the rat and mouse cerebellum. The use of genetic mutants, GABA autoradiography, Golgi staining, ultrastructural characterization, and physiological techniques have now been augmented by a rapidly growing number of immunocytochemical reagents to assess the nature and extent of neuronal differentiation.

Antibodies to the neurotransmitter enzyme glutamic acid decarboxylase (GAD), the key enzyme in GABA synthesis, have been used on tissue sections of the cerebellar cortex with excellent results (Oertel *et al.*, 1982). In dissociated cultures of the cerebral cortex there was an 85–95% overlap of GAD-staining neurons and cells that accumulate [^{3}H]-GABA (Neale *et al.*, 1983). GABA uptake visualized by autoradiography has been used extensively on cerebellar cell cultures to show the survival and maturation of many stellate and/or basket cell neurons as well as a few Purkinje and/or Golgi type II neurons (Lasher, 1974). Granule cells are the smallest and most populous neuronal cell type in most cultures made from neonatal or postnatal rodent cerebellum, and they do not accumulate GABA.

In dissociated cell cultures from neonatal rat cerebellum, all neurons have tetanus and cholera toxin receptors (Raff *et al.*, 1979), A4 antigen (Cohen and Selvendran, 1981), and UC45 antigen (Hogg *et al.*, 1981). However, the expression of other antigens is more complex (Fields *et al.*, 1982). At short times in culture, the proportion of neurons expressing Thy-1 antigen depended most strongly on the age of the rat. In cultures derived from embryonic rats, 5–40% of the neurons were positive for this surface marker. The wide variation in positive cells, rather than being due to a failure of neuronal differentiation in culture, was more likely due to a variation in the survival of the largest neurons. A crude analysis of the Thy-1-positive neurons showed that the smallest neurons were antigen-negative, whereas the largest were all positive. In cultures from neonatal or postnatal day 4 rats, less than 1% of the cells were Thy-1-positive. However, these antigen-negative neurons were not permanently Thy-1-deficient. Like brain tissue as a whole, they slowly acquired the antigen, so that 30–80% of the cells were positive after about 4 weeks in culture (Fields *et al.*, 1982; Fields, 1983b). It is not known why all neurons do not become positive *in vitro* and whether this is also true *in vivo*. The important point is that, even though Thy-1 is neither region-specific nor really specific for the large neurons of the cerebellum, nevertheless, at one stage in development it can be used to identify the most mature cells. In the cerebellum the first neurons to develop, the Purkinje and Golgi cells, are also the largest neurons. Neurons from the brain stem also become Thy-1-positive in cultures, and the antibody recognizes some striking neurons in the olfactory bulb; however, we do not know anything more about their identity (Fields, 1983b). Since Thy-1 is perhaps the most abundant cell surface glycoprotein in brain and excellent monoclonal antisera are commercially available (Mason and Williams, 1980; Fields and Raine, 1982), it is a neuronal antigen that may prove useful in cultures of many regions of brain.

In cultures of postnatal mouse cerebellum, small neurons predominate, but the few large neurons were the only ones labeled by anti-Thy-1 sera or the lectin *Ricinus communis* 120. However, survival of the large neurons was poor in the cultures and they rarely extended processes. The small neurons did not become Thy-1-positive by 14 days *in vitro*, even though granule neurons do acquire antigen *in vivo*. By *in vivo* [³H]thymidine labeling, the large neurons were found to divide at times in development (E11–13) characteristic of Golgi and Purkinje cells (Schnitzer and Schachner, 1981a,b). H-2 antigen was not expressed by mouse cerebellar neurons, whereas NS-4 and tetanus toxin receptors were present on all of them (Schnitzer and Schachner, 1981c).

Subsets of small cerebellar neurons have been identified by monoclonal and conventional sera that bind to gangliosides (Fields, 1983b). In cultures that contain predominantly granule cells, 5–15% of the neurons bound R24, a monoclonal antibody that bound to GD_3 (Pukel et al., 1982). The positive cells did not appear to be particularly immature, for they had long processes and bound tetanus or cholera toxin as well as R24 antibody (Fields, 1983b). A much smaller percentage of astrocytes with glial filaments also bound R24. The antigen, presumably GD_3 itself, when present, was distributed uniformly around the neural cell body, on processes, and at the growing neurite tips.

Giotta et al. (1982) have described a monoclonal antibody, C4/12, that bound to the surface of some but not all cerebellar granule cells, DRG neurons, and a few astrocytes in vitro. In vivo it was expressed in the cerebellar granular layer, cerebrum, and kidney. It was more strongly expressed around the soma than on the processes of granule cells in vitro, and in vivo there was strong labeling in the granular layer but not the molecular layer, which is packed with granule cell axons.

Rougon et al. (1983) also described a monoclonal antibody, anti-NSP-4, that bound to mouse cerebellar cell membranes and to small subsets of cerebellar neurons and astrocytes in vitro, as well as to small dark neurons in DRG cultures. The positive cerebellar neurons in tissue sections appeared to be neuroblasts and migrating granule cells. Positive astrocytes persisted in the granular layer of the adult, but no neurons remained positive. The glycoproteins that bound this monoclonal antibody changed in molecular weight during development, and the authors suggested that these proteins could play a role in cell–cell interactions and recognition during development.

Two other monoclonal antibodies labeled subsets of cerebellar cells (Stallcup et al., 1983). D1.1, which bound to a ganglioside, bound to germinal cells in the external granular layer and other similar germinal regions of embryonic brain. NG2 monoclonal antibody bound to a 300,000-dalton core glycoprotein associated with chondroitin sulfate chains. It was expressed by a small class of cells, perhaps basket and stellate cells, in the molecular layer. Previous work with rabbit and mouse sera showed that NG2 was on cells that had some tetanus toxin receptors and some cells that had glial filaments (Stallcup, 1981). These may be cells that Raff et al. (1983a,b) have interpreted as glial precursor cells or a type of astrocyte.

Most attempts to culture cerebellar neurons underline the need for a better understanding of the growth and survival factors required by large CNS neurons. In explant, microexplant, or reaggregate cell cultures, Purkinje neurons survive better than in dissociated cell cultures, and it may be possible to analyze their cell surface antigens there. In one culture system (Gruol, 1983) the Purkinje cells were identified using a very well-characterized and seemingly absolutely specific cytoplasmic antigen, GMP-dependent protein kinase (Lohmann *et al.*, 1981; Franklin and Gruol, 1983). In these microexplant-style cultures many Purkinje cells survived for long times in culture and were available for physiological studies (Gruol, 1983).

4.3. Ciliary Ganglion Neurons

A determined effort to find monoclonal antibodies specific for ciliary ganglion (CG) neurons has been quite successful (Barald, 1982), even though our current techniques only detect surface antigens that are present at a relatively high density. Four different monoclonal antibodies Barald characterized support the view that neuronal subpopulations differ in surface components early in development and that these differences may persist even in the adult.

After immunizing with cultured chick CG neurons, 10,000 supernatants from 10 fusions were screened before one fusion gave about 10% of the wells positive in a test for antibody binding to CG neurons. Seven wells showed specificity for CG neurons compared to DRG neurons. Four CG neuron-specific antibodies and one antibody that bound to all kinds of neurons were characterized by binding, immunofluorescence, and cytotoxic assays. None of these antibodies bound to nonneuronal cells such as fibroblasts, glia, heart, or liver cells. One antibody bound to all tested PNS and CNS neurons but did not bind to neural crest cells. The most restricted antibody bound only to CG neurons and not to any other neurons or nonneuronal cells except small regions on muscle cells. Three antibodies bound to CG neurons and interesting subpopulations of other cells. Antibody CG-2 bound to all CG neurons and to 12% of spinal cord neurons. Two clones produced antibodies that bound to CG neurons and to a small population (5%) of cranial neural crest cells, but not to any trunk neural crest cells. Since CG neurons develop from the cranial neural crest, Barald proposed that the antigen-positive neural crest cells may be just those cells that normally migrate out and form this ganglion. She found conditions where mixtures of the two CG/cranial neural crest cell antibodies were cytotoxic for cells *in vitro*, and proposed to test her precursor hypothesis by experiments with early embryo cells. The first reported results, which include the use of the antibody to select out positive cranial neural crest cells by fluorescence-activated cell sorting, indicated that the antigen-positive cells have high choline acetyltransferase activity and high-affinity choline uptake. In these properties they resemble CG neurons, despite their nonneuronal morphology (Barald, 1983).

4.4. Sympathetic Ganglion Neurons

Neurons from the rat SCG can be grown in the absence of non-neuronal cells, and they develop adrenergic or cholinergic properties depending on their environment. Chun et al. (1980) have raised monoclonal antibodies to cell surface antigens of SCG neurons. Antibody N10, while it bound to both adrenergic and cholinergic cells, showed more binding to adrenergic cells, and it bound more to membranes of the soma than the processes. The antigen was not found on heart cells, fibroblasts, Schwann cells, or nonneural tissues, but was shared with brain. Two other antibodies were tested for an effect on neuronal function by growing cells in the presence of antibody for several weeks. Neither norepinephrine uptake nor its evoked release was affected. However, one of the two monoclonal antibodies resulted in a 50% decrease in acetylcholine or catecholamine synthesis without affecting cell survival or growth.

4.5. Cholinergic Neurons

Another monoclonal antibody that bound rather selectively to SCG neurons was raised by Kushner (1984) against a cholinergic tissue, the *Torpedo* electric organ. It detected an antigen shared by *Torpedo* synaptosomes and some mammalian neurons, including motor neurons and SCG neurons. The antigen was a non-integral membrane-associated protein of 180,000 daltons, so it was probably not related to the other cholinergic marker, Chol-1 (see Section 3.7).

5. ANTIBODIES THAT AFFECT CELL SORTING OUT OR NEURITE OUTGROWTH

Antibodies to N-CAM affected cell sorting out in aggregates of chick neural retinal cells, the formation of ordered histotypic layers in retina explant cultures, and the diameter but not length of neurite fascicles growing out from DRG explants (Rutishauser et al., 1978a,b; Buskirk et al., 1980). Anti-N-CAM Fab' bound directly to neurites and may have affected the fascicles either by increasing adhesion of neurites to the culture substratum or by blocking N-CAM-mediated side-to-side adhesion of neurites (Rutishauser et al., 1978b). The aggregation inhibited by anti-N-CAM Fab' and the increased fasciculation of neurites are calcium-independent effects, whereas calcium-dependent systems are less tissue-specific and appear to oppose fasciculation (Brackenbury et al., 1981).

Coating glass coverslips with an anti-Thy-1 monoclonal antibody improved the adhesion, survival, and neurite growth of retinal ganglion cells, while other neurons which had no Thy-1 antigen, the amacrine cells, were unaffected. A different monoclonal antibody, although it bound to an antigen (RET-N2) on the same cells, did not enhance process growth (Leifer et al., 1983).

Affinity-purified anti-GM$_1$ antibodies, in contrast, blocked neurite outgrowth from DRG explants (Schwartz and Spirman, 1982). The authors' interpretation was that the effect was on an interaction of NGF with GM$_1$ ganglioside, since when they added 10-fold more NGF to their serum-free medium, the antibodies had much less effect. Inhibition in this system was greatest after 24 hr and much less significant after 48 hr. However, explants of goldfish retina were also sensitive to antiganglioside antibodies (Spirman et al., 1982), and it is unlikely that this effect was due to NGF receptors. Antiganglioside antibodies, and anti-GM$_1$ sera in particular, have been shown to have a number of effects on brain functions and animal behavior when they are injected directly into ventricles or specific brain regions (Karpiak et al., 1981; Rapport, 1981b; Rapport and Huang, 1984; Gregson, 1981). Antiganglioside antibodies, however, are not the only ones that affect behavior. Anti-Thy-1, injected into the hypothalamus, inhibited carbachol-induced drinking behavior but did not affect norepinephrine-induced eating (Williams et al., 1980). However, cell culture models for these specific effects have not been developed yet, and it is unclear how the effects on brain function are related to effects of gangliosides and antibodies on neurite outgrowth (Rapport and Gorio, 1981).

A protein antigen affecting neurite outgrowth was identified by a monoclonal antibody, T61/3/12, isolated by Henke-Fahle and Bonhoeffer (1983) after 20 injections (!) of chick retinal membrane fractions. The antibody bound to the outer and inner plexiform layers and the optic fibers in tissue sections of retina. Dissociated neurons from retina, tectum, or cerebellum bound the antibody on all their surfaces, but fibroblasts, heart cells, or DRG neurons had no visible binding. The presence of this antibody prevented most outgrowth of retinal ganglion cell neurites from explants. Most retinal cell growth cones responded to the addition of this antibody by ceasing their movements, which resumed when antibody was washed away. The antigen was not detected in mouse retina and was somewhat sensitive to Pronase. Since it was not found on DRG cells, it was unlikely to be related to N-CAM. The authors suggested that the T61 antigen might mediate an interaction of the growth cone with the substratum or block the action of a neurite outgrowth-stimulating factor. The sensitivity of neurite outgrowth by neurons from other CNS regions was not reported, but it would be interesting to test whether substrata that allow SCG neurite outgrowth in the absence of NGF (Lander et al., 1983) affect the inhibition of neurite outgrowth and growth cone movements by this antibody.

6. SOME GLIAL AND OTHER MARKERS

6.1. Oligodendrocytes

Cell surface markers (Table III) for these glial cells, which are responsible for CNS myelination, include NS-1 antigen, the lipid galactocerebroside (GalC) and its sulfated derivative (sulfatide) (Schachner, 1974; Raff et al., 1978; Schachner and Willinger, 1979a,b), and a series of O-antigens (O1-O4) defined by monoclonal antibodies (Sommer and Schachner, 1981). Myelin basic protein is another marker for oligodendrocytes; it is cytoplasmic and appears in cells after longer times in culture (Schachner and Willinger, 1979a,b; Mirsky et al., 1980; Bhat et al., 1981). Cholera toxin-binding sites, presumably GM_1 ganglioside, are present on young cultured oligodendrocytes in high concentrations, but as they are also present on neurons they are less useful than the more specific markers (Raff et al., 1979, Schachner and Willinger, 1979b). These markers have been reviewed quite often; for more details and extensive references see Mirsky (1982) and Schachner (1982a,b,c).

GalC was the first marker to be described as oligodendrocyte-specific using cultured cells. It was already known to neurochemists as an abundant glycosphingolipid of brain and isolated myelin (Norton and Autilio, 1966). Furthermore, antisera to whole brain or myelin fractions had been shown to be cytotoxic for the myelin in organotypic cultures due to anti-GalC antibodies (Fry et al., 1974). Therefore, the GalC was presumed to be somewhere on the oligodendroglial cell surface. Sternberger et al. (1978) showed anti-GalC reactivity to be present in oligodendrocytes early in development in vivo, but did not see positive cells, only positive myelin, in older animals. Shortly afterward, GalC-like antigen was shown by indirect immunofluorescence to be on the surface of a subpopulation of dissociated cultured cells from white matter, optic nerve, or in small numbers of cells from most parts of the neonatal rat CNS (Raff et al., 1978, 1979; Schachner and Willinger, 1979a,b). A mon-

Table III. *Positive Antigenic Markers for Nonneuronal Cells*[a]

Marker	Comment	Section
Oligodendrocytes		
Galactocerebroside	Also on Schwann cells	6.1
Sulfatide	Also on Schwann cells	6.1
GM_4 ganglioside	Predicted on chick, human	3.1
GM_3 ganglioside	—	3.3
O-antigens	Detect GalC or sulfatide?	6.1
Myelin-associated proteins	Most are cytoplasmic	6.1
NS-1	Also in PNS nerves	6.1
Schwann cells		
Ran-1	Rat only; also SCG neurons[b]	6.2
Gal-C, sulfatide, myelin basic protein	Expression declines in culture	6.2
Laminin	Also on astrocytes	6.2
C4	Only if axons are present	6.2
Glial precursor cells		
Tetanus toxin receptors	Less than on neurons	3.5
A2B5	Shared with neurons inter alia	3.5
D1.1	Shared with neuroblasts?	4.2
Astrocytes		
RET-G1	Müller cells and cells in cortex	4.1
RET-G2, G3	Müller cells only	4.1
GFA	Cytoplasmic, also in enteric glial cells and some Schwann cells	6.3
C1	Cytoplasmic antigen	6.3
M1	Cytoplasmic and surface	6.3
Ran-2	Also on ependymal and leptomeningeal cells	6.3
Thy-1	Requires long time in culture; not astrocytes only	6.3
SSEA-1	Not all astrocytes	6.3
MI/N1 and 308	Not all human astrocytes	6.3
Ependymal cells		
Ran-2	Also on astrocytes	6.4
Epen-1	Rat and mouse	6.4
Leptomeningeal cells		
Fibronectin	Also on fibroblasts	6.5
Ran-2	Rat only, also on astrocytes	6.3
Fibroblasts		
Fibronectin	Also on leptomeningeal cells	6.5
Thy-1	Also on some neurons	6.5

[a] See text at indicated section for references and full description. Not all exceptions are noted here.
[b] Fields (unpublished observations).

oclonal antibody that reacts with GalC has been described recently, and its reactivity with GalC and sulfatide has been compared with conventional rabbit antisera (Ranscht et al., 1982).

NS-1 antigen was defined by polyclonal mouse antisera raised to a mouse oligodendroglioma. The cytotoxicity of anti-NS-1 for these tumor cells was adsorbed by brain, CNS white matter, or peripheral nerve tissue, so the antigen may be expressed in vivo by both oligodendroglia and Schwann cells. NS-1 was found not only in mouse brain, but in rat, cat, and human brain, but not in chicken brain (Schachner, 1974). It was shown to be a specific marker for oligodendrocytes in culture and did not bind to neurons, astrocytes, or fibroblasts; furthermore, the antigen was probably a lipid (Schachner and Willinger, 1979a,b). NS-1-positive cells had the ultrastructural characteristics of oligodendroglial cells, and positive cells in culture also have surface GalC and cytoplasmic myelin basic protein.

The O1–O4 monoclonal antibodies were produced by immunization of mice with whole white matter (Schachner, 1982a,b). O3 and O4 antibodies may react with sulfatide and O1 and O2 with GalC. Cells in culture develop O3 and O4 binding sites about 1 day before O1 and O2 binding sites appear. Precursor cells evidently coexist with more differentiated cells of the oligodendrocyte lineage, since lysis of O-bearing cells did not prevent their reappearance upon continued culture. It is important to note that the oligodendrocyte-specificity of these antibodies disappears if cells are fixed or tissue sections are examined. Evidently there are O-antigens associated with the cytoskeletal elements of astrocytes in culture (Berg and Schachner, 1981) or Bergmann glia in tissue sections (Sommer and Schachner, 1981). Polyclonal anti-GalC antibodies bind to microtubules in epithelial cell lines (Sakakibara et al., 1981a,b), and the similar properties of the O monoclonal antibodies and polyclonal rabbit anti-GalC or antisulfatide antibodies require that they be used on on live cells whenever possible for maximum oligodendrocyte specificity.

Oligodendroglia in cultures are most likely to be confused with neurons or macrophages. Tetanus toxin receptors can be used to distinguish oligodendrocytes from neurons. Macrophages often show a low level of surface staining with many immunoglobulin reagents since they have Fc receptors, but this can usually be seen to involve obvious pinocytosis, which can be confirmed with live cells by testing for the ingestion of glass beads or carbon particles (Raff et al., 1979).

Quite pure suspensions of young rodent cells with surface GalC have been obtained by fluorescence-activated cell sorting (Bartlett, 1983). Excellent separation has also been obtained with the O4 monoclonal antibody attached to magnetic beads, and after separation these cells could be cultured, with some surviving and growing for several weeks (Meier and Schachner, 1982). Cells of equal or even superior purity and excellent viability were obtained from neonatal rats by exploiting the low adhesiveness of these cells in culture (McCarthy and de Vellis, 1980; Bhat et al., 1981).

Most myelin components and myelin-specific enzymes have been explored for use in culture (Roussel et al., 1981). The reader is referred to recent reviews (Norton, 1983, 1984) for a more complete listing.

6.2. Schwann Cells

Schwann cells, which make myelin and ensheath axons in the PNS, have the surface antigen Ran-1. It was defined by an antiserum raised to a rat glial tumor cell line and is a rat-specific antigen, probably a glycoprotein. Ran-1 was present in brain, peripheral nerve, embryonic tissue, and nearly all rat neural tumor cell lines (Fields et al., 1975; Fields, 1977). In vitro the antigen was found on Schwann cells, but not fibroblasts (Brockes et al., 1977), DRG neurons (Fields et al., 1978), or enteric neurons (Jessen and Mirsky, 1980). SCG neurons are positive (K. Fields, unpublished observations). Less than 1% of the cells in most CNS cultures had Ran-1, and most of them looked like Schwann cells (Raff et al., 1979). However, some cells were large and flat, very like the Ran-1-positive cells found in cultures of the neonatal adrenal medulla (K. Fields, unpublished observations) or enteric ganglia (Jessen and Mirsky, 1980, 1983). Cultures of olfactory bulb have many more Ran-1-positive cells than other parts of the CNS. Adult rat Schwann cells also have this antigen (Fields, 1983a). An otherwise tumor-specific antigen defined by a mouse monoclonal antibody (Peng et al., 1982) is on all Ran-1-positive cells, and it may also bind to the dominant antigenic determinant defined by Ran-1 sera (Fields and Dammerman, 1985).

Schwann cells from young rats in culture, unlike oligodendroglia, quickly abandon GalC and myelin basic protein synthesis (Mirsky et al., 1980), although a low level of sulfatide synthesis is detected in vitro by a sensitive ^{35}S assay (Fryxell, 1980). Sulfatide on the surface of oligodendrocytes, as judged by O3, O4, or polyclonal antibodies (Schachner, 1982c; Ranscht et al., 1982), is characteristic of less fully differentiated cells, and sulfatide may accumulate earlier than GalC in vivo (Ranscht et al., 1982).

Schwann cells in culture express laminin on their cell surface, whether they are grown alone, with fibroblasts, or with neurons (Cornbrooks et al., 1983; McGarvey et al., 1984). In the presence of neurons under conditions that allow myelination, the pattern of Schwann cell surface laminin changes from a punctate to a continuous distribution. At all stages laminin can be used to distinguish Schwann cells from fibroblasts or neurons (Cornbrooks *et al.*, 1983). There has been one report that astrocytes in culture also synthesize laminin (Liesi *et al.*, 1983).

Schwann cells, in cocultures with neurons, expressed a surface antigen, C4, defined by a monoclonal antibody. C4 expression was a property that changed due to Schwann cell-axon interactions, for it required the presence of neurons but did not persist if the Schwann cell made myelin (Cornbrooks and Bunge, 1982).

A polyclonal rabbit serum raised to purified rat Schwann cells was made specific for them by tissue adsorption (Krieder *et al.*, 1981); however, the specific antigens it detects have not been characterized.

6.3. Astrocytes

Astrocytes in culture have been successfully identified for many years by their reactivity with antisera against GFA (Antanitus *et al.*, 1975) or intact glial filament protein (Yen and Fields, 1981). Rat astrocytes, but not oligodendrocytes or neurons, also contain vimentin (Yen and Fields, 1981; Chiu *et al.*, 1981) as do mouse astrocytes and ependymal cells (Schnitzer *et al.*, 1981). Two monoclonal antibodies reacted with intermediate filament elements (C1 and M1) and a surface antigen (M1), but they were not entirely astrocyte-specific *in vitro*. In tissue sections, however, they have been shown to distinguish astrocyte subclasses (Schachner, 1982c).

The rat-specific surface antigen Ran-2 was found on immature and GFA-containing astrocytes, ependymal cells and leptomeningeal cells (Bartlett *et al.*, 1981). Thy-1 antigen was also found on some astrocytes in long-term cultures (Pruss, 1979), as was the mouse H-2 antigen (Schnitzer and Schachner, 1981b). Some, but not all, astrocytes, but no other differentiated CNS cell types, had SSEA-1 (Lagenaur *et al.*, 1982), an early embryonic antigen (Solter and Knowles, 1978). Two monoclonal antibodis (MI/N1 and 308) react with some, but not all, human astrocytes in cultures and may be related to SSEA-1 (Dickson *et al.*, 1983).

At present there is no specific marker for all astrocytes. Glial filaments are used most often, but these generally develop postnatally, and immature astrocytes are negative as are protoplasmic astrocytes *in vivo*. All anti-GFA antisera so far tested also react both *in vivo* and *in vitro* with at least two other types of cells in the PNS: enteric glial cells and Schwann cells associated with adult C-type fibers (Jessen and Mirsky,

1980, 1983; Yen and Fields, 1981, 1983; Fields, 1983a) as well as Schwann cells in the olfactory nerve (Barber and Lindsay, 1982).

6.4. Ependymal Cells

Ependymal cells from neonatal rats are usually identified in cultures by their waving cilia (Abney *et al.*, 1981). They expressed the Ran-2 antigen but not GFA, GalC, Thy-1, Ran-1, or fibronectin (Bartlett *et al.*, 1981). Recently, an ependymal cell-specific monoclonal antibody, Epen-1, was described, which bound only to the ependymal cells in dissociated cell suspensions from adult mice or rats and in cultures or tissue sections from mice (Tardieu *et al.*, 1983).

6.5. Leptomeningeal Cells and Fibroblasts

These cells are often present in cell cultures and it can be difficult or impossible to distinguish them morphologically from astrocytes at the light microscopic level. Rodent and human fibroblasts can be positively identified by the use of antifibronectin and anti-Thy-1 antibodies, for they are positive for both markers, and in the rat they are known to be Ran-2-negative. Leptomeningeal cells are highly fibronectin-positive, but differ from fibroblasts by being Thy-1-negative (Raff *et al.*, 1979) and Ran-2-positive (Bartlett *et al.*, 1981). In species without Thy-1 or Ran-2 markers, fibronectin expression may be the only available marker, and it will distinguish antigen-negative astrocytes from antigen-positive fibroblasts, leptomeningeal, and endothelial cells (Schachner *et al.*, 1978).

7. CONCLUDING REMARKS

It obviously is not possible to summarize neatly the work of so many independent laboratories, but we may ask whether antigenic markers are proving to be useful in cell culture. Clearly the answer is yes, especially for those markers which are reproducible, widely available, span species differences, and are not very sensitive to developmental or environmental regulation. The markers for the major cell types (tetanus toxin, GFA, GalC, and fibronectin) developed several years ago (Raff *et al.*, 1979; Schachner, 1982b) have proven to be quite reliable and informative. There are also supplementary markers: cholera toxin, N-CAM and its relatives, A2B5 in many situations, and so on, which are or should soon become more widely available. Their use can reduce the uncertainty that always remains when a single marker is used.

Monoclonal antibodies are clearly a major improvement over dwindling supplies and doubtful bleeds of conventional antibodies, and they will increase the confidence of occasional users in the validity of their binding experiments, provided they are used with some appreciation for the limits of the immunological techniques. However, monoclonal antibody regents cannot guarantee the size or chemical class of the antigen in many situations, especially when glycoproteins and glycolipids are both candidates. Several examples were detailed here, hopefully enough to instill some caution and controls in the use of antibodies in new systems.

In addition to the broadly cell type-specific markers, there are an increasing number of antibodies to well-defined differentiation-dependent antigens. Some of these are on the cell surface, but many others are not. All of them are extending the evaluation of differentiation in cell cultures down to the single-cell level. In the case of neuronal subsets and cell surface markers, progress has been fairly slow, but there should be an explosion of subset-specific markers as more extensive and focused screening procedures are adopted. This review has described in some detail two of the most successful examples of subset-specific antibodies—in the ciliary ganglion and in the retina. Other antibodies that label subpopulations, anti-Thy-1 and antiganglioside sera, were also described, although the distinction between positive and negative neuron sets is not well understood. In the arena of glial cell markers, steady progress has been made. The definitions of glial precursor cells in the CNS and differentiated subsets of Schwann cells in the PNS illustrate the new information that came from pursuing the exceptions to broad generalizations: in one case the tetanus toxin- and A2B5-binding nonneurons, and in the other case, the cells in the PNS with reactivity to an astrocyte-specific marker.

Is the new wave of immunological reagents providing a pathway from cell culture to biochemistry and even molecular biology? We have gone into considerable detail in the section on N-CAM and its relatives to illustrate the power of immunological approaches to make a direct connection between function and antigens. In addition, monoclonal antibodies have provided welcome leverage to biochemists in the purification of adhesion molecules, even though separate immunological and even purely biochemical approaches also led to the same highly antigenic glycoproteins.

One of the most encouraging aspects of this now-popular technology is the feeling among seasoned practitioners and new converts alike that it is almost impossible to either predict or put limits on the new information that may arise from tomorrow's new monoclonal antibody.

While we try to look for statistically probable events, there is always the possibility of a scientific jackpot lurking in the spleen of the next mouse.

ACKNOWLEDGMENTS

I thank William Norton for his constant encouragement and innumerable discussions, Rochelle Small for her comments on the manuscript, and Robert Yu for advice on gangliosides. The research in my laboratory is supported by NIH Grant NS-14580 and by generous gifts of antisera from Norman Gregson, George Eisenbarth, Shu-hui Yen, Kenneth Lloyd, and other very cooperative colleagues. Finally, I thank Linda Stein and Jason Fields for their patience and support.

REFERENCES

Abney, E. R., Bartlett, P. P., and Raff, M. C., 1981, Astrocytes, ependymal cells, and oligodendrocytes develop on schedule in dissociated cell cultures of embryonic rat brain, *Develop. Biol.* **83**:301–310.

Abney, E. R., Williams, B. P., and Raff, M. C., 1983, Tracing the development of oligodendrocytes from precursor cells using monoclonal antibodies, fluorescence activated cell sorting and cell culture, *Develop. Biol.* **100**:166–171.

Akagawa, K., Barnstable, C. J., and Hofstein, R., 1983, Identification of cell types in the cultures of rat retina using monoclonal antibodies, *J. Neurochem.* **41**(Suppl.):137B.

Akeson, R., and Hsu, W., 1978, Identification of a high molecular weight nervous system specific cell surface glycoprotein on murine neuroblastoma cells, *Exp. Cell Res.* **115**:367–377.

Antanitus, D. S., Choi, B. H., and Lapham, L. W., 1975, Immunofluorescence staining of astrocytes *in vitro* using antiserum to glial fibrillary acidic protein, *Brain Res.* **89**:363–367.

Barald, K., 1982, Monoclonal antibodies to embryonic neurons: Cell-specific markers for chick ciliary ganglion, in: *Neuronal Development* (N. C. Spitzer, ed.), Plenum Press, New York, pp. 101–120.

Barald, K. F., 1983, Monoclonal antibodies in chick ciliary ganglion isolate a neural crest subpopulation by fluorescence activated cell sorting, *Soc. Neurosci. Abstr.* **9**:103.2.

Barber, P. C., and Lindsay, R. M., 1982, Schwann cells of the olfactory nerves contain glial fibrillary acidic protein and resemble astrocytes, *Neuroscience*, **7**:3077–3090.

Barnstable, C. J., 1980, Monoclonal antibodies that recognize different cell types in the rat retina, *Nature* **286**:231–235.

Barnstable, C. J., 1982, Immunological studies of the retina, in: *Neuroimmunology* (J. Brockes, ed.), Plenum Press, New York, pp. 183–214.

Barnstable, C. J., Akagawa, K., Hofstein, R., and Horn, J. P., 1983, Monoclonal antibodies that label discrete cell types in the mammalian nervous system, *Cold Spring Harbor Symp. Quant. Biol.* **48**:863–876.

Bartlett, P. F., 1983, Oligodendrocyte function studied *in vitro*, in: *Molecular Aspects of Neurological Disorders* (P. L. Austin and P. L. Jeffrey, eds.), Academic Press, New York, pp. 211–220.

Bartlett, P. F., Noble, M. D., Pruss, R. M., Raff, M. C. Rattray, S., and Williams, C. A., 1981, Rat neural antigen-2 (RAN-2)—A cell surface antigen on astrocytes, ependymal cells, Muller cells and leptomeninges defined by a monoclonal antibody, *Brain Res.* **204**:339–351.

Beale, R., and Osborn, N. N., 1982, Localization of the Thy-1 antigen to the surfaces of rat retinal ganglion cells, *Neurochem. Int.* **4**:587–595.

Beale, R., Nicolas, D., Neuhoff, V., and Osborn, N. N., 1982, The binding of tetanus toxin to retinal cells, *Brain Res.* **248**:141–149.

Berg, G. J., and Schachner, M., 1981, Immunoelectronmicroscopic identification of O antigen bearing oligodendroglial cells *in vitro*, *Cell Tissue Res.* **219**:313–325.

Berg, G. J., and Schachner, M., 1982, Electron microscopic localization of A2B5 cell surface antigen in monolayer cultures of mouse cerebellum, *Cell Tissue Res.* **224**:637–645.

Bhat, S., Barbarese, E., and Pfeiffer, S. E., 1981, Requirement for non-oligodendrocyte cell signals for enhanced myelinogenic gene expression in long term cultures of purified oligodendrocytes, *Proc. Natl. Acad. Sci. USA* **78**:1283–1287.

Bock, E., 1978, Nervous system specific proteins, *J. Neurochem.* **30**:4–14.

Bock, E., Yavin, Z., Jørgensen, O. S., and Yavin, E., 1980, Nervous system-specific proteins in developing rat cerebral cells in culture, *J. Neurosci.* **35**:1297–1302.

Brackenbury, R., Thiery, J.-P., Rutishauser, U., and Edelman, G. M., 1977, Adhesion among neural cells of the chick embryo. I. An immunological assay for molecules involved in cell–cell binding, *J. Biol. Chem.* **252**:6835–6840.

Brackenbury, R., Rutishauser, U., and Edelman, G. M., 1981, Distinct calcium-independent and calcium-dependent adhesion systems of chicken embryo cells, *Proc. Natl. Acad. Sci. USA* **78**:387–391.

Brady, R. O., 1981, Sphingolipidoses and other lipid metabolic disorders , in: *Basic Neurochemistry*, 3rd ed. (G. J. Siegel, R. W. Albers, B. W. Agranoff, and R. Katzman, eds.), Little, Brown, Boston, pp. 615–626.

Brockes, J. (ed.), 1982, *Neuroimmunology*, Plenum Press, New York.

Brockes, J. P., Fields, K. L., and Raff, M. C., 1977, A surface antigenic marker for rat Schwann cells, *Nature* **266**:364–366.

Buskirk, D. R., Thiery, J. P., Rutishauser, U., and Edelman, G. M., 1980, Antibodies to a neural cell adhesion molecule disrupt histogenesis in cultured chick retinae, *Nature* **285**:488–489.

Chiu, F.-C., Norton, W. T., and Fields, K. L., 1981, The cytoskeleton of primary astrocytes in culture contains actin, glial fibrillary acidic protein, and the fibroblast-type filament protein, vimentin, *J. Neurochem.* **37**:147–155.

Chun, L. L. Y., Patterson, P. H., and Cantor, H., 1980, Preliminary studies on the use of monoclonal antibodies as probes for sympathetic development, *J. Exp. Biol.* **89**:73–83.

Chuong, C.-M., McClain, D. A., Streit, P., and Edelman, G. M., 1982, Neural cell adhesion molecules in rodent brains isolated by monoclonal antibodies with cross-species reactivity, *Proc. Natl. Acad. Sci. USA* **79**:4234–4238.

Cochran, F. B. Yu, R. K., and Ledeen, R. W., 1982, Myelin gangliosides in vertebrates, *J. Neurochem.* **39**:773–779.

Cohen, J., and Selvendran, S. Y., 1981, A neuronal cell surface antigen is found in the CNS but not in peripheral neurones, *Nature* **291**:421–423.

Cornbrooks, C. J., and Bunge, R. P., 1982, A cell-surface specific monoclonal antibody to differentiating Schwann cells, *Trans. Am. Soc. Neurochem.* **13**:171.

Cornbrooks, C. J., Carey, D. J., McDonald, J. A., Timpl, R., and Bunge, R. P., 1983, *In vivo* and *in vitro* observations on laminin production by Schwann cells, *Proc. Natl. Acad. Sci. USA* **80**:3850–3854.

Crisanti-Combes, P., Lorinet, A. M., Girard, A., Pessac, B., Wasseff, M., and Colothy, G., 1982, Expression of neuronal markers in chick and quail embryo neuroretina cultures infected with Rous sarcoma virus, *Cell Differ.* **11:**45–54.

deBaecque, C., Johnson, A., Naiki, M., Schwarting, G., and Marcus, D. M., 1976, Ganglioside location in cerebellar cortex: An immunoperoxidase study with antibody to GM1 ganglioside, *Brain Res.* **114:**117–122.

Dickson, J. G., Flanigan, T. P., and Walsh, F. S., 1982, Cell surface antigens of human fetal brain and dorsal root ganglion cells in tissue culture, in: *Human Motor Neuron Diseases* (L. P. Rowland, ed.), Raven Press, New York, pp. 435–451.

Dickson, J. G., Flanigan, T. P., Kemshead, J. T., Doherty, P., and Walsh, F. S., 1983, Identification of cell-surface antigens present exclusively on a sub-population of astrocytes in human foetal brain cultures, *J. Neuroimmunol.* **5:**111–123.

Dimpfel, W., Neale, J. H., and Habermann, E., 1975, ^{125}I-labelled tetanus toxin as a neuronal marker on tissue cultures derived from embryonic CNS, *Naunyn-Schmiedebergs Arch. Exp. Pathol. Pharmakol.* **290:**329–333.

Dimpfel, W., Huang, R. T. C., and Habermann, E., 1977, Gangliosides in nervous tissue cultures and binding of ^{125}I-labelled tetanus toxin, a neuronal marker, *J. Neurochem.* **29:**329–334.

Dreyfus, H., Louis, J. C., Harth, S., and Mandel, P., 1980, Gangliosides in cultured neurons, *Neuroscience* **5:**1647–1655.

Dulbecco, R., Unger, M., Bologna, M., Battifora, H., Syka, P., and Okada, S., 1981, Cross-reactivity between Thy-1 and a component of intermediate filaments demonstrated using a monoclonal antibody, *Nature* **292:**772–774.

Edelman, G., 1983, Cell adhesion molecules, *Science* **219:**450–457.

Edelman, G. M., and Chuong, C.-M., 1982, Embryonic to adult conversion of neural cell adhesion molecules in normal and staggerer mice, *Proc. Natl. Acad. Sci. USA* **79:**7036–7040.

Eisenbarth, G. S., Walsh, F. S., and Nirenberg, M., 1979, Monoclonal antibody to a plasma membrane antigen of neurons, *Proc. Natl. Acad. Sci. USA* **76:**1286–1300.

Eisenbarth, G. S., Shimazu, K., Conn, M., Mittler, R., and Wells, S., 1981, Monoclonal antibody F12A2B5: Reaction with a plasma membrane antigen of vertebrate neurons and peptide-secreting endocrine cells, in: *Monoclonal Antibodies to Neural Antigens* (R. McKay, M. C. Raff, and L. F. Reichardt, eds.), Cold Spring Harbor Laboratory, Cold Spring Harbor, N.Y., pp. 209–218.

Fekete, D. M., and Barnstable, C. J., 1983, Subcellular localization of rat photoreceptor-specific antigens, *J. Neurocytol.* **12:**785–803.

Fields, K. L., 1977, Biochemical studies of the common and restricted antigens, two neural cell surface antigens, *Prog. Clin. Biol. Res.* **15:**179–190.

Fields, K. L., 1983a, Differentiated Schwann cells cultured from adult sciatic nerves contain astrocyte-type intermediate filaments, *Soc. Neurosci. Abstr.* **9:**5.6.

Fields, K. L., 1983b, Monoclonal antibodies binding to subsets of rat neurons in cell cultures, *J. Neurochem.* 41 Suppl.: S147.

Fields, K. L., and Dammerman, M., 1985, A monoclonal antibody equivalent to anti-Ran-1 as a marker for Schwann cells, *Neuroscience* (in press).

Fields, K. L., and Raine, C. S., 1982, Ultrastructure and immunocytochemistry of rat Schwann cells and fibroblasts *in vitro*, *J. Neuroimmunol.* **2:**155–166.

Fields, K. L., Gosling, C., Megson, M., and Stern, P. L., 1975, New cell surface antigens in rat defined by tumors of the nervous system, *Proc. Natl. Acad. Sci. USA* **72:**1286–1300.

Fields, K. L., Brockes, J. P., Mirsky, R., and Wendon, L. M. B., 1978, Cell surface antigenic markers for distinguishing different types of rat dorsal root ganglion cells in culture, *Cell* **14**:43–51.

Fields, K. L., Currie, D. N., and Dutton, G. R., 1982, Thy-1 and GABA autoradiography on cerebellar cells in culture, *J. Neurosci.* **2**:663–673.

Finne, J., Finne, U., Deagostini-Bazin, H., and Goridis, C., 1983, Occurrence of α2-8 linked polysialosyl units in a neural cell adhesion molecule, *Biochem. Biophys. Res. Commun.* **112**:482–487.

Fishman, P. H., and Brady, R. O., 1976, Biosynthesis and function of gangliosides, *Science* **194**:904–915.

Franklin, C. F., and Gruol, D. L., 1983, Immunohistochemical identification of developing Purkinje neurons in cultures of rat cerebellum, *Soc. Neurosci. Abstr.* **9**:88.9.

Fredman, P., Magnani, J. L., Nirenberg, M., and Ginsberg, V., 1984, Monoclonal antibody A2B5 reacts with many gangliosides in neuronal tissue, *Arch. Biochem. Biophys.* **233**:661–666.

Fry, J. M., Weissbarth, S., Lehrer, G. M., and Bornstein, M. B., 1974, Cerebroside antibody inhibits sulfatide synthesis and myelination and demyelinates in cord tissue culture, *Science* **183**:540–542.

Fryxell, K. J., 1980, Synthesis of sulfatide by cultured Schwann cells, *J. Neurochem.* **35**:1461–1464.

Ganser, A. L., Kirschner, D. A., and Willinger, M., 1983, Ganglioside localization on myelinated nerve fibers by cholera toxin binding, *J. Neurocytol.* **12**:921–938.

Giotta, G. J., Heitzmann, J., and Cohn, M., 1982, Immunological identification of cerebellar cell lines, *Develop. Brain Res.* **4**:209–222.

Goridis, C., Joher, M. A., Hirsch, M., and Schachner, M., 1978, Cell surface proteins of cultured brain cells and their recognition by anti-cerebellum (anti-NS-4) antiserum, *J. Neurochem.* **31**:531–539.

Gregson, N. A., 1981, Studies with anti-ganglioside antibodies, in: *Chemisms of the Brain* (R. Rodnight, H. S. Bachelard, and W. L. Stahl, eds.), Churchill Livingstone, Edinburgh, pp. 167–175.

Gregson, N. A., and Hammer, C. T., 1980, Antibodies against defined nerve cell components: Gangliosides, *J. R. Soc. Med.* **73**:501–504.

Gregson, N. A., and Hammer, C. T., 1982, Some immunological properties of antisera raised against the trisialoganglioside GT_{1b}, *Mol. Immunol.* **19**:543–550.

Gregson, N. A., Kennedy, M., and Liebowitz, S., 1977, Gangliosides as surface antigens on cells isolated from the rat cerebellar cortex, *Nature* **277**:461–463.

Grumet, M., Hoffman, S., and Edelman, G. M., 1984, Two antigenically related neuronal cell adhesion molecules of different specificities mediate neuron–neuron and neuron–glia adhesion, *Proc. Natl. Acad. Sci. USA* **81**:267–271.

Grunwald, G. B., Trisler, D., and Nirenberg, M., 1983, Monoclonal antibodies with regional specificity in the nervous system, *Soc. Neurosci. Abstr.* **9**:203.19.

Gruol, D. L., 1983, Cultured cerebellar neurons: Endogenous and exogenous components of Purkinje cell activity and membrane response to putative transmitters, *Brain Res.* **263**:223–241.

Hakomori, S.-I., 1984, Monoclonal antibodies directed to cell surface carbohydrates, in: *Monoclonal Antibodies and Functional Cell Lines* (R. H. Kennett, K. B. Bechtol, and T. J. McKearn, eds.), Plenum Press, New York.

Henke-Fahle, S., and Bonhoeffer, F., 1983, Inhibition of axonal growth by a monoclonal antibody, *Nature* **303**:65–67.

Hirn, M., Pierres, M., Deagostini-Bazin, H., Hirsch, M., and Goridis, C., 1981, Monoclonal antibody against cell surface glycoprotein of neurons, *Brain Res.* **214**:433–439.

Hirn, M., Ghandour, M. S., Deagostini-Bazin, H., and Goridis, C., 1983, Molecular heterogeneity and structural evolution during cerebellar ontogeny detected by monoclonal antibody of the mouse cell surface antigen BSP-2, *Brain Res.* **265**:87–100.

Hoffman, S., and Edelman, G. M., 1983, Kinetics of homophilic binding by embryonic and adult forms of the neural cell adhesion molecule, *Proc. Natl. Acad. Sci. USA* **80**:5762–5766.

Hoffman, S., Sorkin, B. C., White, P. C., Brackenbury, R., Mailhammer, R., Rutishauser, U., Cunningham, B. A., and Edelman, G. M., 1982, Chemical characterization of a neural cell adhesion molecule purified from embryonic brain membranes, *J. Biol. Chem.* **257**:7720–7729.

Hogg, N., 1983, Human monocytes are associated with the formation of fibrin, *J. Exp. Med.* **157**:473–485.

Hogg, N., Slusarenko, M., Cohen, J., and Reiser, J., 1981, Monoclonal antibody with specificity for monocytes and neurons, *Cell* **24**:875–884.

Holmgren, J., Elwing, H., Fredman, P., Strannegard, O., and Svennerholm, L., 1980, Gangliosides as receptors for bacterial toxins and Sendai virus, *Adv. Exp. Med. Biol.* **125**:453–470.

Huber, G., and Matus, A., 1984, Differences in the cellular distributions of two microtubule-associated proteins, MAP1 and MAP2, in rat brain, *J. Neurosci.* **4**:151–160.

Jessen, K., and Mirsky, R., 1980, Glial cells in the enteric nervous system contain glial fibrillary acidic protein, *Nature* **286**:736–738.

Jessen, K. R., and Mirsky, R., 1983, Astrocyte-like glia in the peripheral nervous system: An immunohistochemical study of enteric glia, *J. Neurosci.* **3**:2206–2218.

Jones, R. T., Walker, J. H., Richardson, P. J., Fox, G. Q., and Whittaker, V. P., 1981, Immunohistochemical localization of cholinergic nerve terminals, *Cell Tissue Res.* **218**:355–373.

Jørgensen, O. S., 1979, Polypeptides of the synaptic membrane antigens D1, D2, and D3, *Biochim. Biophys.* Acta **581**:153–162.

Jørgensen, O. S., and Bock, E., 1974, Brain specific synaptosomal membrane proteins demonstrated by crossed immunoelectrophoresis, *J. Neurochem.* **23**:879–880.

Jørgensen, O. S., and Møller, M., 1980, Immunocytochemical demonstration of the D2 protein in the presynaptic complex, *Brain Res.* **194**:419–429.

Jørgensen, O. S., and Møller, M., 1983, A testis antigen related to the brain D2 adhesion protein, *Develop. Biol.* **100**:275–286.

Jørgensen, O. S., Delouvee, A., Thiery, J.-P., and Edelman, G. M., 1980, The nervous system specific protein D2 is involved in adhesion among neurites from cultured rat ganglia, *FEBS Lett.* **111**:39–42.

Karpiak, S. E., Mahadik, S. P., Graf, L., and Rapport, M. M., 1981, An immunological model of epilepsy: Seizures induced by antibodies to GM1 ganglioside, *Epilepsia* **22**:189–196.

Kasai, N., and Yu, R. K., 1983, The monoclonal antibody A2B5 is specific to ganglioside GQ_{1c}, *Brain Res.* **277**:155–158.

Kohn, L. D., Consiglio, E., DeWolf, M. S., Grollman, E. F. Ledley, F. D., Lee, G., and Morris, N. P., 1980, Thyrotropin receptors and gangliosides, *Adv. Exp. Med. Biol.* **125**:487–502.

Koulakoff, A., Bizzini, B., and Berwald-Netter, Y., 1982, A correlation between the appearance and the evolution of tetanus toxin binding cells and neurogenesis, *Develop. Brain Res.* **5**:139–147.

Koulakoff, A., Bizzini, B., and Berwald-Netter, Y., 1983, Neuronal acquisition of tetanus toxin binding sites: Relationship with the last mitotic cycle, *Develop. Biol.* **100**:350–357.

Kreider, B. Q., Messing, A., Doan, H., Kim, S. U., Lisak, R. P., and Pleasure, D. E., 1981, Enrichment of Schwann cell cultures from neonatal rat sciatic nerve by differential adhesion, *Brain Res.* **207**:433–444.

Kushner, P. D., 1984, A library of monoclonal antibodies to Torpedo cholinergic synaptosomes, *J. Neurochem.* **43**:775–786.

Lacetti, P., Tombaccini, D., Aloj, S., Grollman, E. F., and Kohn, L. D., 1984, Gangliosides, the thyrotropin receptor, and autoimmune thyroid disease in: *Ganglioside Structure, Function, and Biomedical Potential* (R. W. Ledeen, R. K. Yu, M. M. Rapport, and K. Suzuki, eds.), Plenum Press, New York, pp. 355–367.

Lagenaur, C., Schachner, M., Solter, D., and Knowles, B., 1982, Monoclonal antibody against SSEA-1 is specific for a subpopulation of astrocytes in mouse cerebellum, *Neurosci. Lett.* **31**:181–184.

Lander, A. D., Tomaselli, K., Calof, A. L., and Reichardt, L. F., 1983, Studies on extracellular matrix components that promote neurite outgrowth, *Cold Spring Harbor Symp. Quant. Biol.* **48**:611–623.

Lasher, R. S., 1974, The uptake of [^{3}H]GABA and differentiation of stellate neurons in cultures of dissociated newborn rat cerebellum, *Brain Res.* **69**:235–254.

Ledeen, R. W., Yu, R. K., and Eng, L. F., 1973, Gangliosides of human myelin: Sialosylgalactosylceramide (G7) as a major component, *J. Neurochem.* **21**:829–839.

Ledeen, R. W., Yu, R. K., Rapport, M. M., and Suzuki, K. (eds.), 1984, *Ganglioside Structure, Function and Biomedical Potential*, Plenum Press, New York.

Lee, V. M,. Greene, L. A., and Shelanski, M. L., 1981, Identification of neural and adrenal medullary surface membrane glycoproteins recognized by antisera to cultured rat sympathetic neurons and PC12 pheochromocytoma cells, *Neuroscience* **6**:2773–2786.

Leifer, D., Lipton, S. A., and Barnstable, C. J., 1983, A monoclonal antibody to Thy-1 enhances process regeneration by differentiated rat retinal ganglion cells in culture, *Soc. Neurosci. Abstr.* **9**:5.10.

Liesi, P., Dahl, D., and Vaheri, A., 1983, Laminin is produced by early rat astrocytes in primary culture, *J. Cell Biol.* **96**:920–924.

Lietzke, R., and Unsicker, K., 1983, Tetanus toxin binding to different morphological phenotypes of cultured rat and bovine adrenal medullary cells, *Neurosci. Lett.* **38**:233–238.

Lohmann, S. M., Walter, U., Miller, P. E., Greengard, P., and DeCamilli, P., 1981, Immunohistochemical localization of cyclic GMP-dependent protein kinase in mammalian brain, *Proc. Natl. Acad. Sci. USA.* **78**:653–657.

McCarthy, K. D., and de Vellis, J., 1980, Preparation of separate astroglial and oligodendroglial cell cultures from rat cerebral tissue, *J. Cell Biol.* **85**:890–902.

McGarvey, M. N., Baron-Van Evercooren, A., Kleinman, H. K., and Dubois-Dalcq, M., 1984, Synthesis and effects of basement membrane components in cultured rat Schwann cells, *Develop. Biol.* **105**:18–28.

McGuire, J. C., Greene, L. A., and Furano, A. V., 1978, NGF stimulates incorporation of fucose or glucosamine into an external glycoprotein in cultured rat PC12 pheochromocytoma cells, *Cell* **15**:357–365.

Marangos, P. J., Polak, J. M., and Pearse, A. G. E., 1982, Neuron-specific enolase, a probe for neurons and neuroendocrine cells, *Trends Neurosci.* **5**:193–196.

Mason, D. W., and Williams, A. F., 1980, The kinetics of antibody binding to membrane antigens in solution and at the cell surface, *Biochem. J.* **187**:1–20.

Meier, D., and Schachner, M., 1982, Immunoselection of oligodendrocytes by magnetic beads. II. In vitro maintenance of immunoselected oligodendrocytes, *J. Neurosci. Res.* **7**:135–145.

Mirsky, R., 1982, The use of antibodies to define and study major cell types in the central and peripheral nervous system, in: *Neuroimmunology* (J. Brockes, ed.), Plenum Press, New York, pp. 141–181.

Mirsky, R., Wendon, L. M. B., Black, P., Stolkin, C., and Bray, D., 1978, Tetanus toxin: A cell surface marker for neurons in culture, *Brain Res.* **148:**251–259.

Mirsky, R., Winter, J., Abney, E. R., Pruss, R. M., Gavrilovic, J., and Raff, M. C., 1980, Myelin-specific proteins and glycolipids in rat Schwann cells and oligodendrocytes in culture, *J. Cell Biol.* **84:**483–494.

Morris, R. J., 1982, The surface antigens of nerve cells, in: *Neuroscience Approached Through Cell Culture*, Volume I (S. E. Pfeiffer, ed.), CRC Press, Boca Raton, Florida, pp. 1–49.

Naiki, M., Marcus, D. M., and Ledeen, R., 1974, Properties of antisera to ganglioside GM1 and asialo GM1, *J. Immunol.* **113:**84–93.

Neale, E. A., Oertel, W. H., Bowers, L. M., and Weise, V. K., 1983, Glutamate decarboxylase immunoreactivity and ^{3}H-aminobutyric acid accumulation within the same neurons in dissociated cell cultures of cerebral cortex, *J. Neurosci.* **3:**376–382.

Norton, W. T., 1983, Recent advances in the neurobiology of oligodendroglia, *Adv. Cell. Neurobiol.* **4:**3–55.

Norton, W. T. (ed.) 1984, *Oligodendroglia*, Plenum Press, New York.

Norton, W. T., and Autilio, L. A., 1966, The lipid composition of purified bovine brain myelin, *J. Neurochem.* **13:**213–222.

Obata, K., Momoko, M., and Handa, S., 1977, Effects of glycolipids on *in vitro* development of neuromuscular junctions, *Nature* **266:**369–371.

Oertel, W. H., Mugnaini, E., Schmechel, D. E., Tappaz, M. L., and Kopin, I. J., 1982, The immunocytochemical demonstration of gamma-aminobutyric acid-ergic neurons–Methods and application, in: *Cytochemical Methods in Neuroanatomy* (S. L. Palay and V. Chan-Palay, eds.), Liss, New York, pp. 297–329.

Ostermann, E., Sternberger, N. H., and Sternberger, L. A., 1983, Immunocytochemistry of brain-reactive monoclonal antibodies in peripheral tissues, *Cell Tissue Res.* **228:**459–473.

Peng, W. W., Bressler, J. P., Tiffany-Castiglioni, E., and de Vellis, J., 1982, Development of a monoclonal antibody against a tumor-associated antigen, *Science* **215:**1102–1104.

Pfenninger, K. H., 1978, Organization of neuronal membranes, *Annu. Rev. Neurosci.* **1:**445–471.

Pruss, R. M., 1979, Thy-1 antigen on astrocytes in long-term cultures of rat central nervous system, *Nature* **280:**688–689.

Pukel, C. S., Lloyd, K. O., Travassos, L. R., Dippold, W. G., Oettgen, H. F., and Old, L. J., 1982, G_{D3}, a prominent ganglioside of human melanoma: Detection and characterization by mouse monoclonal antibody, *J. Exp. Med.* **155:**1133–1147.

Raff, M. C., Mirsky, R., Fields, K. L., Lisak, R. P., Dorfman, S. H., Silberberg, D. H., Gregson, N. A., Liebowitz, S., and Kennedy, M. C., 1978, Galactocerebroside is a specific cell-surface antigenic marker for oligodendrocytes in culture, *Nature* **274:**813–816.

Raff, M. C., Fields, K. L., Hakomori, S.-I., Mirsky, R. M., Pruss, R., and Winter, J., 1979, Cell-type-specific markers for distinguishing and studying neurons and the major classes of glial cells in culture, *Brain Res.* **174:**283–308.

Raff, M. C., Miller, R. H., and Noble, M., 1983a, A glial progenitor cell that develops *in vitro* into an astrocyte or an oligodendrocyte depending on culture medium, *Nature* **303:**390–396.

Raff, M. C., Abney, E. R., Cohen, J., Lindsay, R., and Noble, M., 1983b, Two types of astrocytes in cultures of developing rat white matter: Differences in morphology, surface gangliosides, and growth characteristics, *J. Neurosci.* **3:**1289–1300.

Rauscht, B., Clapshaw, P. A., Price, J., Noble, M., and Seifert, W., 1982, Development of oligodendrocytes and Schwann cells studied with a monoclonal antibody against galactocerebroside, *Proc. Natl. Acad. Sci. USA* **79**:2709–2713.

Rapport, M. M., 1981a, Introduction to the biochemistry of gangliosides, in: *Gangliosides in Neurological and Neuromuscular Function, Development, and Repair* (M. M. Rapport and A. Gorio, eds.), Raven Press, New York, pp. xv–xix.

Rapport, M. M., 1981b, Specificity of antiganglioside serum in the perturbation of CNS functions, in: *Gangliosides in Neurological and Neuromuscular Function, Development, and Repair* (M. M. Rapport and A. Gorio, eds.), Raven Press, New York, pp. 91–97.

Rapport, M. M., and Gorio, A. (eds.), 1981, *Gangliosides in Neurological and Neuromuscular Function, Development and Repair*, Raven Press, New York.

Rapport, M. M., and Huong, Y.-Y. 1984, Present status of the immunology of gangliosides, in: *Ganglioside Structure, Function and Biomedical Potential* (R. W. Ledeen, R. K., Yu, M. M. Rapport, and K. Suzuki, eds.), Plenum Press, New York, pp. 15–25.

Revesz, T., and Greaves, M., 1975, Ligand-induced redistribution of lymphocyte membrane ganglioside GM1, *Nature* **257**:103–106.

Richardson, P. J., 1983, Presynaptic distribution of the cholinergic-specific antigen Chol-1 and 5′-nucleotidase in rat brain, as determined by complement-mediated release of neurotransmitters, *J. Neurochem.* **41**:640–648.

Rodman, J. S., and Akeson, R., 1981, A new antigen common to the rat nervous and immune systems. II. Molecular characterization, *J. Neurosci. Res.* **6**:179–192.

Rohrer, H., and Schachner, M., 1980, Surface proteins of cultured mouse cerebellar cells, *J. Neurochem.* **35**:792–803.

Roisen, F. J., Bartfeld, H., and Rapport, M. M., 1981, Ganglioside mediation of *in vitro* neuronal maturation, in: *Gangliosides in Neurological and Neuromuscular Function, Development, and Repair* (M. M. Rapport and A. Gorio, eds.), Raven Press, New York, pp. 135–150.

Rothbard, J. B., Brackenbury, R., Cunningham, B. A., and Edelman, G. M., 1982, Difference in the carbohydrate structures of neural cell-adhesion molecules from adult and embryonic chicken brains, *J. Biol. Chem.* **257**:11064–11069.

Rougon, G., Deagostini-Bazin, H., Hirn, M., and Goridis, C., 1982, Tissue and developmental stage-specific forms of a neural cell surface antigen linked to differences in glycosylation of a common polypeptide, *EMBO J.* **1**:1239–1244.

Rougon, G., Hirsch, M. R., Hirn, M., Guenet, J. L., and Goridis, C., 1983, Monoclonal antibody to neural cell surface protein: Identification of a glycoprotein family of restricted cellular localization, *Neuroscience* **10**:511–520.

Roussel, G., Labourdette, G., and Nussbaum, J. L., 1981, Characterization of oligodendrocytes in primary cultures from brain hemispheres of newborn rats, *Develop. Biol.* **81**:372–378.

Rutishauser, U., 1983, Molecular and biological properties of a neural cell adhesion molecule, *Cold Spring Harbor Symp. Quant. Biol.* **48**:501–514.

Rutishauser, U., Thiery, J.-P., Brackenbury, R., Sela, B.-A., and Edelman, G. M., 1976, Mechanisms of adhesion among cells from neural tissues of the chick embryo, *Proc. Natl. Acad. Sci. USA* **73**:577–581.

Rutishauser, U., Thiery, J.-P., Brackenbury, R., and Edelman, G. M., 1978a, Adhesion among neural cells. III. Relationship of the surface molecule CAM to cell adhesion and the development of histotypic patterns, *J. Cell Biol.* **79**:371–381.

Rutishauser, U., Gall, E. W., and Edelman, G. M,. 1978b, Adhesion among neural cells of the chick embryo. IV. Role of the cell surface molecule CAM in the formation of neurite bundles in cultures of spinal ganglia, *J. Cell Biol.* **79**:382–393.

Sadoul, R., Hirn, M., Deagostini-Bazin, H., Rougon, G., and Goridis, C., 1983, Adult and embryonic mouse neural cell adhesion molecules have different binding properties, *Nature* **304**:347–349.

Sakakibara, K., Iwamori, M., Uchida, T., and Nagai, Y., 1981a, Immunohistochemical localization of galactocerebroside in kidney, liver, and lung of golden hamster, *Experientia* **37**:712–714.

Sakakibara, K., Momoi, T., Uchida, T., and Nagai, Y., 1981b, Evidence for an association of glycosphingolipid with a colchicine-sensitive microtubule-like cytoskeletal structure of cultured cells, *Nature* **293**:76–78.

Salton, S. R. J., Richter-Landsberg, C., Greene, L. A., and Shelanski, M. L., 1983a, Nerve growth factor-inducible large external (NILE) glycoprotein: Studies of a central and peripheral neuronal marker, *J. Neurosci.* **3**:441–454.

Salton, S. R. J., Shelanski, M. L., and Greene, L. A., 1983b, Biochemical properties of the nerve growth factor-inducible large external (NILE) glycoprotein, *J. Neurosci.* **3**:2420–2430.

Sarthy, P. V., Curtis, B. M., and Catterall, W. A., 1983, Retrograde labeling, enrichment, and characterization of retinal ganglion cells from the neonatal rat, *J. Neurosci.* **3**:2532–2544.

Schachner, M., 1974, NS-1 (nervous system antigen-1), a glial cell-specific antigenic component of the cell surface, *Proc. Natl. Acad. Sci. USA* **71**:1795–1799.

Schachner, M., 1982a, Cell type-specific surface antigens in the mammalian nervous system, *J. Neurochem.* **39**:1–8.

Schachner, M., 1982b, Immunological analysis of cellular heterogeneity in the cerebellum, in: *Neuroimmunology* (J. Brockes, ed.), Plenum Press, New York, pp. 215–250.

Schachner, M., 1982c, Glial antigens and the expression of neuroglial phenotypes, *Trends Neurosci.* **5**:225–228.

Schachner, M., and Willinger, M., 1979a, Developmental expression of oligodendrocyte specific cell surface markers: NS-1 (nervous system antigen-1), cerebroside, and basic protein of myelin, in: *The Menarini Series on Immunopathology* (P.-A. Miescher, L. Bolis, S. Gorini, T. A. Lambo, G. J. V. Nossal, and G. Torrigiani, eds.), Volume 2, pp. 37–60.

Schachner, M., and Willinger, M., 1979b, Cell type-specific cell surface antigens in the cerebellum, *Prog. Brain Res.* **51**:23–44.

Schachner, M., Wortham, K. A., Carter, L. D., and Chaffee, J. K., 1975, NS-4 (nervous system antigen-4), a cell surface antigen of developing and adult mouse brain and sperm, *Develop. Biol.* **44**:313–325.

Schachner, M., Schoonmaker, G., and Hynes, R. O., 1978, Cellular and subcellular localization of LETS protein in the nervous system, *Brain Res.* **158**:149–158.

Schnitzer, J., and Schachner, M., 1981a, Expression of Thy-1, H-2, and NS-4 cell surface antigens and tetanus toxin receptors in early postnatal and adult mouse cerebellum, *J. Neuroimmunol.* **1**:429–456.

Schnitzer, J., and Schachner, M., 1981b, Characterization of isolated mouse cerebellar cell populations *in vitro*, *J. Neuroimmunol.* **1**:457–470.

Schnitzer, J., and Schachner, M., 1981c, Developmental expression of cell type-specific markers in mouse cerebellar cells *in vitro*, *J. Neuroimmunol.* **1**:471–487.

Schnitzer, J., and Schachner, M., 1982, Cell type specificity of a neural cell surface antigen recognized by the monoclonal antibody A2B5, *Cell Tissue Res.* **224**:625–636.

Schnitzer, J,. Franke, W. W., and Schachner, M,. 1981, Immunocytochemical demonstration of vimentin in astrocytes and ependymal cells of developing and adult mouse nervous system, *J. Cell Biol.* **90**:435–447.

Schwartz, M., and Spirman, N., 1982, Sprouting from chicken embryo dorsal root ganglia induced by nerve growth factor is specifically inhibited by affinity-purified anti-ganglioside antibodies, *Proc. Natl. Acad. Sci. USA* **79**:6080–6083.

Seyfried, T. N., Yu, R. K., and Miyazawa, N., 1982, Differential cellular enrichment of gangliosides in the mouse cerebellum: Analysis using neurological mutants, *J. Neurochem.* **38**:551–559.

Solter, D., and Knowles, B. B., 1978, Monoclonal antibody defining a stage-specific mouse embryonic antigen (SSEA-1), *Proc. Natl. Acad. Sci. USA* **75**:5565–5569.

Sommer, I., and Schachner, M., 1981, Monoclonal antibodies (O1 to O4) to oligodendrocyte cell surfaces: An immunocytological study in the central nervous system, *Develop. Biol.* **83**:311–327.

Spirman, N., Sela, B.-A., and Schwartz, M., 1982, Anti-ganglioside antibodies inhibit neuritic outgrowth from regenerating goldfish retinal explants, *J. Neurochem.* **39**:874–877.

Stallcup, W. B., 1981, The NG2 antigen, a putative lineage marker: Immunofluorescence localization in primary cultures of rat brain, *Develop. Biol.* **83**:154–165.

Stallcup, W. B., Arner, L. S., and Levine, J. M., 1983, An antiserum against the PC12 cell line defines cell surface antigens specific for neurons and Schwann cells, *J. Neurosci.* **3**:68.

Stallcup, W. B., Beasley, L., and Levine, J., 1983, Cell surface molecules that characterize different stages in the development of cerebellar interneurons, *Cold Spring Harbor Symp. Quant. Biol.* **48**:761–774.

Sternberger, N. H., Itoyama, Y., Kies, M. W., and Webster, H. d., 1978, Immunocytochemical method to identify basic protein in myelin-forming oligodendrocytes of newborn rat C.N.S., *J. Neurocytol.* **7**:251–263.

Sweadner, K. J., 1983, Post-translational modification and evoked release of two large surface proteins of sympathetic neurons, *J. Neurosci.* **3**:2504–2517.

Tardieu, M., Noseworthy, J. H., Perry, L., Che, M., Greene, M. I., and Weiner, H. L., 1983, Generation of a monoclonal antibody (Epenl) which binds selectively to murine ependymal cells, *Brain Res.* **277**:339–346.

Thiery, J.-P., Brackenbury, R., Rutishauser, U., and Edelman, G. M., 1977, Adhesion among neural cells of the chick embryo. II. Purification and characterization of a cell adhesion molecule from neural retina, *J. Biol. Chem.* **252**:6841–6845.

Trisler, G. D., 1982, Are molecular markers of cell position involved in the formation of neural circuits?, *Trends Neurosci.* **5**:306–310.

Trisler, G. D., Schneider, M. D., and Nirenberg, M., 1981, A topographic gradient of molecules in retina can be used to identify neuron position, *Proc. Natl. Acad. Sci. USA* **78**:2145–2149.

van Heyningen, W. E., 1974, Gangliosides as membrane receptors for tetanus toxin, cholera toxin and serotonin, *Nature* **249**:415–417.

Vulliamy, T., and Messenger, E. A., 1981, Tetanus toxin: A marker of amphibian neuronal differentiation *in vitro*, *Neurosci. Lett.* **22**:87–90.

Vulliamy, T., Rattray, S., and Mirsky, R., 1981, Cell-surface antigen distinguishes sensory and autonomic peripheral neurones from central neurones, *Nature* **291**: 418–420.

Walsh, F. S., 1980, Identification and characterization of plasma membrane antigens of neurons and muscle cells using monoclonal antibodies, in: *Synaptic Constituents in Health and Disease* (M. Brzin, D. Skit, and H. Bachelard, eds.) Pergamon Press, Elmsford, New York, pp,. 285–320.

Williams, A. F., Barclay, A. N., Letarte-Muirhead, M., and Morris, R. J., 1977, Rat Thy-1 antigens from thymus and brain: Their tissue distribution, purification and chemical composition, *Cold Spring Harbor Symp. Quant. Biol.* **41**:51–61.

Williams, C. A., Barna, J., and Schupf, N., 1980, Antibody to Thy-1 antigen injected into rat hypothalamus selectively inhibits carbamylcholine induced drinking, *Nature* **283**:82–84.

Willinger, M., and Schachner, M,. 1980, GM1 ganglioside as a marker for neuronal differentiation in mouse cerebellum, *Develop. Biol.* **74**:101–117.

Yen, S.-H., and Fields, K. L., 1981, Antibodies to neurofilament, glial filament and fibroblast intermediate filament proteins bind to different cell types in the nervous system, *J. Cell Biol.* **88**:115–126.

Yen, S.-H., and Fields, K. L., 1983, Schwann cells contain a protein similar to the CNS astroglial filament protein, *Soc. Neurosci. Abstr.* **9**:71.4.

Yu, R. K., and Ando, S., 1980, Structures of some new complex gangliosides of fish brain, *Adv. Exp. Med. Biol.* **125**:33–45.

3

Neuronotrophic Factors

J. REGINO PEREZ-POLO

1. INTRODUCTION

At the heart of developmental neurobiology is the attempt to rationalize the exquisite specificity of the vertebrate nervous system. That is, throughout the sequence of events that constitute neuronal development, neuroblasts become postmitotic, migrate, extrude neurites that follow tortuous but precise paths throughout the organism, and finally establish synaptic contacts among themselves and with nonneuronal target tissues. In addition, maturation events take place that result in the evolution of electrically excitable membranes and the myelination of axons by oligodendrocytes in the CNS or by Schwann cells in the PNS. Lastly, the repertoire of the neurotransmitters to be released or of the appropriate receptors to respond to these must be selected in concert with the events mentioned above.

At the turn of the century, Forssman, Ramón y Cajal, and Tello elaborated the concept of neuronotropic substances as an explanation for the directionality and specificity of axonal growth seen in the developing nervous system (Ramón y Cajal, 1928). Thus, neuronotrophic substances (NTF) are extracellular substances that stimulate neuronal metabolism and allow neuronal differentiation to take place, whereas neuronotropic substances orient growing neurites. The discovery and subsequent purification of an NTF substance, the nerve growth factor

J. REGINO PEREZ-POLO • Department of Human Biological Chemistry and Genetics, University of Texas Medical Branch, Galveston, Texas 77550.

protein (NGF), by Levi-Montalcini (1982) allowed for the manipulation of some of the variables associated with neuronal development.
As a result of many of the subsequent studies using NGF and antisera
to NGF, both *in vivo* and *in vitro* (Levi-Montalcini and Angeletti, 1968;
Hendry, 1976, 1980; Mobley *et al.*, 1977; Purves and Nja, 1978; Varon
and Bunge, 1978; Black, 1980; Greene and Shooter, 1980; Thoenen and
Barde, 1980; Vinores and Guroff, 1980; Harper and Thoenen, 1981;
Oppenheim *et al.*, 1982; Yankner and Shooter, 1982), the role of NGF
as a neuronotrophic or permissive factor took center stage and only
more recently has its neuronotropic activity been explored (Campenot,
1977; Letourneau, 1978; Gundersen and Barrett, 1980; Campenot,
1982a,b; Levi-Montalcini, 1983). Rather, neuronotropic factors are now
believed to be associated with neuronal substrata and are often called
neurite-promoting factors (NPF) (Varon *et al.*, 1968; Patterson, 1978; Varon
and Bunge, 1978). Neuronotrophic or permissive factors modulate "programmed cell death," neurite pruning, and *perhaps* synaptogenic maturation during development (Purves and Nja, 1978; Black, 1980; Hendry, 1980; Campenot, 1982b; Hendry *et al.*, 1983; Perez-Polo and Haber,
1983). Clearly, a case could be made that *neuronotropic* activity is excluded
from this definition, but it will be included in the concept of developmental neurite pruning discussed here.

2. CELL DEATH, NEURITE PRUNING, AND SYNAPSE
MATURATION

Neuronal specificity in development can be explained in terms of
a spectrum of restrictive events under epigenetic control that allow for
the elaboration of highly specific neuronal networks and that, in addition, display some degree of variability from organism to organism.
This is a case of functional specificity without obligatory architectorial
rigidity, where the major restrictive influence is "programmed neuronal
cell death." Although the description of cell death as a part of developmental processes in the nervous system has been labeled "programmed," this is a loose interpretation of the word since neuroblasts
do not have strict cell-specific genomic instructions as to the developmental sequelae that take place (Stent, 1981). Both in the PNS and in
the CNS there is ample evidence that concurrent with development there
is an ongoing process by which neuroblasts proceed to die in large numbers as access to neuron-specific NTFs is restricted (Cowan, 1973; Hamburger, 1980). In some instances as many as 30% of the neuroblasts will
die in a period of a few days (Hendry, 1976). The extent of neuron

survival is dependent on the availability of appropriate NTFs to the neuroblasts (Fig. 1). That is, surrounding nonneuronal cells will synthesize and secrete NTFs in response to hormonal cues (Perez-Polo et al., 1977, 1984) or perhaps in response to ongoing neuronal attrition in a manner similar to lesion-induced NTF synthesis in the CNS and PNS (Ebendal et al., 1980; Bjorklund and Stenevi, 1981; Nieto-Sampedro et al., 1982, 1983; Longo et al., 1983; Manthorpe et al., 1983; Skene and Shooter, 1983). In highly vascularized regions, NTFs might be available from blood vessels directly or the hormonal signals that trigger NTF synthesis might be bloodborne (Harper and Thoenen, 1980; Perez-Polo et al., 1980; Beck and Perez-Polo, 1982).

The mobilization of neuronal metabolism by NTFs will result in the extension of profuse networks of neurites that become oriented toward innervation targets that also secrete NTFs. Not all neurites will successfully contact the target tissue, and as innervation proceeds, there is a concomitant decrease in extracellular NTF levels as well as a diminishing requirement by the neurons for the NTF in order to survive (Thoenen and Barde, 1980). It should be emphasized that even in the case of the much-studied and well-characterized NGF effect on sympathetic and embryonic sensory ganglia, there is no common time period during development for these events (Barde et al., 1980). Thus, different neuronal structures may exhibit a different temporal pattern of dependence on an NTF common to the proper development of these neurons.

As extracellular NTF levels drop, those redundant neurites that have not successfully innervated target tissue will be retracted resulting in a reduction in the degree of arborization, or pruning, of the neuritic tree (Hamburger, 1980; Campenot, 1982a,b; Perez-Polo and Haber, 1983). Based on the evidence that in vivo treatment with antisera to NGF results in dramatic changes in synaptic population and function in superior cervical ganglia, one could propose that NTFs are likely to be instrumental in synapse maturation and in some cases, like the requirements of the superior cervical ganglion for NGF, may also be required for synapse maintenance (Nja and Purves, 1978; Purves and Lichtman, 1978,; Purves and Nja, 1978).

After innervation and as part of the maintenance of the neuron, there is retrograde transport of NTF to the neuronal soma following specific uptake of the NTF at nerve endings (Hendry et al., 1974a,b, 1982, 1983; Stockel and Thoenen, 1975; Hendry, 1980; Hendry and Hill, 1980). The specific and saturable transport of an NTF in vivo has been suggested as one of the requirements defining a neuronotrophic activity (Hendry et al., 1983; Lyons and Perez-Polo, 1983). Also, the name retrophins has been suggested for this class of neuronotrophic factors (Hen-

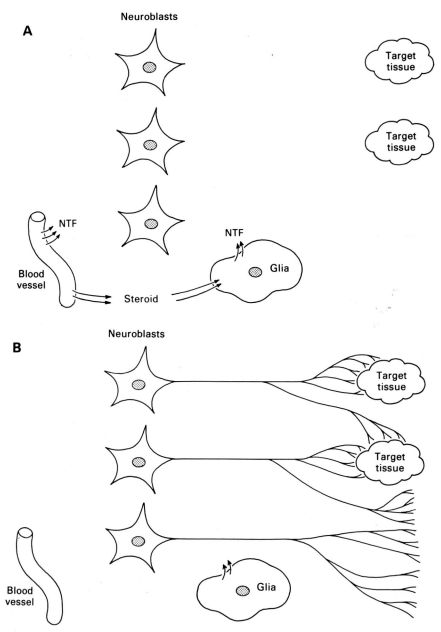

Figure 1. Proposed role of neuronotrophic factor (NTF) in neuronal cell death and neurite pruning during development. (From Perez-Polo and Haber, 1983.)

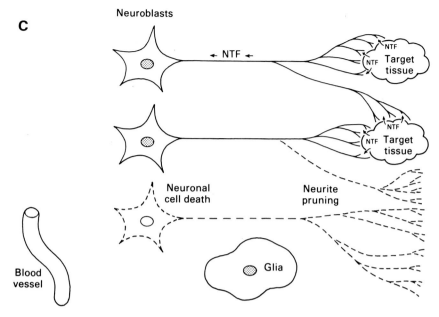

Figure 1. (*continued*)

dry and Hill, 1980). For NGF, this target to soma uptake and transport has been well characterized *in vivo* where [^{125}I]β-NGF has been shown to be transported from the rat iris to the superior cervical ganglion (Hendry *et al.*, 1974a,b, 1982, 1983; Stockel *et al.*, 1974b; Stockel and Thoenen, 1975; Hendry, 1977; Schwab, 1977; Johnson *et al.*, 1978; Hendry and Hill, 1980). Subsequent denervation results, in this case, in a dramatic increase in the synthesis of NGF by the rat iris (Ebendal *et al.*, 1980). This emphasizes the role of an NTF in maintenance of a functioning neuronal innervation pattern and speaks to the permanence and bidirectional nature of this intercellular communication. Thus, in the case of NGF, it would appear that in early development NGF acts as an extracellular trophic factor, and in adulthood it travels across cell boundaries and is retrogradely transported (Fig. 2).

The significance of developmental and chronic NTF insufficiencies on clinical manifestations of neurological disorders is not established at this point; although the topic has been discussed and explored experimentally for NGF, definitive results are lacking (Burdman and Goldstein, 1964; Bill *et al.*, 1969; Waghe *et al.*, 1970; Kumar *et al.*, 1970; Russel and Rubenstein, 1972; Schenkein *et al.*, 1974; Siggers, 1976; Siggers *et al.*, 1975, 1976; Fabricant *et al.*, 1979; Perez-Polo *et al.*, 1980, 1982c;

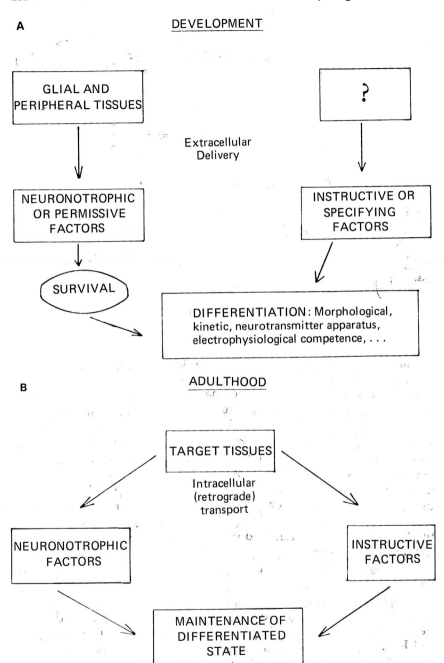

Figure 2. Proposed differences in transport of NTFs in (A) developing nervous system and (B) adult nervous system.

Schwartz and Breakefield, 1980; Edgar *et al.*, 1981). Also, there is much interest in the study of NTFs as possible agents that might allow CNS regeneration to take place or accelerate ongoing PNS regeneration (Cowan, 1973; Baxter, 1983; Giuffrida-Stella, and Lajtha, 1983; Levi-Montalcini, 1983; Perez-Polo *et al.*, 1983b; Skene and Shooter, 1983; Varon and Lundborg, 1983).

3. NEURONOTROPHIC ACTIVITY: *IN VIVO* VS. *IN VITRO* ASPECTS

Given that the discovery and characterization of neuronotrophic factors are largely carried out using *in vitro* assays, it is prudent to explore the limitations of this approach. Implicit to the action of any neuronotrophic activity is the concept that it is not likely to be the sole determinant of all of the properties characterizing a particular class of neurons. For example, although NGF will stimulate neurotransmitter synthesis in sympathetic ganglia *in vivo*, glucocorticoid levels and transsynaptic activity will have potent effects as to whether adrenergic or cholinergic activity is expressed (Patterson, 1978; Chun and Patterson, 1977a,b; MacDonnell *et al.*, 1977; Black, 1980; Hendry *et al.*, 1982; Bohn *et al.*, 1981; Otten *et al.*, 1981; Walicke and Patterson, 1981). Similar effects have been reported for sensory ganglia where transsynaptic activity decreases levels of substance P but increases the levels of norepinephrine in the superior cervical ganglia (Bohn *et al.*, 1981; Kessler and Black, 1981, 1982). Thus, the classical approach of perturbing the organism through the application of exogenous NTFs or antibodies to a given NTF, in order to determine the spectrum of activity of a given NTF on a particular neuronal population, may result in misleading conclusions. In addition, the level of interaction of different neuronal systems may also result in secondary effects if the NTF target is not defined using other localization criteria. Nevertheless, the use of well-characterized NTFs and anti-NTFs when the *in vivo* targets are well established has been shown to be a powerful tool as in the case of NGF (Aloe and Levi-Montalcini, 1979; Gorin and Johnson, 1979; Johnson *et al.*, 1980).

In the early stages of the purification and characterization of NTFs, *in vitro* systems have been used almost exclusively. Their advantages are that some uniformity of the preparation and control of the cellular environment can be achieved with this simpler system. This is particularly true given the development of defined media that will selectively support the culture of specific cell populations in the absence of added serum (Bottenstein, 1983). Thus, *in vitro* preparations for the study of

NTFs are more practical. However, it must be emphasized that all *in vitro* systems consist of "recuperating or regenerating" neurons. Thus, results obtained *in vitro* may not necessarily be applicable to neuronal development. Since electrophysiological function is also disrupted in explanting and in some cases dissociating neuronal cultures, this may also play a modulatory role on NTF characterization *in vitro* given the trophic character of transsynaptic activity (Stockel *et al.*, 1974a,b; Coughlin *et al.*, 1978; Bohn *et al.*, 1981; Kessler and Black, 1981, 1982; see Chapter 10). In some instances it has been demonstrated that requirements of explanted ganglia differ significantly from those of dissociated cells from the same ganglia (Helfand *et al.*, 1978; Meyer *et al.*, 1979). However, for purposes of NTF purification alone, there is little doubt that *in vitro* systems are optimal.

4. CLONAL MODEL SYSTEMS

Transformed clonal cell lines have been useful for the purification of NTFs and dissection of the multicompartmental effect of NTFs. Given the homogeneous character of these *in vitro* cellular populations and their ability to survive in culture without NTFs, certain types of metabolic studies are feasible that would be difficult to carry out using neuronal explants or dissociated primary cultures.

4.1. Neuroblastoma

Two clonal systems that have been useful for the study of neuronotrophic activities and factors are PNS-derived neuroblastoma lines of murine and human origin. Since these are transformed cell lines that do not require neuronotrophic factors in order to survive *in vitro*, some caution must be exercised in extrapolating insights gained with these systems to *in vivo* situations. Also, they are not as useful in the determination of effects of neuronotrophic factors on cellular proliferation since this aspect of their metabolism is most assuredly modified. Lastly, it must be kept in mind that given the presumed sympathetic origin of these neuroblastoma tumors (Abell *et al.*, 1970), they should only be suitable for the study of neuronotrophic factors acting on the PNS. However, for PNS-targeted neuronotrophic factors, these neuroblastoma systems are useful for the study of neurotransmitter synthesis regulation, cell attachment, neurite elongation, and tropic effects as well as neuronal recuperation and regeneration (Perez-Polo *et al.*, 1979, 1982a,b, 1983b; Reynolds and Perez-Polo, 1981; Schulze and Perez-Polo, 1982; Perez-Polo, 1984a,b,c; Perez-Polo and Werrbach-Perez, 1984).

Murine neuroblastoma lines share a common ancestry to a spontaneous tumor in an A/J mouse called the C1300 tumor (Stewart *et al.*, 1959). Continuous cell lines (Augusti-Tocci and Sato, 1969; McMorris *et al.*, 1973) derived from the C1300 tumor have been principally used to study agents that induce morphological differentiation (Augusti-Tocci and Sato, 1969; Schubert *et al.*, 1969) or activate neurotransmitter metabolism (Augusti-Tocci and Sato, 1969; Klebe and Ruddle, 1969; Schubert *et al.*, 1969; Amano *et al.*, 1972; Anagnoste *et al.*, 1972; McMorris *et al.*, 1973; Narotzky and Bondareff, 1974; Breakfield *et al.*, 1975; Zwiller *et al.*, 1975; Donnelly *et al.*, 1976; Waymire and Gilmer-Waymire, 1978). In addition, electrophysiological studies have been carried out in an effort to characterize ionic mechanisms responsible for the generation of action potentials (Catterall, 1982). A disadvantage of the murine neuroblastoma is its genetic instability in culture as expressed by its high degree of aneuploidy or tetraploidy (McMorris *et al.*, 1973; Warter *et al.*, 1974). In addition, although of presumed sympathetic origin, there are no murine neuroblastoma clones that respond to NGF, suggesting that critical regulatory properties have been lost on transformation and adaptation to *in vitro* growth and maintenance.

There are a number of human neuroblastoma clonal lines that are nearly diploid and display stable chromosomes (Waris *et al.*, 1973; Reynolds and Perez-Polo, 1975; Seeger *et al.*, 1977; Perez-Polo *et al.*, 1979; Ross *et al.*, 1981). In studies carried out with NGF, a number of these cell lines have been identified that have receptors to NGF, extend neurites, and develop the capability to generate action potentials in response to NGF (Fig. 3) (Waris *et al.*, 1973; Kuramoto *et al.*, 1977, 1981; Reynolds and Perez-Polo, 1981; Perez-Polo *et al.*, 1982a; Sonnenfeld and Ishii, 1982). In addition, they can become postmitotic and hypertrophied when exposed to NGF (Perez-Polo *et al.*, 1979, 1982a) and can transport, synthesize, and accumulate catecholamines (Biedler *et al.*, 1978; Perez-Polo *et al.*, 1982b; Perez-Polo and Werrbach-Perez, 1984). Their properties are summarized in Tables I and II.

4.2. Rat Pheochromocytoma

Another clonal line that has been used in the characterization of the NGF response is the rat pheochromocytoma cell line PC12 (Tischler and Greene, 1975; Greene and Tischler, 1976; see Chapter 8). In addition,

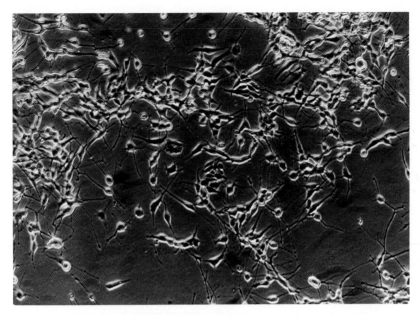

Figure 3. Response of human neuroblastoma IMR-32 to 5-day exposure to murine 7S-NGF
(1 μg/ml). Phase contrast.

this cell line has been useful in the characterization of a neuronotrophic
activity secreted by rat glioma cells in culture that is different from NGF
(Barde *et al.*, 1978; Edgar *et al.*, 1979). Like their neuroblastoma counterparts, PC12 extend functional neurites in response to NGF (Greene
and Tischler, 1976) and take up, synthesize, and storie catecholamines
(Dichter *et al.*, 1977). In contrast to the NGF-responsive human neuroblastoma clones, PC12 can be induced by NGF to synthesize acetylcholine (Greene and Rein, 1977; Schubert *et al.*, 1977; Edgar and Thoenen,
1978; Rieger *et al.*, 1980; Greene and Rukenstein, 1981). This may be due
to their adrenal medullary origin. PC12 cells have NGF receptors on
their cell surface whose properties are similar to those of neuroblastoma
and embryonic chick sensory ganglia (Herrup and Thoenen, 1979; Yankner and Shooter, 1979; Calissano and Shelanski, 1980; Landreth and
Shooter, 1980; Lyons *et al.*, 1983). PC12 cells have been most useful in
the characterization of the effects of NGF on neurotransmitter-synthesizing enzymes, characterization of the NGF surface receptor, and the
precise morphological response to NGF exposure (Yankner and Shooter,
1979).

Table I. Agents That Induce Morphological Differentiation in Human Neuroblastoma
Cell Lines

Inducer	Cell line	Reference
Nerve growth factor	MJB	Kolber et al. (1974)
	NMB	Brodeur and Goldstein (1976)
	NGP	Goldstein and Brodeur (1974)
	SK-N-SH-SY5Y	Perez-Polo et al. (1979)
	LAN-1	Haskell et al. (1983)
	KA-9	Schulze and Perez-Polo (1982)
	IMR-32	Reynolds and Perez-Polo (1981)
5-Bromodeoxyuridine	IMR-32	Prasad and Kumar (1975)
	NMB	Goldstein and Brodeur (1974)
	NGP	Goldstein and Brodeur (1974)
Serum-free media	IMR-32	Prasad and Kumar (1975)
Papaverine	IMR-32	Prasad and Kumar (1975)
R020-1724	IMR-32	Prasad and Kumar (1975)
X-rays	IMR-32	Prasad and Kumar (1975)
Prostaglandin E_1	IMR-32	Prasad and Kumar (1975)
Dibutyryl cAMP	IMR-32	Miyoke et al. (1975)
	NB-1	Prasad and Kumar (1975)
Sodium butyrate	IMR-32	Prasad and Kumar (1975)

5. ASSAY SYSTEMS

The purpose of assay systems is to provide an efficient screening
paradigm for the copurification of NTFs and neuronotrophic activity
prior to further characterization of the biological effects of an NTF. The
advantages and disadvantages of tissue explants vs. dissociated cell cultures have been extensively described elsewhere (Barde et al., 1983).

5.1. Cell Attachment

Effects of NGF on rates of cell attachment have been reported for
PC12 (Schubert and Whitlock, 1977; Schubert et al., 1978; Landreth et

Table II. Response of Human Neuroblastoma Clones to NGF

Line	NGF receptors	Neurite elongation	Increased attachment rate	Electrically excitable	Dopaminergic metabolism
IMR-32	ND	+	ND	+	+ +
LAN-1	+ +	+ +	ND	ND	ND
SY5Y	+	+ +	+	+	+
KA	+	+ +	+	ND	+

Table III. Effect of NGF on Attachment of SY5Y Human Neuroblastoma Cells[a]

Treatment	Percent attachment after 45 min (N)	p vs. control
Control	38 ± 3 (8)	
NGF (3.6 nM)	65 ± 4 (4)	$p < 0.001$
NGF + anti-NGF	35 ± 8 (4)	NS
Anti-NGF	36 ± 8 (3)	NS
EGF (6 nM)	45 ± 3 (4)	$p < 0.01$
Insulin (37 nM)	39 ± 1 (4)	NS
Cytochrome c (19 nM)	39 ± 1 (4)	NS
Bu₂cAMP (1 mM)	26 ± 3 (4)	$p < 0.001$
Bu₂cAMP + NGF	40 ± 2 (4)	NS
S180-conditioned medium	70 ± 3 (4)	$p < 0.001$
Theophylline (1 mM)	25 ± 5 (4)	$p < 0.025$
Theophylline + NGF	36 ± 1 (3)	NS
Bu₂cGMP (1 mM)	25 ± 3 (4)	$p < 0.001$

[a] Effect of 7S-NGF, nerve growth factor protein (1.7 μg/ml), on the attachment of SK-N-SH-SY5Y neuroblastoma cells to culture dishes. Anti-NGF, rabbit antiserum to mouse submaxillary gland β-NGF; EGF, epidermal growth factor; Bu₂cAMP, dibutyryl cAMP; S180, mouse sarcoma line S180; Bu₂cGMP, dibutyryl cGMP.

al., 1980), sensory ganglia (Varon *et al.*, 1974), human neuroblastoma (Schulze and Perez-Polo, 1982), and anaplastic glioma cells (Vinores and Koestner, 1981). It was suggested that the proportion of cells attaching to culture dishes might be predictive of survival (Varon *et al.*, 1974) or be a prerequisite to neurite elongation (Schubert and Whitlock, 1977) and thus be a useful, easily carried out assay for NTF activity (Varon *et al.*, 1974). However, discrepancies of the effects observed for PC12 cells (Schubert *et al.*, 1978; Landreth *et al.*, 1980), the complex nature of the attachment process, and the lack of a quantifiable relationship between rates of attachment and morphological effects of NGF and dibutyryl cAMP (Table III) make this assay difficult to evaluate at this time.

5.2. Cell Survival

Given that all of the effects of NTFs on target neurons are dependent on survival of neurons, it is logical that many neuronotrophic activities are defined in terms of the effect of an NTF on the proportion of dissociated neurons that will adapt to tissue culture and survive in a well-defined period of time. Although simple in concept, there are a number of factors that can have profound consequences on observed survival curves and hence interpretation of results. For sensory neurons, it has been demonstrated that whereas NGF is required for the *in vitro* survival

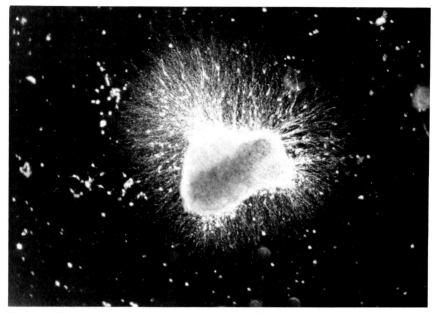

Figure 4. Response of explanted embryonic day 9 chick sensory ganglia after 1-day exposure to 7S-NGF (10 ng/ml). Darkfield illumination.

of neurons derived from embryos at early stages of development (Levi-Montalcini and Angeletti, 1968), an activity secreted by C6 rat glioma cells in culture, that is not NGF, is required by *in vitro* sensory neurons from older embryos (Barde *et al.*, 1980). Another difficulty is that all neurons have complex nutrient and hormonal requirements *in vitro* that in the past have been satisfied through the use of calf serum, fetal calf serum, and horse serum either alone or in combination. Although defined media for neurons have been developed (Bottenstein, 1983; see Chapter 1), their use is not yet widespread.

5.3. Neurite Outgrowth

It was the development of the now-classical bioassay for NGF activity that allowed NGF to be purified (Cohen *et al.*, 1954). Explanted 8- or 9-day-old chick embryo sensory ganglia will, in the presence of NGF, extend a neurite halo (Fig. 4). Attempts at quantitation of this response have been described elsewhere (Varon *et al.*, 1972). Similar quantitation of response to NTFs has been carried out for retinal explants (Adler, 1982) as well as for sympathetic and parasympathetic explants (Manthorpe et al., 1982). A major advantage of the explant assays is that in coculture experiments it is possible to determine qualitatively the presence of tropic as well as trophic effects (Ebendal and Jacobson, 1977; Adler, 1982). The use of dissociated neuronal targets and of clonal lines allows the determination of the percentage of neurite-bearing cells or in some instances the weighted average length of extended neurites. A major difficulty of this assay is the counting of fibers and the difficulty of making quantitative measurements when neurons aggregate in response to the neuronotrophic activity (Reynolds and Perez-Polo, 1981).

5.4. Neurotransmitter Synthesis

The stimulatory effect of NTFs on neurotransmitter synthesis provides an easily quantitated biochemical assay for neuronotrophic activity applicable to target neurons whose endogenous neurotransmitters are well known (Stockel et al., 1974a; Otten and Thoenen, 1976, 1977; Chun and Patterson, 1977b; MacDonnell et al., 1977; Nagaiah et al., 1977; Rohrer et al., 1978; Otten et al., 1979). Thus, NTFs acting on sympathetic ganglia can be assayed by measuring tyrosine hydroxylase levels in NTF-stimulated ganglia in the presence of antibodies to NGF (Pollack and Muhlach, 1982). However, given the overlap in the response of neurons to different NTFs, assignment of an induction in neurotransmitter metabolism to a specific NTF may not be straightforward (Yankner and Shooter, 1979; Lucas et al., 1981).

5.5. Radioassays

If, as is the case for NGF (Hendry et al., 1974a,b) and ciliary neuronotrophic factor (Hendry and Hill, 1980; Hendry et al., 1983), retrograde transport of the NTF from the nerve terminals to the cell body takes place in a specific and saturable fashion, then labeling of partially purified fractions with ^{125}I might provide partial characterization of the physicochemical properties of the factor prior to purification to homogeneity (Hendry and Hill, 1980; Hendry et al., 1983). In the case of the ciliary ganglion-directed NTF, Hendry and co-workers injected a partially purified preparation of ^{125}I-labeled ciliary NTF intraocularly and recovered from ciliary ganglia sufficient $[^{125}I]$-NTF to determine the isoelectric point of the transported species (Hendry et al., 1983). The advantage of this approach is that characterization of the NTF molecular species can be obtained in vivo prior to complete purification.

Table IV. Cell Lines That Synthesize NGF

Cell type	Species	Reference
Nontransformed		
Glia	Human	Ebendal and Jacobson (1975), Norrgren *et al.* (1980)
Fibroblast	Chick	Young *et al.* (1975)
Transformed		
Neuroblastoma (N2a)	Mouse	Murphy *et al.* (1975), Schwartz and Costa (1978)
Sarcoma (S180)	Mouse	Barklis and Perez-Polo (1981)
Fibroblast (3T3, L)	Mouse	Oger *et al.* (1974), Pantazis *et al.* (1977)
Glioma (C6)	Rat	Murphy *et al.* (1974), Perez-Polo *et al.* (1977), Schwartz and Costa (1977), Schwartz *et al.* (1977)

6. FACTOR CHARACTERIZATION

6.1. Sources of Activity

Some tissues contain neuronotrophic activity that can act on the neurons innervating that tissue. Also, it has been shown that lesions to the CNS or PNS will result in the secretion of neuronotrophic and neurotoxic activity (Nieto-Sampedro *et al.*, 1982, 1983; Longo *et al.*, 1983; Manthorpe *et al.*, 1983). However, these lesion-induced factors have not been purified. Since explanted tissues such as iris appear to respond to the *in vitro* environment by markedly increasing the amounts of NGF secreted into their surroundings (Ebendal *et al.*, 1980), it is not surprising that many transformed and nontransformed cells *in vitro* will synthesize and secrete NGF (Table IV). In many cases, it would apear that a particular cell type is secreting more than one NTF (Monard *et al.*, 1975; Barde *et al.*, 1978; Helfand *et al.*, 1978; Ebendal *et al.*, 1980; Harper and Thoenen, 1980; Barker *et al.*, 1982; Dribin and Barrett, 1982). Given the unknown consequences of cell transformation or of adapting cells to cell culture, it is difficult to assign biological significance to NTF secretion by cells in culture although the lesion-mediated induction of neuronotrophic activity could have practical significance as a useful strategy for NTF purification.

Established glial cell lines, for example, also secrete a variety of NTFs and there is evidence that steroids stimulate secretion of NGF and NTFs (Ishii and Shooter, 1975; Perez-Polo *et al.*, 1977, 1983a; Arenander and de Vellis, 1981).

Table V. Properties of Nerve Growth Factor

Species	Tissue	Quaternary structure	Active species	Reference
Mouse	Submaxillary gland	$\alpha_2\beta_2\gamma$	β	Shooter and Greene (1980), Varon et al. (1972)
Snake	Venom	$\gamma\beta$, No α	β	Perez-Polo et al. (1978, 1982c)
Guinea pig	Prostate	β, No γ	β	Chapman et al. (1981), Harper et al. (1979)
Human	Placenta	$\alpha\beta$, No γ	β	Beck and Perez-Polo (1982), Blum el al. (1980)
Bovine	Seminal plasma	?	β	Harper and Thoenen (1980)
Bovine	Seminal vesicle	β, No γ	β	Hofman and Unsicker (1982)

6.2. Purification and Characterization

NGF is found in very low levels in those neurons that respond to it as well as in their inervation targets. However, a number of tissues, both exocrine and endocrine, have been found to have high levels of NGF (Table V). As a result, much of what is hypothesized about NTF action is extrapolated from what is known about NGF. Only two other NTF species have been purified to date. One is an NTF found in pig brain that increased the survival of dissociated chick sensory ganglia *in vitro* and has been shown to have neurite-promoting effects on rat retinal explants (Barde *et al.*, 1982, 1983). The other NTF is secreted by rat Schwannoma RN-22 and induces neurite outgrowth of dissociated chick ciliary ganglia *in vitro* (Davis *et al.*, 1984; Manthorpe *et al.*, 1984). As can be seen from the properties of both of these NTFs (Table VI), their molecular properties are very different. Perhaps their common property is that they were both purified by two-dimensional polyacrylamide gel electrophoresis, a process calling for boiling the sample in 1% SDS (Barde *et al.*, 1983; Davis *et al.*, 1984; Manthorpe *et al.*, 1984). In addition, present yields are so low as to make *in vivo* experiments or careful biochemical analysis difficult.

It is interesting that whereas NGF is both a neuronotrophic factor, insofar as it is necessary for survival, and is also neurite-promoting, the ciliary NTF activity can be dissociated into two very different molecular species (Table VI). Ciliary neuronotrophic factors as described by Manthorpe *et al.* (1984) consist of a purified polyornithine-binding neurite-promoting factor (PNPF) and a soluble survival-promoting trophic factor. The fact that PNPF is of rodent glial origin and the survival-pro-

Table VI. Properties of Purified Neuronotrophic Factors

Factor	Source	Chemical properties		Reference
		M_r	pI	
β-NGF	Mouse submaxillary gland	26,500	9.4	Shooter and Greene (1980)
Ciliary ganglia PNPF[a]	Rat Schwannoma RN-22-conditioned media	200,000	5.5	Davis *et al.* (1984)
Ciliary ganglia NTF	Chick eye	20,000	5.0	Manthorpe *et al.* (1984)
Retinal NTF	Pig brain	12,300	10.1	Barde *et al.* (1983)

[a] PNPF, polyornithine-binding neurite-promoting factor; NTF, neuronotrophic factor.

moting factor is obtained from chick tissue may account for these differences.

Coculturing of neuronal explants with presumptive target tissues or in the presence of media conditioned by these tissues has been useful in demonstrating the existence of a number of neuronotrophic and gliotrophic activities *in vitro* (Monard *et al.*, 1973, 1975; Lim and Mitsunobu, 1975; Young *et al.*, 1975; Westermark, 1976; Couglin and Rathbone, 1977; Lim *et al.*, 1977, 1981; Helfand *et al.*, 1978; Ebendal, 1979; Kato *et al.*, 1979; Brockes *et al.*, 1980; Dribin and Barrett, 1980; Obata and Tanaka, 1980; Chan and Haschke, 1981; Coughlin *et al.*, 1981; Manthorpe *et al.*, 1981; Riopelle and Cameron, 1981; Dribin, 1982; Henderson *et al.*, 1982; Longo *et al.*, 1982; Muller and Seifert, 1982). In most cases neuronotrophic activity has been defined in terms of increased neuronal survival, neurite elongation, or increased neurotransmitter synthesis (Varon *et al.*, 1967; Godfrey *et al.*, 1980; McLennan *et al.*, 1980). In many cases the activities described are not specific in terms of the neuronal populations found to be responsive, and the converse is also true in that synergistic effects for various neuronotrophic activities on NGF activity have been reported (Edgar *et al.*, 1979, 1981; Vinores and Guroff, 1980). A comparison of some of the various activities reported for other putative NTFs is shown in Table VII. Direct comparisons of biological and biochemical properties would be difficult at this point, since assay conditions vary and these are partially purified factors.

Except for the experiments of Hendry *et al.* (1983) with a partially purified fraction, little is known about the *in vivo* effects of these various

Table VII. Non-NGF Neuronotrophic Activities[a]

NTF source	Target tissue	Effect	Reference
Embryonic extract (chick)	Sympathetic (chick); ciliary	Neurite outgrowth	Ebendal et al. (1982)
Eye extract (chick)	Ciliary ganglion (chick); sensory ganglia (mouse)	Survival	Manthorpe et al. (1982)
Cardiac extract (bovine)	Ciliary ganglion (chick)	Survival	Hendry et al. (1983)
Brain extract (chick)	Cerebral cortical neurons (chick)	Neuroblast proliferation	Barakat et al. (1982)
Brain extract (fish)	Retinal neurons (fish)	Neurite outgrowth	Johnson and Turner (1982)
Glial cerebellar cells (mouse)	Cerebellum (mouse)	NGF antigen	Schwartz et al. (1982)
Lesioned PNS and CNS glial-conditioned fluid (rat)	Spinal neurons (chick)	Survival; neurotoxicity	Manthorpe et al. (1982)
HCM (chick)	Sympathetic, parasympathetic, sensory neurons (chick)	Neurite outgrowth	Riopelle and Cameron (1981)
Schwannoma RN-22-conditioned media (rat)	Retinal neurons (chick)	Neurite outgrowth	Adler (1982)
Glial-conditioned media (rat)	Hippocampal neurons (rat)	Survival; neurite outgrowth	Muller and Seifert (1982)
Muscle-conditioned media (rat)	Spinal neurons (rat)	Neurite outgrowth	Dribin and Barrett (1982)
Heart cell-conditioned media (chick)	Cerebral cortical neurons (chick)	Neurite outgrowth	Kligman (1982)
Heart cell-conditioned media (mice)	Sympathetic neurons (mouse)	Neurite outgrowth	Coughlin and Kessler (1982)

[a] This is not an inclusive list. See also Varon and Adler (1981) and Barde et al. (1983).

NTFs. However, it is clear that biochemical, cell culture, and immunological tools equal to the task are available and it would seem likely that there will be a large array of NTFs available for *in vivo* experiments likely to provide new answers to developmental questions and perhaps a new understanding of neuronal regeneration.

ACKNOWLEDGMENTS

I wish to thank C. Beck, M. Blum, K. Huebner, B. Haskell, C. R. Lyons, C. P. Reynolds, R. W. Stach, E. Tiffany-Castiglioni, and K. Werrbach-Perez for their collaboration and B. Dzambo for manuscript preparation. Some of this work was supported by grants from the National Institutes of Health and The Robert A. Welch Foundation.

REFERENCES

Abell, M. R., Hart, W. R., and Olson, J. R., 1970, Tumors of the peripheral nervous system, *Hum. Pathol.* **1**:503–551.

Adler, R., 1982, Regulation of neurite growth in purified retina neuronal cultures: Effects of PNPF, a substratumbound, neurite-promoting factor, *J. Neurosci. Res.* **8**:165–177.

Aloe, L., and Levi-Montalcini, R., 1979, Nerve growth factor-induced transformation of immature chromaffin cells *in vitro* into sympathetic neurons: Effect of antiserum to nerve growth factor, *Proc. Natl. Acad. Sci. USA* **76**:1246–1250.

Amano, T., Richelson, E., and Nirenberg, M., 1972, Neurotransmitter synthesis by neuroblastoma clones, *Proc. Natl. Acad. Sci. USA* **69**:258–263.

Anagnoste, B., Freedman, L. S., Goldstein, M., Broome, J., and Fuxe, K., 1972, Dopamine-beta-hydroxylase activity in mouse neuroblastoma tumors and in cell cultures, *Proc. Natl. Acad. Sci. USA* **69**:1883–1886.

Arenander, A. T., and de Vellis, J., 1981, Glial-released proteins II. Two-dimensional electrophoretic identification of proteins regulated by hydrocortisone, *Brain Res.* **224**:105–116.

Augusti-Tocci, G., and Sato, G., 1969, Establishment of functional clonal lines of neurons from mouse neuroblastoma, *Proc. Natl. Acad. Sci. USA* **64**:311–315.

Barakat, I., Sensenbrenner, M., and Labourdette, G., 1982, Stimulation of chick neuroblast proliferation in culture by brain extracts, *J. Neurosci. Res.* **8**:303–314.

Barde, Y. A., Lindsay, R. M., Monard, D., and Thoenen, H., 1978, New factor released by cultured glioma cells supporting survival and growth of sensory neurones, *Nature* **274**:818.

Barde, Y. A., Edgar, D., and Thoenen, H., 1980, Sensory neurons in culture: Changing requirements for survival factors during embryonic development, *Proc. Natl. Acad. Sci. USA* **77**:1199–1203.

Barde, Y. A., Edgar, D., and Thoenen, H., 1982, Purification of a new neurotrophic factor from mammalian brain, *EMBO J.* **1**:549–553.

Barde, Y. A., Edgar, D., and Thoenen, H., 1983, New neurotrophic factors, *Annu. Rev. Physiol.* **45**:601–612.

Barker, D. L., Wong, R. G., and Kater, S. B., 1982, Separate factors produced by the CNS of the snail *Helisoma* stimulate neurite outgrowth and choline metabolism in cultured neurons, *J. Neurosci. Res.* **8:**419–432.

Barklis, E., and Perez-Polo, J. R., 1981, S-180 cells secrete nerve growth factor protein similar to 7S-nerve growth factor, *J. Neurosci. Res.* **6:**21–36.

Baxter, C. F., 1983, Some thoughts concerning the study of intrinsic and extrinsic factors that promote neuronal injury and recovery, *Birth Defects Orig. Artic. Ser.* **19:**241–245.

Beck, C. E., and Perez-Polo, J. R., 1982, Human beta nerve growth factor does not cross react with antibodies to mouse beta nerve growth factor in a two-site radioimmunoassay, *J. Neurosci. Res.* **8:**137–152.

Biedler, J. L., Roffler-Tarlov, S., Schachner, M., and Freedman, L. S., 1978, Multiple neurotransmitter synthesis by human neuroblastoma cell lines and clones, *Cancer Res.* **38:**3751–3757.

Bill, A. H., Seibert, E. S., Beckwith, J. B., and Hartmann, J. R., 1969, Nerve growth factor and nerve growth-stimulating activity in sera from normal and neuroblastoma patients, *J. Natl. Cancer Inst.* **43:**1221–1230.

Bjorklund, A., and Stenevi, U., 1981, In vivo evidence for a hippocampal adrenergic neuronotrophic factor specifically released on septal deafferentation, *Brain Res.* **229:**403–428.

Black, I. B., 1980, Developmental regulation of neurotransmitter phenotype, *Curr. Top. Develop. Biol.* **15:**27–40.

Blum, M., Beck, C. E., and Perez-Polo, J. R., 1980, Absence of arginine-esteropeptidase activity in human nerve growth factor, *Proc. for 10th Annual Meeting of Society for Neuroscience* **6:**376.

Bohn, M. C., Goldstein, M., and Black, I. B., 1981, Role of glucocorticoids in expression of the adrenergic phenotype in rat embryonic adrenal gland, *Develop. Biol.* **82:**1–10.

Bottenstein, J., 1983, Growth requirements of neural cells *in vitro*, in: *Advances in Cellular Neurobiology*, Volume 4 (S. Fedoroff and L. Hertz, eds.), Academic Press, New York, pp. 333–380.

Breakefield, X. O., Neale, E. A., Neale, J. H., and Jacobowitz, D. M., 1975, Localized catecholamine storage associated with granules in murine neuroblastoma cells, *Brain Res.* **92:**237–256.

Brockes, J. P., Lemke, G. E., and Balzer, D. R., Jr., 1980, Purification and preliminary characterization of a glial growth factor from the bovine pituitary, *J. Biol. Chem.* **255:**8374–8377.

Brodeur, G. M., and Goldstein, M. N., 1976, Histochemical demonstration of an increase in acetylcholinesterase in established lines of human and mouse neuroblastomas by nerve growth factor, *Cytobios* **16:**133–138.

Burdman, J. A., and Goldstein, M. A., 1964, Long-term tissue culture of neuroblastomas. III. In vitro studies of a nerve growth-stimulating factor in sera of children with neuroblastoma, *J. Natl. Cancer Inst.* **33:**123–133.

Calissano, P., and Shelanski, M. L., 1980, Interaction of nerve growth factor with pheochromocytoma cells: Evidence for tight binding and sequestration, *Neuroscience* **5:**1033–1039.

Campenot, R. B., 1977, Local control of neurite development by nerve growth factor, *Proc. Natl. Acad. Sci. USA* **74:**4516–4519.

Campenot, R. B., 1982a, Development of sympathetic neurons in compartmentalized cultures. I. Local control of neurite growth by nerve growth factor, *Develop. Biol.* **93:**1–12.

Campenot, R. B., 1982b, Development of sympathetic neurons in compartmentalized cultures. II. Local control of neurite survival by nerve growth factor, *Develop. Biol.* **93**:13–21.

Catterall, W. A., 1982, Sodium channels in electrically excitable cells, *Cell* **30**:672–674.

Chan, K. Y., and Haschke, R. H., 1981, Action of a trophic factor(s) from rabbit corneal epithelial culture on dissociated trigeminal neurons, *J. Neurosci.* **1**:1155–1162.

Chapman, C. A., Banks, B. E. C., Vernon, C. A. and Walker, J. M., 1981, The isolation and characterization of nerve growth factor from the prostate gland of the guinea-pig, *Eur. J. Biochem.* **115**:347–351.

Chun, L. Y., and Patterson, P. H., 1977a, Role of nerve growth factor in the development of rat sympathetic neurons *in vitro*. I. Survival, growth, and differentiation of catecholamine production, *J. Cell Biol.* **75**:694–704.

Chun, L. Y., and Patterson, P. H., 1977b, Role of nerve growth factor in the development of rat sympathetic neurons *in vitro*. II. Developmental study, *J. Cell Biol.* **75**:705–711.

Cohen, S., Levi-Montalcini, R., and Hamburger, V., 1954, A nerve growth-stimulating factor isolated from sarcomas 37 and 180, *Proc. Natl. Acad. Sci. USA* **40**:1014–1018.

Coughlin, M. D., and Kessler, J. A., 1982, Antiserum to a new neuronal growth factor: Effects on neurite outgrowth, *J. Neurosci. Res.* **8**:289–302.

Coughlin, M. D., and Rathbone, M. P., 1977, Factors involved in the stimulation of parasympathetic nerve outgrowth, *Develop. Biol.* **61**:131–139.

Coughlin, M. D., Dibner, M. D., Boyer, D. M., and Black, I. B., 1978, Factors regulating development of an embryonic mouse sympathetic ganglion, *Develop. Biol.* **66**:513–528.

Coughlin, M. D., Bloom E. M., and Black, I. B., 1981, Characterization of a neuronal growth factor from mouse heart-cell-conditioned medium, *Develop. Biol.* **82**:56–68.

Cowan, W. M., 1973, Neuronal death as a regulative mechanism in the control of cell number in the nervous system, in: *Development and Aging in the Nervous System* (M. Rockstein, ed.), Academic Press, New York, pp. 19–34.

Davis, G. E., Manthorpe, M., and Varon, S., 1984, Further purification of rat Schwannoma neurite promoting factor, *Trans. ASN* **15**:181.

Dichter, M. A., Tischler, A. S., and Greene, L. A., 1977, Nerve growth factor-induced increase in electrical excitability and acetylcholine sensitivity of a rat pheochromocytoma cell line, *Nature* **268**:501–504.

Donnelly, C. H., Richelson, E., and Murphy, D. L., 1976, Properties of monoamine oxidase in mouse neuroblastoma N1E-115 cells, *Biochem. Pharmacol.* **25**:1639–1643.

Dribin, L. B., 1982, On the species and substrate specificity of conditioned medium enhancement of neuritic outgrowth from spinal cord explants, *Develop. Brain Res.* **3**:300–304.

Dribin, L. B., and Barrett, J. N., 1980, Conditioned medium enhances neuritic outgrowth from rat spinal cord explants, *Develop. Biol.* **74**:184–195.

Dribin, L. B., and Barrett, J. N., 1982, Two components of conditioned medium increase neuritic outgrowth from rat spinal cord explants, *J. Neurosci. Res.* **8**:271–280.

Ebendal, T., 1979, Stage-dependent stimulation of neurite outgrowth exerted by nerve growth factor and chick heart in cultured embryonic ganglia, *Develop. Biol.* **72**:276–290.

Ebendal, T., and Jacobson, C.-O., 1975, Human glial cells stimulating outgrowth of axons in cultured chick embryo ganglia, *Zoon.* **3**:169–172.

Ebendal, T., and Jacobson, C.-O., 1977, Tissue explants affecting extension and orientation of axons in cultured chick embryo ganglia, *Exp. Cell Res.* **105**:379–387.

Ebendal, T., Olson, L., Seiger, A., and Hedlund, K.-O., 1980, Nerve growth factors in the rat iris, *Nature* **286**:25–28.

Ebendal, T., Hedlund, K.-O., and Norrgren, G., 1982, Nerve growth factors in chick tissues, *J. Neurosci. Res.* **8**:153–164.

Edgar, D. H., and Thoenen, H., 1978, Selective enzyme induction in a nerve growth factor-responsive pheochromocytoma cell line (PC12), *Brain Res.* **154**:186–190.

Edgar, D., Barde, Y.-A., and Thoenen, H., 1979, Induction of fiber outgrowth and choline acetyltransferase in PC12 pheochromocytoma cells by conditioned media from glial cells and organ extracts, *Exp. Cell Res.* **121**:353–361.

Edgar, D., Barde Y.-A., and Thoenen, H., 1981, Subpopulations of cultured chick sympathetic neurones differ in their requirements for survival factors, *Nature* **289**:294–295.

Fabricant, R. N., Todaro, G. J., and Eldridge, R., 1979, Increased levels of a nerve growth factor cross-reacting protein in "central" neurofibromatosis, *Lancet* **1**:4–7.

Guiffrida-Stella, A. M., and Lajtha, A., 1983, Perspectives for neural regeneration with changes in macromolecular metabolism, *Birth Defects Orig. Artic. Ser.* **19**:23–32.

Godfrey, E. W., Schrier, B. K., and Nelson, P. G., 1980, Source and target cell specificities of a conditioned medium factor that increases choline acetyl transferase activity in cultured spinal cord cells, *Develop. Biol.* **77**:403–418.

Goldstein, M. N., and Brodeur, G. M., 1974, Human neuroblastomas *in vitro*: Activation of the membrane pump for catecholamines by 5-bromodeoxyuridine, *Proc. Int. Cancer Congr.* **1**:178–183.

Gorin, P. D., and Johnson, E. M., 1979, Experimental autoimmune model of nerve growth factor deprivation: Effects on developing peripheral sympathetic and sensory neurons, *Proc. Natl. Acad. Sci. USA* **76(10)**:5382–5386.

Greene, L. A., and Rein, G., 1977, Synthesis, storage, and release of acetylcholine by a noradrenergic pheochromocytoma cell line, *Nature* **268**:349–351.

Greene, L. A., and Rukenstein, A., 1981, Regulation of acetylcholinesterase activity by nerve growth factor, *J. Biol. Chem.* **256**:6363–6367.

Greene, L. A., and Shooter, E. M., 1980, The nerve growth factor: Biochemistry, synthesis, and mechanism of action, *Annu. Rev. Neurosci.* **3**:353–402.

Greene, L. A., and Tischler, A. S., 1976, Establishment of a noradrenergic clonal line of rat adrenal pheochromocytoma cells which respond to nerve growth factor, *Proc. Natl. Acad. Sci. USA* **73**:2424–2428.

Gunderson, R. W., and Barrett, J. N., 1980, Characterization of the turning response of dorsal root neurites toward nerve growth factor, *J. Cell Biol.* **87**:546–554.

Hamburger, V., 1980, Trophic interactions in neurogenesis: A personal historical account, *Annu. Rev. Neurosci.* **3**:269–278.

Harper, G. P., and Thoenen, H., 1980, Nerve growth factor: Biological significance, measurement, and distribution, *J. Neurochem.* **34**:5–16.

Harper, G. P., and Thoenen, H., 1981, Target cells, biological effects, and mechanism of action of nerve growth factor and its antibodies, *Annu. Rev. Pharmacol. Toxicol.* **21**:205–229.

Harper, G. P., Barde, Y. A., Burnstock, G., Carstairs, J. R., Dennison, M. E., Suda, K., and Vernon, C. A., 1979, Guinea pig prostate is a rich source of nerve growth factor, *Nature* **279**:160–162.

Haskell, B. E., Carney, D. H., Thompson, W. C., and Perez-Polo, J. R., 1983, Effects of retinoic acid on NGF responsive cells, *Am. Soc. Neurochem.* **14**:183.

Helfand, S. L., Riopelle, R. J., and Wessells, N. K., 1978, Non-equivalence of conditioned medium and nerve growth factor for sympathetic, parasympathetic, and sensory neurons, *Exp. Cell Res.* **113**:39–45.

Henderson, C. E., Huchet, M., and Changeux, J-P., 1982, Neurite outgrowth from embryonic chicken spinal neurons if promoted by media conditioned by muscle cells, *Proc. Natl. Academy of Science* **78(4)**:2625–2629.

Hendry, I. A., 1976, Control in the development of the vertebrate sympathetic nervous system, *Annu. Rev. Neurosci.* **2**:149–194.

Hendry, I. A., 1977, The effect of the retrograde axonal transport of nerve growth factor on the morphology of adrenergic neurons, *Brain Res.* **134**:213–223.

Hendry, I. A., 1980, Retrograde axonal transport, in: *Proteins of the Nervous System*, 2nd ed. (R. A. Bradshaw and D. M. Schneider, eds.), Liss, New York, pp. 183–211.

Hendry, I. A., and Hill, C. E., 1980, Retrograde axonal transport of target tissue-derived macromolecules, *Nature* **287**:647–649.

Hendry, I. A., Stach, R., and Herrup, K., 1974a, Characteristics of the retrograde axonal transport system for nerve growth factor in the sympathetic nervous system, *Brain Res.* **82**:117–128.

Hendry, I. A., Stockel, K., Thoenen, H., and Iversen, L. L., 1974b, The retrograde axonal transport of nerve growth factor, *Brain Res.* **68**:103–121.

Hendry, I. A., Hill, C. E., and Bonyhady, R. E., 1982, The interactions between developing autonomic neurones and their target tissues, *Ciba Found. Symp.* **83**:194–206.

Hendry, I. A., Bonyhady, R. E., and Hill, C. E., 1983, The role of target tissues in development and regeneration—Retrophins, *Birth Defects Orig. Artic. Ser.* **19**:263–276.

Herrup, K., and Thoenen, H., 1979, Properties of the nerve growth factor receptor of a clonal line of rat pheochromocytoma (PC12) cells, *Exp. Cell Res.* **121**:71–78.

Hofmann, H-D., and Unsicker, K., 1982, The seminal vesicle of the bull: A new and very rich source of nerve growth factor, *Eur. J. Biochem.* **128**:421–426.

Ishii, D. N., and Shooter, E. M., 1975, Regulation of nerve growth factor synthesis in mouse submaxillary glands by testosterone, *J. Neurochem.* **25**:843–851.

Johnson, E. M., Andres, R. Y., and Bradshaw, R. A., 1978, Characterization of the retrograde transport of nerve growth factor using high specific activity (^{125}I) nerve growth factor, *Brain Res.* **150**:319–331.

Johnson, E. M., Jr., Gorin, P. D., Brandeis, L. D., and Pearson, J., 1980, Dorsal root ganglion neurons are destroyed by exposure in utero to maternal antibody to nerve growth factor, *Science* **210**:916–918.

Johnson, J. E., and Turner, J. E., 1982, Growth from regenerating goldfish retinal cultures in the absence of serum or hormonal supplements: Tissue extract effects, *J. Neurosci. Res.* **8**:315–329.

Kato, T., Chiu, T. C., Lim, R., Troy, S. S., and Turriff, D. E., 1979, Multiple molecular forms of glia maturation factor, *Biochim. Biophys. Acta* **579**:216–227.

Kessler, J. A., and Black, I. B., 1981, Similarities in development of substance P and somatostatin in peripheral sensory neurons: Effects of capsaicin and nerve growth factor, *Proc. Natl. Acad. Sci. USA* **78**:4644–4647.

Kessler, J. A., and Black, I. B., 1982, Regulation of substance P in adult rat sympathetic ganglia, *Brain Res.* **234**:182–187.

Klebe, R. J., and Ruddle, F. H., 1969, Neuroblastoma: Cell culture analysis of a differentiating stem cell system, *J. Cell Biol.* **43**:69a.

Kligman, D., 1982, Neurite outgrowth from cerebral cortical neurons is promoted by medium conditioned over heart cells, *J. Neurosci. Res.* **8**:281–287.

Kolber, A. R., Goldstein, M. N., and Moore, B. W., 1974, Effect of nerve growth factor on the expression of colchicine-binding activity and 14-3-2 protein in an established line of human neuroblastoma, *Proc. Natl. Acad. Sci. USA* **71**:4203–4207.

Kumar, S., 1973, Nerve growth factor, *Nature* **244**:471.

Kuramoto, T., Perez-Polo, J. R., and Haber, B., 1977, Membrane properties of a human neuroblastoma, *Neurosci. Lett.* **4**:151–159.

Kuramoto, T., Werrbach-Perez, K., Perez-Polo, J. R., and Haber, B., 1981, Membrane properties of a human neuroblastoma II. Effects of differentiation, *J. Neurosci. Res.* **6**:441–449.

Landreth, G. E., and Shooter, E. M., 1980, Nerve growth factor receptors on PC12 cells: Ligand-induced conversion from low to high-affinity states, *Proc. Natl. Acad. Sci. USA* **77**:4751–4755.

Landreth, G., Cohen, P., and Shooter, E. M., 1980, Ca^{2+} transmembrane fluxes and nerve growth factor action on a clonal cell line of rat pheochromocytoma, *Nature* **283**:202–204.

Letourneau, P. C., 1978, Chemotactic response of nerve fiber elongation to nerve growth factor, *Develop. Biol.* **66**:183–196.

Levi-Montalcini, R., 1982, Developmental neurobiology and the natural history of nerve growth factor, *Annu. Rev. Neurosci.* **5**:341–362.

Levi-Montalcini, R., 1983, The nerve growth factor–target cells interaction: A model system for the study of directed axonal growth and regeneration, *Birth Defects Orig. Artic. Ser.* **19**:3–22.

Levi-Montalcini, R., and Angeletti, P. U., 1968, Nerve growth factor, *Physiol. Rev.* **48**:534–569.

Lim, R., and Mitsunobu, K., 1975, Partial purification of a morphological transforming factor from pig brain, *Biochim. Biophys. Acta* **400**:200–207.

Lim, R., Troy, S. S., and Turriff, D. E., 1977, Fine structure of cultured glioblasts before and after stimulation by a glia maturation factor, *Exp. Cell Res.* **106**:357–372.

Lim, R., Nakagawa, S., Arnason, B. G., and Turriff, D. E., 1981, Glia maturation factor promotes contact inhibition in cancer cells, *Proc. Natl. Acad. Sci. USA* **78**:4373–4377.

Longo, F. M., Manthorpe, M., and Varon, S., 1982, Spinal cord neuronotrophic factors (SCNTFs). I. Bioassay of Schwannoma and other conditioned medium, *Develop. Brain Res.* **3**:277–294.

Longo, F. M., Manthorpe, M., Skaper, S. D., Lundborg, G., and Varon, S., 1983, Neuronotrophic activities in fluid accumulated *in vivo* within silicone nerve regeneration chambers, *Brain Res.* **261**:109–117.

Lucas, C. A., Czlonkowska, A., and Kreutzberg, G. W., 1981, Regulation of acetylcholinesterase activity in the pheochromocytoma PC12 clonal nerve cell line by C6 glioma conditioned medium and brain homogenates, *Biol. Cell* **41**:91–96.

Lyons, C. R., and Perez-Polo, J. R., 1983, Nerve growth factor: Structure and synthesis, in: *Neurology and Neurobiology*, Volume 6 (P. W. Coates, R. R. Markwald, and A. D. Kenney, eds.), Liss, New York, pp. 167–174.

Lyons, C. R., Stach, R. W., and Perez-Polo, J. R., 1983, Binding constants of isolated NGF-receptors from different species, *Biochem. Biophys. Res. Commun.* **115**:368–374.

MacDonnell, P. C., Tolson, N., and Guroff, G., 1977, Selective *de novo* synthesis of tyrosine hydroxylase in organ cultures of rat superior cervical ganglia after in vivo administration of nerve growth factor, *J. Biol. Chem.* **252**:5859–5863.

McLennan, I. S., Hill, C. E., and Hendry, I. A., 1980, Glucocorticosteroids modulate transmitter choice in developing superior cervical ganglion, *Nature* **283**:206–207.

McMorris, F. A., Nelson, P. G., and Ruddle, F. H., 1973, Contributions of clonal systems to neurobiology, *Neurosci. Res. Prog. Bull.* **11**:411–536.

Manthorpe, M., Skaper, S. D., and Varon, S., 1981, Neuronotrophic factors and their antibodies: In vitro microassays for titration and screening, *Brain Res.* **230**:295–306.

Manthorpe, M., Skaper, S. D., Barbin, G., and Varon, S., 1982, Cholinergic neuronotrophic factors: Concurrent activities on certain nerve growth factor-responsive neurons, *J. Neurochem.* **38**:415–421.

Manthorpe, M., Nieto-Sampedro, M., Skaper, S. D., Lewis, E. R., Barbin, G., Longo, F. M., Cotman, C. W., and Varon, S., 1983, Neuronotrophic activity in brain wounds of the developing rat: Correlation with implant survival in the wound cavity, *Brain Res.* **267**:47–56.

Manthorpe, M., Barbin, G., and Varon, S., 1984, Purification of the ciliary neuronotrophic factor from chick embryo eye, *Trans. ASN* **15**:180.

Meyer, T., Burkhart, W., and Jockusch, H., 1979, Choline acetyltransferase induction in cultured neurons: Dissociated spinal cord cells are dependent on muscle cells, organotypic explants are not, *Neurosci. Lett.* **11**:59–62.

Miyoke, S., Kitamura, T., and Shima, Y., 1975, Morphological differentiation of NB-1 human neuroblastoma line using (BUT) cAMP, *Neurol. Surg.* **3**:407–411.

Mobley, W. C., Server, A. C., Ishii, D. N., Riopelle, R. J., and Shooter, E. M., 1977, Nerve growth factor, *New Engl. J. Med.* **297**:1096–1104, 1149–1158, 1211–1218.

Monard, D., Solomon, F., Rentsch, M., and Gysin, R., 1973, Glia-induced morphological differentiation in neuroblastoma cells, *Proc. Natl. Acad. Sci. USA* **70**:1894–1897.

Monard, D., Stockel, K., Goodman, R., and Thoenen, H., 1975, Distinction between nerve growth factor and glial factor, *Nature* **258**:444–445.

Muller, H. W., and Seifert, W., 1982, A neurotrophic factor (NTF) released from primary glial cultures supports survival and fiber outgrowth of cultured hippocampal neurons, *J. Neurosci. Res.* **8**:195–204.

Murphy, R. A., Pantazis, N. J., Arnason, B. G. W., and Young, M., 1975, Secretion of a nerve growth factor by mouse neuroblastoma cells in culture, *Proc. Natl. Acad. Sci. USA* **72(5)**:1895–1898.

Nagaiah, K., MacDonnell, P., and Guroff, G., 1977, Induction of tyrosine hydroxylase synthesis in rat superior cervical ganglia *in vitro* by nerve growth factor and dexamethasone, *Biochem. Biophys. Res. Commun.* **75**:832–837.

Narotzky, R., and Bondareff, W., 1974, Biogenic amines in cultured neuroblastoma and astrocytoma cells, *J. Cell Biol.* **63**:64–70.

Nieto-Sampedro, M., Lewis, E. R., Cotman, C. W., Manthorpe, M., Skaper, S. D., Barbin, G., Longo, F. M., and Varon, S., 1982, Brain injury causes a time dependent increase in neuronotrophic activity at the lesion site, *Science* **217**:860–861.

Nieto-Sampedro, M., Manthorpe, M., Barbin, G., Varon, S., and Cotman, C. W., 1983, Injury-induced neuronotrophic activity in adult rat brain: Correlation with survival of delayed implants in the wound cavity, *J. Neurosci.* **3**:2219–2229.

Nja, A., and Purves, D., 1978, The effects of nerve growth factor and its antiserum on synapses in the superior cervical ganglion of the guinea pig, *J. Physiol.* **277**:53–75.

Norrgren, G., Ebendal, T., Belew, M., Jacobson, C-O., and Porath, J., 1980, Release of nerve growth factor by human glial cells in culture, *Exp. Cell Res.* **130**:31–39.

Obata, K., and Tanaka, H., 1980, Conditioned medium promotes neurite growth from both central and peripheral neurons, *Neurosci. Lett.* **16**:27–33.

Oger, J., Arnason, B. G. W., Pantazis, N., Lehrich, J. and Young, M., 1974, Synthesis of nerve growth factor by L and 3T3 cells in culture, *Proc. Natl. Acad. Sci. USA* **71(4)**:1554–1558.

Oppenheim, R. W., Manderdrut, J. L., and Wells, D. J., 1982, Reduction of naturally-occuring cell death in the thoracolumbar preganglionic cell column of the chick embryo by nerve growth factor and hemicholinium-3, *Develop. Brain Res.* **3**:134–139.

Otten, U., and Thoenen, H., 1976, Modulatory role of glucocorticoids on nerve growth factor-mediated enzyme induction in organ cultures of sympathetic ganglia, *Brain Res.* **111**:438–441.

Otten, U., and Thoenen, H., 1977, Effect of glucocorticoid on nerve growth factor-mediated enzyme induction in organ cultures of rat sympathetic ganglia: Enhanced response and reduced time requirement to initiate enzyme induction, *J. Neurochem.* **29**:69–75.

Otten, U., Baumann, J. B., and Girard, J., 1979, Stimulation of the pituitary–adrenocortical axis by nerve growth factor, *Nature* **282**:413–414.

Otten, U., Goedert, M., Baumann, J. B., and Girard, J., 1981, Stimulation of the pituitary–adrenocortical axis and induction of tyrosine hydroxylase by nerve growth factor are not dependent on mouse submaxillary gland isorenin, *Brain Res.* **217**:207–211.

Pantazis, N. J., Blanchard, M. H., Arnason, B. G. W. and Young, M., 1977, Molecular properties of the nerve growth factor secreted by L cells, *Proc. Natl. Acad. Sci. USA* **74(4)**:1492–1496.

Patterson, P. H., 1978, Environmental determination of autonomic neurotransmitter functions, *Annu. Rev. Neurosci.* **1**:1–12.

Perez-Polo, J. R., 1984, Neuroblastoma: Maturation and differentiation, in: *Transmembrane Potentials and Characteristics of Immune and Tumor Cells* (R. C. Niemtzow, ed.), CRC Press, Boca Raton, Florida, in press.

Perez-Polo, J. R., and Haber, B., 1983, Neuronotrophic interactions, in: *The Clinical Neurosciences*, Volume 5 (R. N. Rosenberg, ed.), Churchill Livingstone, Edinburgh, pp. V37–V51.

Perez-Polo, J. R., and Werrbach-Perez, K., 1984, Effects of nerve growth factor on the in vitro response of neurons to injury, in: *Recent Achievements in Restorative Neurology* (J. Eccles and M. R. Dimitrijevic, eds.), Karger, Basel, in press.

Perez-Polo, J. R., Hall, K., Livingston, K., and Westlund, K., 1977, Steroid induction of nerve growth factor synthesis in cell culture, *Life Sci.* **21**:1535–1544.

Perez-Polo, J. R., Bomar, H., Beck, C. and Hall, K., 1978, Nerve growth factor from *Crotalus adamenteus*, *J. Biol. Chem.* **253(17)**:6140–6148.

Perez-Polo, J. R., Werrbach-Perez, K., and Tiffany-Castiglioni, E., 1979, A human clonal cell line model of differentiating neurons, *Develop. Biol.* **71**:341–355.

Perez-Polo, J. R., Beck, C. E., and Blum, M., 1980, Biochemical correlates of behavior: What is a neurochemist to measure?, in: *Perspectives in Schizophrenia Research* (C. Baxter and T. Melnechuk, eds.), Raven Press, New York, pp. 237–246.

Perez-Polo, J. R., Reynolds, C. P., Tiffany-Castiglioni, E., Ziegler, M., Schulze, I., and Werrbach-Perez, K., 1982a, NGF effects on human neuroblastoma lines: A model system, in: *Proteins in the Nervous System: Structure and Function* (B. Haber, J. R. Perez-Polo, and J. D. Coulter, eds.), Liss, New York, pp. 285–299.

Perez-Polo, J. R., Tiffany-Castiglioni, E., Ziegler, M., and Werrbach-Perez, K., 1982b, Effect of nerve growth factor on catecholamine metabolism in a human neuroblastoma clone (SY5Y), *Develop. Neurosci.* **5**:418–423.

Perez-Polo, J. R., Beck, C., Reynolds, C. P., and Blum, M., 1982c, Human nerve growth factor: Comparative aspects, in: *Growth and Maturation Factors* (G. Guroff, ed.), Wiley, New York, pp. 129–163.

Perez-Polo, J. R., Schulze, I., and Werrbach-Perez, K., 1983a, The synthesis of nerve growth factor, in: *Neurology and Neurobiology*, Volume 4 (L. Battistini, G. A. Hashim, and A. Lajtha, eds.), Liss, New York, pp. 285–299.

Perez-Polo, J. R., Tiffany-Castiglioni, E., and Werrbach-Perez, K., 1983b, Model clonal system for study of neuronal cell injury, *Birth Defects Orig. Artic. Ser.* **19**:201–220.

Perez-Polo, J. R., Schulze, I., and Werrbach-Perez, K., 1983, The synthesis of nerve growth factor, in: *Clinical and Biological Aspects of the Peripheral Nervous System Diseases* (L. Battistini, G. Hashim, and A. Lajtha, eds.), Liss, New York, pp. 285–299.

Pollack, E. D., and Muhlach, W. L., 1982, Target control of neuronal development during formation of the spinal reflex arc: An operant model, *J. Neurosci. Res.* **8**:343–355.

Prasad, K. N., and Kumar, S., 1975, Role of cyclic AMP in differentiation of human neuroblastoma cells in culture, *Cancer* **36**:1338–1343.

Purves, D., and Lichtman, J. W., 1978, Formation and maintenance of synaptic connections in autonomic ganglia, *Physiol. Rev.* **58**:821–862.

Purves, D., and Nja, A., 1978, Trophic maintenance of synaptic connections in autonomic ganglia, in: *Neuronal Plasticity* (C. W. Cotman, ed.), Raven Press, New York, pp. 27–47.

Ramón y Cajal, S., 1928, *Degeneration and Regeneration of the Nervous System* (R. M. Macey, trans.), Oxford University Press, London.

Reynolds, C. P., and Perez-Polo, J. R., 1975, Human neuroblastoma: Glial induced morphological differentiation, *Neurosci. Lett.* **1**:91–97.

Reynolds, C. P., and Perez-Polo, J. R., 1981, Induction of neurite outgrowth in the IMR-32 human neuroblastoma cell line by nerve growth factor, *J. Neurosci. Res.* **6**:319–325.

Rieger, F., Shelanski, M. L., and Greene, L. A., 1980, The effects of nerve growth factor on acetylcholinesterase and its multiple forms in cultures of rat PC12 pheochromocytoma cells: Increased total specific activity and appearance of the 16S molecular form, *Develop. Biol.* **76**:238–243.

Riopelle, R. J., and Cameron, D. A., 1981, Neurite growth promoting factors of embryonic chick—Ontogeny, regional distribution, and characteristics, *J. Neurobiol.* **12**:175–186.

Rohrer, H., Otten, U., and Thoenen, H., 1978, On the role of RNA synthesis in the selective induction of tyrosine hydroxylase by nerve growth factor, *Brain Res.* **159**:436–439.

Ross, R. A., Biedler, J. L., Spengler, B. A., and Reis, D. J., 1981, Neurotransmitter-synthesizing enzymes in 14 human neuroblastoma cell lines, *Cell. Mol. Neurobiol.* **1**:301–312.

Russel, D. S., and Rubenstein, L. J., 1972, *Pathology of Tumors of the Nervous System*, Williams and Wilkins, Baltimore, pp. 284–304.

Schenkein, K., Bueker, E. D., Helson, L., Axelrod, F., and Dancis, J., 1974, Increased nerve-growth-stimulating activity in disseminated neurofibromatosis, *New Engl. J. Med.* **290**:613–614.

Schubert, D., and Whitlock, C., 1977, Alteration of cellular adhesion by nerve growth factor, *Proc. Natl. Acad. Sci. USA* **74**:4055–4058.

Schubert, D., Humphreys, S., Baroni, C., and Cohn, M., 1969, In vitro differentiation of a mouse neuroblastoma, *Biochemistry* **64**:316–323.

Schubert, D., Hienemann, S., and Kidokoro, Y., 1977, Cholinergic metabolism and synapse formation by a rat nerve cell line, *Proc. Natl. Acad. Sci. USA* **74**:2579–2583.

Schubert, D., LaCorbiere, M., Whitlock, C., and Stallcup, W., 1978, Alterations in the surface properties of cells responsive to nerve growth factor, *Nature* **273**:718–723.

Schulze, I., and Perez-Polo, J. R., 1982, Nerve growth factor and cyclic AMP: Opposite effect on neuroblastoma substrate adhesion, *J. Neurosci. Res.* **8**:393–411.

Schwab, M. E., 1977, Ultrastructural localization of a nerve growth factor–horseradish peroxidase (NGF-HRP) coupling product after retrograde axonal transport in adrenergic neurons, *Brain Res.* **130**:190–196.

Schwartz, J. P., and Breakefield, X. O., 1980, Altered nerve growth factor in fibroblasts from patients with familial dysautonomia, *Proc. Natl. Acad. Sci. USA* **77**:1154–1158.

Schwartz, J. P. and Costa, E., 1977, Regulation of nerve growth factor content in C6 glioma cells by beta-adrenergic receptor stimulation, *Nauyn-Schimedeberg's Arch. Pharmacol.* **300**:123–129.

Schwartz, J. P., Chuang, D-M., and Costa, E., 1977, Increase in nerve growth factor content of C6 glioma cells by the activation of a beta-adrenergic receptor, *Brain Res.* **137**:369–375.

Schwartz, J. P., Ghetti, B., Truex, L. and Schmidt, M. J., 1982, Increase of a nerve growth factor-like protein in the cerebellum of PCD mutant mice, *J. Neurosci. Res.* **8**:205–211.

Seeger, R. C., Rayner, S. A., Banerjee, A., Chung, H., Laug, W. E., Neustein, H. B., and Benedict, W. F., 1977, Morphology, growth, chromosomal pattern, and fibrinolytic activity of two new human neuroblastoma cell lines, *Cancer Res.* **37**:1364–1371.

Siggers, D. C., 1976, Nerve growth factor and some inherited neurological conditions, *Proc. R. Soc. Med.* **69**:183–184.

Siggers, D. C., Boyer, S. H., and Eldrige, R., 1975, Nerve growth factor in disseminated neurofibromatosis, *New Engl. J. Med.* **292**:1134.

Siggers, D. C., Rogers, J. G., Boxer, S. H., Margolet, L., Dorkin, H., Banerjee, S. P., and Shooter, E. M., 1976, Increased nerve growth factor beta-chain crossreacting material in familial dysautonomia, *New Engl. J. Med.* **295**:629–634.

Skene, J. H., and Shooter, E. M., 1983, Denervated sheath cells secrete a new protein after nerve injury, *Proc. Natl. Acad. Sci. USA* **80**:4169–4173.

Sonnenfeld, K. H., and Ishii, D. N., 1982, Nerve growth factor effects and receptors in cultured human neuroblastoma cell lines, *J. Neurosci. Res.* **8**:375–391.

Stent, G. S., 1981, Strength and weaknesses of the genetic approach to the development of the nervous system, in: *Studies in Development Neurobiology* (W. M. Cowan, ed.), Oxford University Press, London, p. 288–321.

Stewart, H. L., Snell, K. C., Dunham, L. J. and Schlyen, S. M., 1959, *Transplantable and Transmissible Tumors of Animals*, Armed Forces Institute of Pathology, Washington, D.C., p. 337.

Stockel, K., and Thoenen, H., 1975, Retrograde axonal transport of nerve growth factor: Specificity and biological importance, *Brain Res.* **85**:337–341.

Stockel, K., Solomon, F., Paravicini, U., and Thoenen, H., 1974a, Dissociation between effects of nerve growth factor on tyrosine hydroxylase and tubulin synthesis in sympathetic ganglia, *Nature* **250**:150–151.

Stockel, K., Paravicini, U., and Thoenen, H., 1974b, Specificity of the retrograde axonal transport of nerve growth factor, *Brain Res.* **76**:413–422.

Thoenen, H., and Barde, Y.-A., 1980, Physiology of nerve growth factor, *Physiol. Rev.* **60**:1284–1335.

Tischler, A. S., and Greene, L. A., 1975, Nerve growth factor-induced process formation of cultured rat pheochromocytoma cells, *Nature* **258**:341–342.

Varon, S., and Adler, R., 1981, Trophic and specifying factors directed to neuronal cells, in: *Advances in Cellular Neurobiology*, Volume 2 (S. Fedoroff and L. Herz, eds.), Academic Press, New York, p. 115–163.

Varon, S. S., and Bunge, R. R., 1978, Trophic mechanisms in the peripheral nervous system, *Annu. Rev. Neurosci.* **1**:327–361.

Varon, S., and Lundborg, G., 1983, In vivo models for peripheral nerve regeneration and the presence of neuronotrophic factors, *Birth Defects Orig. Artic. Ser.* **19**:221–240.

Varon, S., Nomura, J., and Shooter, E. M., 1967, The isolation of the mouse nerve growth factor protein in a high molecular weight form, *Biochemistry* **6**:2202–2209.

Varon, S., Nomura, J., and Shooter, E. M., 1968, Reversible dissociation of the mouse nerve growth factor protein into different subunits, *Biochemistry* **7**:1296–1303.

Varon, S., Nomura, J., Perez-Polo, J. R., and Shooter, E. M., 1972, The isolation and assay of the nerve growth factor proteins, in: *Methods of Neurochemistry*, volume 3 (R. Fried, ed.), Dekker, New York, pp. 203–229.

Varon, S., Raiborn, C., and Burnham, P. A., 1974, Selective potency of homologous ganglionic non-neuronal cells for the support of dissociated ganglionic neurons in culture, *Neurobiology* **4**:231–252.

Vinores, S., and Guroff, G., 1980, Nerve growth factor: Mechanism of action, *Annu. Rev. Biophys. Bioeng.* **9**:223–257.

Vinores, S. A., and Koestner, A., 1981, Effect of nerve growth factor producing cells on anaplastic glioma cells, *J. Neurosci. Res.* **6**:389–401.

Waghe, M., Kumar, S., and Steward, J. K., 1970, Nerve growth factor in human sera, *J. Pediatr. Surg.* **5**:14–17.

Walicke, P. A., and Patterson, P. H., 1981, On the role of cyclic nucleotides in the transmitter choice made by cultured sympathetic neurons, *J. Neurosci.* **1**:333–342.

Waris, T., Rechardt, L., and Waris, P., 1973, Differentiation of neuroblastoma cells induced by nerve growth factor *in vitro, Experientia* **29**:1128–1129.

Warter, S., Hermetet, J. C., and Cieselski-Treska, J., 1974, Cytogenetic characterization of C1300 neuroblastoma cells, *Experientia* **30**:291–292.

Waymire, J. C., and Gilmer-Waymire, K., 1978, Adrenergic enzymes in cultured mouse neuroblastoma: Absence of detectable aromatic-L-amino-acid decarboxylase, *J. Neurochem.* **31**:693–698.

Westermark, B., 1976, Density dependent proliferation of human glia cells stimulated by epidermal growth factor, *Biochem. Biophys. Res. Commun.* **69**:304–310.

Yankner, B. A., and Shooter, E. M., 1979, Nerve growth factor in the nucleus: Interaction with receptors on the nuclear membrane, *Proc. Natl. Acad. Sci. USA* **76**:1269–1273.

Yankner, B. A., and Shooter, E. M., 1982, The biology and mechanism of action of nerve growth factor, *Annu. Rev. Biochem.* **51**:845–868.

Young, M., Oger, J., Blanchard, M. H., Asdourian, H., Amos, H., and Arnason, B. G. W., 1975, Secretion of a nerve growth factor by a primary chick fibroblast culture, *Science* **187**:361–362.

Zwiller, J., Treska-Ciesielski, J., Mack, G., and Mandel, P., 1975, Uptake of noradrenaline by an adrenergic clone of neuroblastoma cells, *Nature* **254**:443–444.

4

Hormonal Regulation of the Proliferation and Differentiation of Astrocytes and Oligodendrocytes in Primary Culture

RUSSELL P. SANETO and JEAN DE VELLIS

1. INTRODUCTION

One of the most challenging questions in contemporary biology is what controls the orchestration of events which lead to the orderly proliferation and differentiation of cells in the CNS. Evidence has accumulated suggesting that hormones are involved in this critical process. After the discovery of the association of hypothyroidism with mental retardation, thyroidectomy of rats at birth was found to produce irreversible morphological changes with impaired behavior (Eayrs, 1964) as well as marked biochemical alterations in the developing brain (Balazs *et al.*, 1971). Glucocorticoids have also been shown to affect brain development (Balazs, 1974) in addition to regulating the activity of a developmentally

RUSSELL P. SANETO and JEAN DE VELLIS • Departments of Anatomy and Psychiatry, UCLA School of Medicine, and Mental Retardation Research Center, Laboratory of Biomedical and Environmental Sciences, University of California, Los Angeles, California 90024.

expressed enzyme, glycerol phosphate dehydrogenase (GPDH) (de Vellis and Inglish, 1968). Furthermore, induced sexual differentiation of the brain by sex steroids implicates hormones as regulatory agents (McEwen *et al.*, 1979). Thus, hormones seem to be a primary agent in the orchestration of brain proliferation and differentiation.

The complexity within the CNS has limited elucidation of how and where hormones have their effet. The intimate networks of cellular processes and complex cytoarchitecture combined with the multiple homeostatic controls make *in vivo* study of hormonal actions on specific areas or cell types extremely difficult. To circumvent *in vivo* complexities, researchers have sought to minimize uncontrollable variables and delivery mechanisms by the use of cell culture.

The use of cell culture to dissect hormonally regulated phenomena in the CNS is of recent vintage. Almost 20 years ago Hamburgh (1966) reported that thyroid hormone precociously increased the formation of myelin in brain explant cultures. Later, steroids were shown to have effects on glial cell growth in primary neural cultures (Vernadakis, 1971) and to be involved in the regulation of GPDH in the rat glioma cell line C6 (de Vellis *et al.*, 1971) and primary cell culture (de Vellis *et al.*, 1975). These *in vitro* studies provided support for three important concepts in developmental neurobiology. First, hormones regulate glial proliferation and differentiation; second, certain hormones act directly on brain cells during development and their action can be analyzed and studied *in vitro*; and third, specific events observed *in vitro* correspond to *in vivo* events, and therefore cell culture can be used to study normal glial proliferation and differentiation.

Until recently, quantitative data concerning hormonal action on the CNS had eluded neurobiologists. The only available cell culture models allowing the study of cellular function were clonal cell lines of tumor origin. They represent a useful system to study hormonal action because they provide a genetically homogeneous cell population that can be easily grown and maintained. Unfortunately, their tumorigenic state clouds meaningful correlation of *in vitro* findings to responses of normal cells *in vivo*. Nevertheless, combining results from primary cultures of explant, dissociated, and reaggregated cells with those of clonal cell lines may help neurobiologists to correlate *in vitro* and *in vivo* responses.

Explant cultures retain much of their three-dimensional tissue organization; dissociated cell cultures form a simplified two-dimensional network; reaggregate cultures recreate histotypic organization. The importance of tissue organization in hormonal responsiveness is typified by the studies of Moscona and colleagues on hydrocortisone-inducible retinal glutamine synthetase. The induction is observed in organ and aggregate cultures but not in dissociated cell cultures (Morris and Moscona, 1971), indicating the need for tissue organization for the expression of cellular function. However, the study of hormonal action in these primary cultures is complicated by tissue heterogeneity and complexity. A better model system to circumvent the unknowns of using transformed cells and the heterogeneity of mixed primary cultures would be cultures of homogeneous populations of each of the main brain cell types. Such cultures would allow cellular specificity of hormonal action to be studied, selection of a specific brain area, and manipulation of the developmental time of culture initiation. Recently, our laboratory and others have developed methods for culturing nearly pure populations of astrocytes and oligodendrocytes (see Chapter 1). Coupled with other culture methods, isolated primary cultures may better help elucidate the molecular and cellular events involved in hormonal regulation of normal proliferation and differentiation of specific neural cell populations.

1.1. Glial Cell Classification

Since the first account of neuroglia was mentioned by Dutrochet in 1824, the description of glial properties, except for myelination, has been largely morphological. The concept that glia play a passive role can be traced to Virchow (1860) who conceived of glia as a form of connective tissue within the CNS and named them "nerve glue" or neuroglia. Only recently have glia been appreciated as having a dynamic function and relationship to neurons.

Although some controversy exists, neurons and glia probably arise from distinct stem cells (His, 1889; Skoff et al., 1976). The introduction of metallic impregnation by Ramón y Cajal (1909) and del Rio Hortega (1919) demonstrated that neuroglia consisted of three cell types: astrocytes, oligodendrocytes, and microglia. However, some controversy remained about the exact origin of these cells until Kershman (1938) established that astrocytes and oligodendrocytes were of neuroectodermal and microglia of both mesodermal and ectodermal origin. This chapter will focus only on mammalian astrocytes and oligodendrocytes.

The identification of astrocytes and oligodendrocytes has, until recently, relied on metallic staining techniques developed in the early 1900s (Ramón y Cajal, 1913; del Rio Hortega, 1928). The advent of electron microscopy in the 1950s and 1960s has further delineated these cell types. Interestingly, electron microscopy is still the most reliable method for distinguishing the different glial cell types. Recently, biochemical and immunological techniques have been developed to identify specific cell types (see Chapter 2), yet the small number of definitive markers and the lack of markers for specific situations (e.g., stem cell detection) can make absolute definition of cell type by biochemical and immunological methods a problem.

Although expressing morphological variation, astrocytes are classically defined as two morphological types: fibrous and protoplasmic. Fibrous astrocytes (Figs. 1 and 2A) are found predominantly in white matter and are recognized by bushylike processes. Protoplasmic astrocytes (Fig. 2B) are more prevalent in gray matter and in relation to capillaries. They have a clearer cytoplasm and processes that are more branched than fibrous astrocytes. They are specialized forms of astrocytes, e.g., the Bergman glia whose cell body is found in the Purkinje cell layer of the cerebellum and possess one process. These cells extend outward toward the pia mater and often branch into two or more processes in a shape resembling a fork (Penfield, 1932). However, all astrocytes possess in common several cytological features. In 1932, Penfield described astrocytes as cells with a light, irregular, oval nucleus and larger cell body than that of the oligodendrocyte. Although still used as a distinguishing feature together with the presence of glycogen granules (Kruger and Maxwell, 1966), the main criteria today are bundles of 90-Å filaments located in the cytoplasm around the nucleus and in the processes (Palay, 1958; Kruger and Maxwell, 1966).

Oligodendrocytes (Fig. 1) are found in both gray and white matter but are far more numerous in the latter. They are usually found in close association with myelinated axons. Like astrocytes, they bear processes, although fewer in number, and have a highly variable cell shape (Mugnaini and Walberg, 1964). The roughly globular cell soma, more dense than the astrocyte, contains a small round nucleus characterized by clumps of dense heterochromatin. The abundant cytoplasm, usually darker staining than the nucleus, contains distinctive organelle configurations: stacked cisternae of rough endoplasmic reticulum and a prominent perinuclear Golgi (Peters *et al.*, 1976). The major criterion for distinguishing the oligodendrocyte from the astrocyte is the lack of 90-Å glial filaments and the presence of 240-Å microtubules (Mugnaini and Walberg, 1964).

1.2. Primary Culture

To circumvent the cellular heterogeneity of the CNS, a variety of cell separation techniques have been used. Bulk isolation procedures such as velocity sedimentation (Barkley *et al.*, 1973; Cohen *et al.*, 1978), density gradient centrifugation (Poduslo and Norton, 1972; Szuchet *et al.*, 1980; Farooq *et al.*, 1981), differential centrifugation (Fewster and

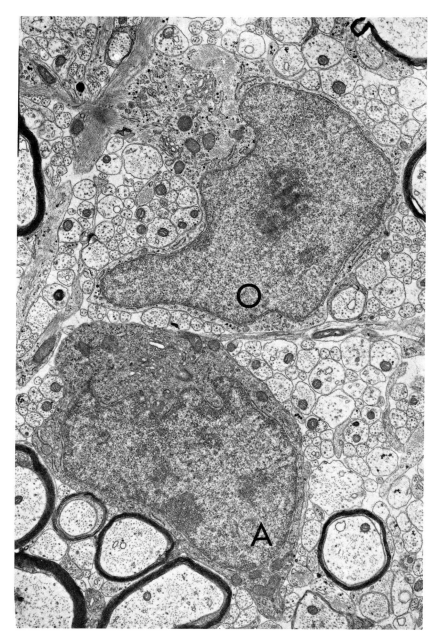

Figure 1. A section from the myelinating white matter of a kitten contains a fibrous astrocyte (A) and an oligodendrocyte (O). The nucleus of the astrocyte has homogeneous chromatin with a denser rim and a central nucleolus. The nucleus and cytoplasm of the oligodendrocyte are denser and more heterogeneous than of the astrocyte. Note the prominent filaments within the astrocyte. (Courtesy of Dr. Cedric S. Raine.)

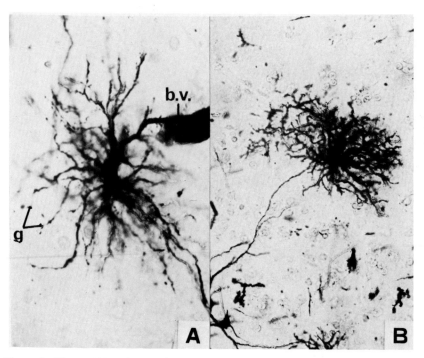

Figure 2. Fibrous (A) and protoplasmic (B) astrocytes in white matter of adult cerebral cortex. Note numerous gliosomes (g) in the processes of the fibrous astrocyte and the vascular end foot on the blood vessel (b.v.). Cells are stained with Golgi stain. (From Carpenter and Sutin, 1983.)

Mead, 1968a; Gebicke-Härter *et al.*, 1981), electronic sorting (Campbell *et al.*, 1977), and immunoselection (Meier and Schachner, 1982; Meier *et al.*, 1982) have been developed and the DNA, RNA, lipid, and protein content of each cell type have been determined (Fewster and Mead, 1968a,b; Poduslo and Norton, 1972; Fewster *et al.*, 1973). However, these preparations have drawbacks such as low yield, possible contamination with other cell types, and cellular damage during tissue disruption and isolation which may induce alterations in membrane integrity and loss of cellular processes (Marchbanks, 1970). A better system to dissect the developmental events within glial subpopulations would be the long-term culture of homogeneous populations of primary oligodendrocytes and astrocytes.

Although mixed primary cultures of oligodendrocytes and astrocytes have been developed since 1965 (Shein, 1965), only recently have essentially pure cultures of oligodendrocytes (McCarthy and de Vellis, 1980; Szuchet *et al.*, 1980; Bhat *et al.*, 1981; Gebicke-Härter *et al.*, 1981) and astrocytes (Booher and Sensenbrenner, 1972; Massarelli *et al.*, 1974; Moonen *et al.*, 1975; Schousboe *et al.*, 1977; Hertz *et al.*, 1978; Morrison and de Vellis, 1981; Chapter 1) been utilized to study glial physiology. With the exception of a few studies which facilitate the separation and enrichment of specific cell types by immunological methods (Meier and Schachner, 1982; Meier *et al.*, 1982) and physical methods (Szuchet *et al.*, 1980; Szuchet and Stefansson, 1980; Farooq *et al.*, 1981), a widely utilized method uses mixed glial cultures initially before cell separation.

Mixed glial cultures contain a bed layer of large polygon-shaped, phase-gray cells with small phase-dark, process-bearing cells lying on top (Fig. 3). By ultrastructural, biochemical, and immunological criteria, the large polygonal cells are astrocytes and the small phase-dark cells are oligodendrocytes (Shein, 1965; Breen and de Vellis, 1974; Raff *et al.*, 1978; McCarthy and de Vellis, 1980; Abney *et al.*, 1981). There are reports that these mixed glial cultures contain up to 15% fibroblast contamination (Hansson *et al.*, 1980); however, this contamination can be minimized to less than 1% by careful removal of the meninges before initiation of the culture (McCarthy and de Vellis, 1980). The initial plating density affects the appearance of oligodendrocytes in mixed culture. If plating is too sparse, oligodendrocytes fail to appear. Additionally, the developmental time at which the tissue is placed into culture can affect the presence or absence of cell types such as neurons (Booher and Sensenbrenner, 1972; McCarthy and de Vellis, 1980). Thus, depending on the age of the tissue, plating density, and area cultured, the types of cells present within the culture may vary.

As noted, there are several approaches for preparing homogeneous cultures of oligodendrocytes or astrocytes. Our method results in pure populations of these cells derived from the same starting material (McCarthy and de Vellis, 1980). This method takes advantage of two observations: (1) the absence of viable neurons in cultures prepared from postnatal rat cortex and (2) the stratification of astrocytes and oligodendrocytes in culture. When the mixed culture is placed on a rotary shaker for 15–18 hr (37°C, 250 rpm, stroke diameter 1.5 in.), the shear forces preferentially remove the overlaying oligodendrocytes. The contaminating astrocytes found in the suspended fraction are usually present in clumps which are easily removed by filtration. Once the filtered suspension is replated, the oligodendrocyte cultures are approximately 98% homogeneous (Fig. 3). The shaking and filtration procedures can be repeated if astrocyte contamination is still present. Bhat *et al.* (1981) find that osmotic shock can also eliminate astrocyte contamination after the mixed culture has been shaken. The remaining astrocyte culture (Fig.

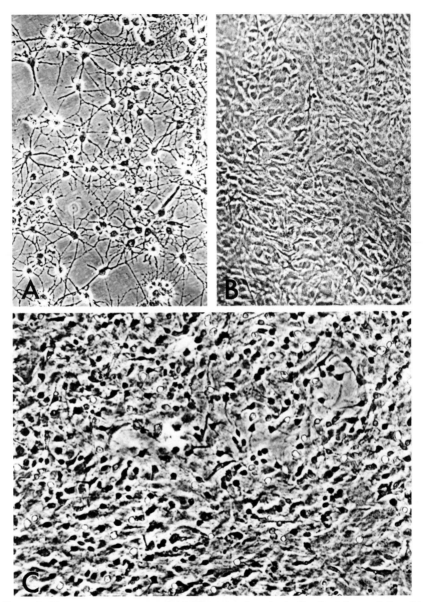

Figure 3. Phase-contrast micrograph of a dissociated cerebral cell culture from a 2-day-old rat after 9 days in culture (C). The phase-dark cells have been identified as oligodendrocytes; they are resting on top of a bed layer of polygonal flat cells. The bed layer cell type has been identified as an astrocyte. The top phase-contrast micrographs are purified cultures of oligodendrocytes (A) and astrocytes (B).

3) is 98–99% pure by morphological, biochemical, and immunological criteria (McCarthy and de Vellis, 1980; Morrison and de Vellis, 1981).

The age of the animal when the culture is initiated may be important in what developmental events have already occurred or been programmed for within the cell type under study. In addition, the time and method of culture may profoundly influence the expression of differentiated functions; thus, care must be taken in comparing data obtained with different methodologies.

1.3. Basic Modes of Hormone Action

Those hormones that affect the proliferation and differentiation of glial cells fall into two categories: steroid hormones and peptide hormones. These hormones have been studied extensively and their modes of action have, to a great extent, been studied in nonneural tissues. The role of hormones has only recently been seen as important in controlling biochemical and cellular functions in the CNS.

1.3.1. *Steroid Hormones.* Steroid hormones influence a variety of cellular events in a number of tissues. The CNS represents a rich target organ for steroids; all five of the major classes of steroid hormones elicit biological responses (McEwen *et al.*, 1979). The basic mechanism of steroid action seems to be similar regardless of the type of steroid or target tissue. Because of their lyophilic nature, all steroid hormones are thought to passively diffuse across the cell membrane and bind to specific soluble cytoplasmic receptors. The hormone–receptor complex then undergoes transformation to an "activated" state which has a high affinity for nuclear chromosomal sites. Interaction of the hormone–receptor complex with specific chromatin receptor sites stimulates the increased production of specific mRNAs (Yamamoto and Alberts, 1976).

1.3.2. *Peptide Hormones.* Peptide hormone actions on cellular events are more diverse. For the purpose of this review we will classify amino acids and peptides as peptide hormones. One group of peptide hormones binds to the cell surface and subsequently stimulates an increase in the intracellular level of cAMP. The increase in intracellular cAMP then acts as a "secondary messenger" by stimulating a protein kinase(s), which may result in the phosphorylation of other protein kinases. At the end of this cascade of phosphorylations, a specific protein(s) is phosphorylated which presumably alters cellular function (Prasad, 1977). A second group of peptide hormones, such as thyroid hormones, alters the level and pattern of gene expression through their interaction with low-capacity, high-affinity nuclear binding sites (Schwartz and Oppenheimer, 1978). Subsequently, RNA synthesis increases (Tata *et al.*, 1963), presumably the consequence of increased activity of a DNA-dependent RNA polymerase (Viarengo *et al.*, 1975). A third group of peptide hormones, such as epidermal growth factor and fibroblast growth factor (Gospodarowicz, 1981), have multiple cellular or biochemical expressions, but the primary cellular event which elicits these responses remains unknown.

The hormonal modulation of intracellular events within the CNS influences both proliferation and differentiation. Different model systems have been employed to study both the specific expression of hormonal action and the cell type in which hormonal action takes place. The final aim of any *in vitro* study is the elucidation of an *in vivo* process. The remainder of this chapter will describe attempts to understand the hormonal regulation of proliferation and differentiation of glial cells utilizing primary cultures of CNS tissue.

2. HORMONAL INFLUENCES ON PROLIFERATION

The application of electron microscopy coupled with autoradiography has enabled a more detailed understanding of gliogenesis. Recent studies (Skoff *et al.*, 1976) have substantiated the early work of His (1889) and Ramón y Cajal (1909) who proposed that neuroglia and neurons arise from distinct stem cells in the neuroectoderm. Radial glia, which are postulated to transform into astrocytes, have been detected in the cerebellum as early as day 15 in the mouse and day 17 in the rat (del Cerro and Swarz, 1976; Levitt and Rakic, 1980). This corresponds to the time when astrocytes undergo the majority of their proliferation while microneurons and perhaps macroneurons begin to migrate toward their final distinations (Rakic, 1971; del Cerro and Swarz, 1976). Depending on the brain region, this proliferative phase lasts until the first postnatal month. After this time, astrocytes still exhibit a slow rate of turnover within the stable population of mature astrocytes (Kaplan and Hinds, 1980).

Using the rat corpus callosum and optic nerve as a model system of oligodendrocyte gliogenesis, morphologically identifiable oligodendrocytes are not found until 2–3 days after birth (Mori and Leblond, 1970; Skoff *et al.*, 1976). However, oligodendrocyte proliferation is seen to occur between the beginning and the ending of axonal myelination. A wide range of morphological types of oligodendrocytes have been described. These have been grouped into three basic types—light, medium, and dark (Mori and Leblond, 1970). Oligodendrocytes are thought to progress through the sequence of light to medium to dark as they differentiate. Systematic counts (Mori and Leblond, 1970) and autoradiography (Paterson *et al.*, 1970) have shown that light oligodendrocytes transform into medium, which in turn give rise to dark oligodendrocytes. Although controversy still exists, apparently only the oligodendroblast, the heretofore undefined stem cell, and perhaps the light oligodendrocyte undergo proliferation. Interestingly, even though the adult brain contains almost entirely dark oligodendrocytes, some proliferation still occurs, indicating that a small population remains undifferentiated in the adult (Dalton *et al.*, 1968).

These animal studies indicate that specific stages exist during development where astrocytes and oligodendrocytes undergo the majority of their proliferation. These developmental stages are distinct but overlapping for each cell type. In addition, the stage of differentiation influences the capacity to proliferate. The mature astrocyte can undergo cell division, the dark oligodendrocyte cannot. Thus, how these cell types respond to extracellular stimuli may depend on what critical period they are in. This suggests that there are probably multiple signals that affect proliferation, and these signals may differ for astrocytes and oligodendrocytes.

Hormones have been shown to influence cellular proliferation. Animals treated with hydrocortisone were found to have decreased cell numbers compared to normal control animals (Balazs *et al.*, 1971). Estradiol treatment in cerebellar explants has been shown to increase [^{3}H]uridine incorporation into RNA and cell migration out of the explant, suggesting cellular proliferation (Vernadakis, 1971). However, the heterogeneity of CNS tissue in these systems makes cellular specificity of hormonal action difficult to elucidate. The use of primary CNS cultures of purified cell populations has eliminated cellular heterogeneity and increased the understanding of hormonal influence on cellular proliferation.

2.1. Oligodendrocytes

2.1.1. Influence of Culture Conditions. Unlike astrocytes, oligodendrocytes require special conditions to grow in culture. Labourdette *et al.* (1980) and others (McCarthy and de Vellis, 1978, 1980) have reported that without a high initial plating density, oligodendrocytes fail to appear in mixed culture. The increase in oligodendrocytes appears to result from the differentiation of precursor cells, as well as proliferation of maturing oligodendrocytes (Bologa *et al.*, 1982b, 1984). Although a high cell density is needed, once in mixed culture, oligodendrocytes can be seen growing as isolated cells (McCarthy and de Vellis, 1980). This indicates that oligodendrocytes do not require intimate contact with astrocytes for proliferation. However, for the expression of oligodendrocytes in mixed culture, a certain level of astrocyte and/or oligodendrocyte stem cell conditioning of the medium may be necessary. Neurons are present early in the culture process but soon degenerate and are not found in mixed cultures from postnatal animals (McCarthy and de Vellis, 1980). Neurons are known to stimulate Schwann cell proliferation (Bunge et al., 1981), and perhaps the initial presence of neurons in close proximity to oligodendrocytes is necessary for oligodendrocyte proliferation (Bologa et al., 1982a, 1983). Thus, some sort of interaction, between oligodendrocytes and astrocytes and/or neurons, may be necessary for oligodendrocyte proliferation.

2.1.2. *Hormonal Influence on Proliferation.* Various means have been used to increase the proliferation of oligodendrocytes in mixed culture. Labourdette et al. (1979) demonstrated that replacing fetal calf serum with newborn calf serum increased the yield of oligodendrocytes. However, another investigation found no difference in oligodendrocyte yield using calf serum or fetal calf serum (McMorris, 1983). Serum batches are known to vary from batch to batch, which may account for the variation in data. The addition of newborn and adult rat brain extracts increases the number of oligodendrocytes in mixed culture, with adult extracts having a greater effect (Pettmann et al., 1980a,b; Witter and Debuch, 1982). Insulin also increases the number of oligodendrocytes in mixed primary cultures (McMorris, 1983). Whether these added factors have a direct effect on oligodendrocyte proliferation or on astrocyte modulation of oligodendrocyte proliferation cannot be determined from these studies.

The detailed study of oligodendrocyte physiology requires the separation of oligodendrocytes from astrocytes, in large enough numbers to investigate different biochemical parameters, and long-term maintenance in culture. Data on oligodendrocyte proliferation and maintenance in mixed and purified culture have been conflicting and not easily interpreted. Many studies have reported that oligodendrocytes are rarely observed in mixed cell cultures after 3 weeks (Booher and Sensenbrenner, 1972; Moonen et al., 1975; Bock et al., 1977; Pettman et al., 1980a). However, we have maintained oligodendrocytes in mixed culture for several months, but it was evident that the oligodendrocyte population was not proliferating (Saneto and de Vellis, unpublished observation). This may indicate that in addition to initial plating densities being critical for oligodendrocyte appearance in culture, the density of oligodendrocytes in mixed culture may influence their proliferation (Bologa *et al.*, 1984). Furthermore, the culture procedure or the age of animal used may influence oligodendrocyte proliferation.

The *in vitro* requirements for maintenance and proliferation of purified oligodendrocytes remain uncertain. Meier and Schachner (1982) have shown that a fibroblast "feeder layer" enhances mouse oligodendrocyte survival in culture, However, other studies have shown that isolated populations of oligodendrocytes from lamb and cat can be maintained for extended periods of time without a feeder layer (Szuchet *et al.*, 1980; Gebicke-Härter *et al.*, 1981). Highly enriched cultures of oligodendrocytes from postnatal rats can also be maintained in culture for long periods of time without a feeder layer (Bressler *et al.*, 1983). The difference in results is hard to explain. Meier and Schachner isolated oligodendrocytes from cerebellum whereas the other studies used cerebrum. The variation in results seen may be a function of species, developmental stage, plating density of the oligodendrocytes being isolated, or culture methods.

Once the proliferation of oligodendrocytes occurs in mixed culture, very little, if any, proliferation takes place upon further purification (Szuchet *et al.*, 1980; Gebicke-Härter *et al.*, 1981; Meier and Schachner, 1982). Under optimal conditions we have not seen more than a doubling of cell number in highly enriched oligodendrocyte cultures (Saneto and de Vellis, unpublished data). The culture methods currently employed may either miss the proliferative stage in development or the culture environment may not possess the critical milieu needed for proliferation. This may account for the lack of effect on purified oligodendrocytes of known mitogenic factors such as fibroblast growth factor, epidermal growth factor, bovine pituitary extracts, or myelin basic protein (Pruss *et al.*, 1982). These data, coupled with the *in vivo* evidence of mature oligodendrocytes not undergoing proliferation, make the selection in purified culture of mature oligodendrocytes a possible explanation for lack of proliferation.

2.1.3. Future Directions. The unknown components found in serum make interpretation of the data uncertain. Serum is manufactured by pooling sera from many animals, so batches have inherent variation depending on the age, sex, nutrition, and physiological state of the animals used to procure sera. Serum also contains enzymes which may metabolize hormones and, hence, change their effects. In addition, the levels of hormones in different batches of sera have been found to vary over a 23-fold range (Esber *et al.*, 1973). These facts may account for the variation in data reported. To better elucidate the factor(s) responsible for oligodendrocyte proliferation, a growth or maintenance medium that does not contain serum would be of great potential value (see Chapter 1).

The degree of interplay between genome and environment leading to the expression of a cellular event remains an important question in developmental biology. *In vivo* and *in vitro* evidence indicates that a window of oligodendrocyte proliferation exists during development. Whether this interval is preprogrammed within the genome or a function of external signals may be best investigated in culture, by manipulation of the hormonal milieu and the age of the cultured oligodendrocytes. The ontological development of oligodendrocytes and astrocytes suggests that astrocytes might influence oligodendrocyte proliferation. Recently, we have begun to investigate possible intercellular interactions by characterizing what types of proteins are secreted from specific cell types under differing culture conditions (Arenander and de Vellis, 1982). We hope to identify proteins that may signal and modulate proliferation and other events. Such information would be important in elucidating the regulation of development.

2.2. Astrocytes

In vivo studies indicate that astrocytes can undergo proliferation throughout the life span of the animal. This proliferation capability, coupled with the ease of culture manipulation, has facilitated the study of astrocyte proliferation (Shein, 1965; Booher and Sensenbrenner, 1972; McCarthy and de Vellis, 1980; Morrison and de Vellis, 1981). For instance, purified cultures of astrocytes can be simply initiated by plating a suspension of brain cells at a low cell density (Labourdette *et al.*, 1980). It is not surprising, therefore, that much more information about the regulatory agents of astrocyte proliferation is known than that of the oligodendrocyte.

2.2.1. *Chemically Defined Medium.* The unknown factors and variation in serum batches make the identification of components necessary for proliferation difficult. To circumvent this problem many laboratories have initiated attempts to formulate serumless media (sse Chapter 1). Our laboratory has developed a serumless medium that allows the proliferation of astrocytes (Morrison and de Vellis, 1981). We found that a basal medium, Dulbecco's modified Eagle's medium and F-12 medium used in a 1:1 (v:v) mixture, allowed purified astrocytes in culture to proliferate at a very slow rate followed by a decrease within a few days. However, when putrescine, prostaglandin $F_{2\alpha}$, insulin, hydrocortisone, and fibroblast growth factor were added to this basal medium, the astrocytes proliferate exponentially. Each of the components, with the exception of prostaglandin $F_{2\alpha}$, when added separately had little influ-

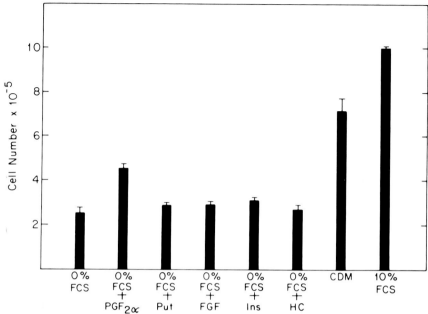

Figure 4. Response to individual supplements in chemically defined medium. Cells were plated at 5×10^4 per 35-mm dish in serum-supplemented medium. Eighteen hours later the cells were washed and converted to serum-free medium, serum-free medium plus one of the five supplements, chemically defined medium (CDM; all supplements), or serum-supplemented medium (10% fetal calf serum). The medium was changed on day 3. On day 5, cultures were trypsinized and the cells were counted; values are expressed as cell number per 35-mm dish. Put, putrescine; Ins, insulin; HC, hydrocortisone.

ence on proliferation. Together these components induced proliferation nearly equal to that of serum-containing medium.

The added components have all been linked to cellular proliferation in CNS and non-CNS cells *in vivo*. Prostaglandins are present in the CNS and are produced in both neurons and glia (Coceani and Pace-Asciak, 1976). Interestingly, the rate of release of prostaglandins correlates with the level of neuronal activity, which may indicate one of the ways neuronal elements might regulate glial proliferation (Coceani and Pace-Asciak, 1976). Hydrocortisone has previously been mentioned to have profound effects on brain development (Balazs, 1974). The polypeptide, fibroblast growth factor, is present both in the pituitary and in whole brain (Gospodarowicz, 1981). Although the primary function of fibroblast growth factor in the CNS is not known, its presence in the brain and mitogenic effect on several glial cell lines (Westermark and

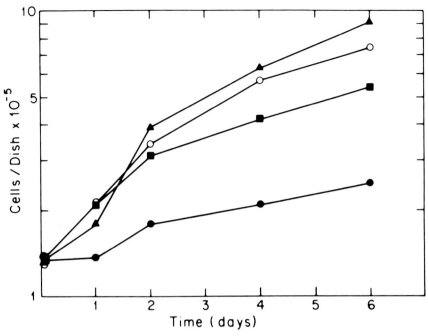

Figure 5. Growth curve for astrocytes. Cells were grown in one of the following media: serum-free (●), serum-supplemented (▲), chemically defined (○), or chemically defined medium without hydrocortisone (■). Data represent cell number per 35-mm dish; day 0, end of the serum preincubation. S.E.M. was less than 10% for all points.

Wasteson, 1975; see Chapter 1) indicate a possible role in glial proliferation *in vivo*. Insulin has specific receptors in most brain areas (Havrankova *et al.*, 1978; Pacold and Blackard, 1979) and is found in amounts 10–100 times those in plasma (Havrankova *et al.*, 1978). Our results with purified cultures of astrocytes and those of McMorris (1983) with oligodendrocytes in mixed cultures strongly indicate a role for insulin in proliferation of CNS glia. The polyamines, of which putrescine is a precursor, are involved in proliferation in a variety of cell types (Tabor and Tabor, 1976). Although the polyamine level in the CNS fluctuates in response to injury or tumor growth (Kremzner, 1973), its primary effect *in vivo* is not known. Whether or not any of these compounds are the actual substances involved in glial proliferation *in vivo* remains speculation at present. However, their action in primary culture certainly suggests that possibility.

    Our original description of chemically defined medium for astrocytes (Morrison and de Vellis, 1981) noted that serum might be needed

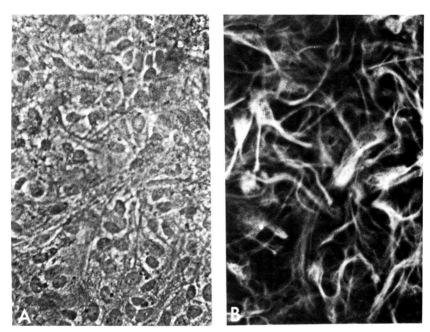

Figure 6. GFA immunofluorescence of purified astrocyte cultures grown for 5 days in serum-supplemented medium. The same field from a representative culture as visualized by phase-contrast microscopy (A) and indirect immunofluorescence for GFA (B).

for cellular attachment. We later found that preincubation of fibronectin in the culture dishes brought the plating efficiency and level of proliferation to those found in serum-containing cultures (Morrison and de Vellis, 1983). Astrocytes do not express fibronectin on their cell surfaces (Schachner *et al.*, 1978), but *in vitro* attachment is enhanced by its presence. Capillaries are known to express fibronectin and the close association between astrocytes and capillaries *in vivo* indicates a possible interaction during cellular proliferation.

A difficulty in primary culture analysis has been the proper identification of cell types. Fortunately, the recent improvements in immunological, biochemical, and morphological techniques have made this task possible (see Chapter 2). The presence of the astrocyte marker, glial fibrillary acidic protein (GFA), and absence of the fibroblast marker, fibronectin (Schachner *et al.*, 1978), suggested that the cells undergoing proliferation in our media were astrocytes (Figs. 6 and 7). A biochemical marker in astrocytes *in vivo* is glutamine synthetase (Norenberg and Martinez-Hernandez, 1979). We found this enzyme present and indu-

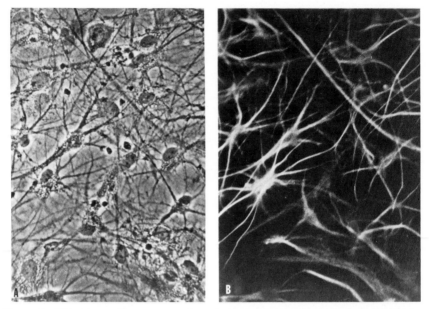

Figure 7. GFA immunofluorescence of purified astrocyte cultures grown for 5 days in chemically defined medium. The same field from a representative culture as visualized by phase-contrast microscopy (A) and indirect immunofluorescence for GFA (B).

cible by hydrocortisone in astrocytes grown in defined medium (Morrison and de Vellis, 1983). This evidence coupled with the immunological data indicates that the cells undergoing proliferation are astrocytes.

A distinction must be made between optimal proliferation and proliferation comparable to serum-supplemented conditions. Our chemically defined medium allows growth comparable to serum-supplemented medium. This is not necessarily optimal growth. The synergism of specific surface interactions between cells, soluble components, and matrix components necessary for proliferation makes absolute defining of optimal conditions extremely difficult. However, comparable increases in cell number in our chemically defined medium with serum-supplemented medium allow adequate cell numbers for experimentation in a highly controllable environment.

2.2.2. *Known Peptide Mitogens.* There are a wide variety of defined factors that stimulate the proliferation of astrocytes in culture. Several groups have reported that epidermal growth factor stimulates thymidine uptake and increases astrocyte cell number (Heldin *et al.*, 1977; Leutz and Schachner, 1981; Simpson *et al.*, 1983). The addition of epidermal growth factor to our chemically defined medium, which includes optimal concentrations of fibroblast growth factor, increases cell number over twofold. These data indicate that epidermal growth factor must stimulate astrocyte proliferation in a manner distinct from that of fibroblast growth factor. In addition to epidermal growth factor, platelet-derived growth factor stimulates both DNA synthesis and proliferation of a human glial cell line (Ek *et al.*, 1982). However, the influence of these mitogens on a variety of cell types raises questions regarding their specificity and importance during cellular development *in vivo*. Further investigation is needed to determine their primary biological function in the CNS.

2.2.3. *Mitogenic Activities.* The adult CNS possesses several endogenous mitogenic activities for astrocytes. Activities have been isolated from the pituitary (Brockes *et al.*, 1980) and whole brain (Pettmann *et al.*, 1980a,b; Kato *et al.*, 1981; Morrison *et al.*, 1982), which differ widely in their biochemical properties. The factor purified from the pituitary needs serum to be active and loses activity in the presence of reducing agents. A mitogen purified from bovine or pig brain (Lim *et al.*, 1973; Pettman *et al.*, 1980b; Kato *et al.*, 1981) induces both morphological changes and proliferation in astrocytes. A partially purified factor from adult rat brain is active in the presence of reducing agents and does not induce morphological change (Saneto *et al.*, 1982). In addition, brain extracts have been found to contain a number of activities that are differentially expressed during development (Morrison *et al.*, 1982). This variation in developmental expression of mitogenic activities and the biochemical differences between factors indicate a multiplicity of specific mitogens that influence astrocytes. The finding of multiple mitogenic activities raises the question of whether unique endogenous mitogens exist for astrocytes. Further studies are needed to elucidate whether these activities are genetically related to one another or to other known growth factors and what their target cell specificities are.

2.2.4. *Future Directions.* Purification of the mitogenic activities found in whole brain extracts may help elucidate the possible controlling agents of cellular proliferation during development. Where these factors are synthesized and their genetic relationship will help define the primary function(s) of these mitogenic activities. Further information about how these factors relate to abnormal proliferation of astrocytes in disease and trauma may help in the control of these adverse effects.

3. HORMONAL INFLUENCES ON DIFFERENTIATION

Control of the developmental process involves selective interactions between the genome and environmental stimuli. The expression of this

interaction in terms of morphological changes has already been described (see Section 1.1). In brief, the oligodendrocyte becomes recognizable late in brain development, just prior to postnatal myelination.
These cells then develop through a light phase, followed by a medium
phase, and subsequently a dark phase of fairly long duration (Vaughn,
1969). Mori and Leblond (1970) suggest that progression through these
morphological types represents maturation or differentiation events.
The most described marker of oligodendrocyte differentiation, myelination, probably occurs during the active light and medium stages,
whereas the function of the dark phase may only be for myelin maintenance (Imamoto et al., 1978).

The most described parameter of astrocyte differentiation is also
one of morphology. In the optic nerve of the rat, immature astrocytes
are characterized by the presence of a few 90-Å filaments with many
microtubules. During differentiation the number of glial filaments (90
Å) increases while the number of microtubules decreases (Peters and
Vaughn, 1967).

The lack of isolated populations of oligodendrocytes and astrocytes
has limited most of the data concerning differentiation to be centered
around myelination for the oligodendrocyte and morphological differentiation for the astrocyte. However, with the advent of purified populations of cells in primary culture, the dynamic properties and functions
of these cell types are beginning to be elucidated.

3.1. Oligodendrocytes

Animal studies suggest the involvement of hormones in myelination. Estradiol treatment in early postnatal life was demonstrated by
histological methods to influence the precocious appearance of myelin
(Curry and Heim, 1966). Estradiol or cortisol treatment during early
postnatal life has been found to increase levels of cerebrosides (Casper
et al., 1967), which have been shown to increase concomitantly with
myelination (Norton and Poduslo, 1973). Additionally, thyroid hormone
has been implicated in the myelination process. Hypothyroidism early
in life produces incomplete myelination (Balazs et al., 1971) and reduced
amounts of several myelin-associated components: cerebrosides, sulfatides, and myelin-associated glycoprotein (Balazs et al., 1969). How
these hormones act to affect myelination is not known. However, one
of these hormones, cortisol, has been extensively investigated in our
laboratory using whole animal, primary cultures, and tumor cell lines to
study its effect on oligodendrocytes. Integrated data from these exper-

iments show that cortisol regulates a specific oligodendrocyte function, the induction of GPDH.

3.1.1. GPDH

3.1.1a. Control of Induction by Hydrocortisone. *In vivo* studies show that GPDH (ED 1.1.18) is regulated by hormones of the pituitary. When hypophysectomized and adrenalectomized animals are assayed, they are found to have about 40% of the specific activity of GPDH seen in normal adults. The injection of adrenocorticotrophic hormone or hydrocortisone in hypophysectomized rats or hydrocortisone injection into adrenalectomized rats restored GPDH levels to those of normal adult rats (de Vellis and Inglish, 1968). These observations show that glucocorticoid hormones influence the expression of GPDH.

The developmental expression of GPDH activity corresponds with myelination, its activity rapidly increasing between days 10 and 30 (de Vellis *et al.*, 1967). Whether hydrocortisone actually controlled the expression of GPDH was only hypothesized. The rise in GPDH activity is known to correspond to pituitary–adrenal axis functionality, suggesting the probable control of enzyme expression by hydrocortisone (de Vellis and Inglish, 1968, 1973). Additional evidence of hormonal control is the precocious appearance of GPDH activity after injection of hydrocortisone into an animal before the pituitary–adrenal axis has become operational (de Vellis and Inglish, 1973). These results suggest that hydrocortisone controls the *in vivo* expression and maintenance of GPDH activity during development.

3.1.1b. Mechanism of GPDH Induction. To further dissect the mechanism of hydrocortisone induction of GPDH activity *in vivo*, a simpler and more controllable system was needed. It was fortuitously found that in the C6 rat glioma cell line, GPDH was induced by hydrocortisone. The amount of tissue continuously available and the homogeneity of the cell population make this model system highly attractive. We found that GPDH was inducible in C6 cells by physiological amounts of hydrocortisone (de Vellis and Inglish, 1973). Elucidation of the possible mechanism of induction was accomplished by using specific inhibitors of DNA synthesis, mRNA processing, RNA polymerase, and protein synthesis. Only the DNA synthesis inhibitor had no effect on the induction (de Vellis *et al.*, 1971; de Vellis and Kukes, 1973; de Vellis and Brooker, 1973). The same results were demonstrated in explant and dissociated cell culture (Breen and de Vellis, 1974, 1975). These results indicated that hydrocortisone induced GPDH activity by *de novo* synthesis, which required RNA synthesis. This was confirmed by purifying the enzyme, raising antibodies to it, and showing that increasing antibody concentrations produced a linear loss of enzyme activity (Mc-

Table I. Regulation of Enzyme Activities in Astrocytes Grown in Serum-Supplemented and Chemically Defined Medium[a]

	Enzyme activity[b]	
Enzyme/treatment	Serum-supplemented	Chemically defined
Glutamine synthetase		
+ hydrocortisone	4.92 ± 0.46	12.16 ± 1.07
− hydrocortisone	3.35 ± 0.89	3.28 ± 0.67
GPDH		
+ hydrocortisone	2.82 ± 0.37	2.99 ± 0.98
− hydrocortisone	2.18 ± 0.71	2.59 ± 0.33

[a] The final concentration of hydrocortisone was 1.0 μM.
[b] Enzyme activity is expressed as nmoles substrate hydrolyzed per min per mg protein.

Ginnis and de Vellis, 1974). Thus, the induction of GPDH was the result of an increase in the number of enzyme molecules rather than an increase in their activity. We further demonstrated that the time course of GPDH inducibility in cultures of both dissociated and explant cultures from 20-day rat fetuses matched the developmental profile of the enzyme *in vivo* (Breen and de Vellis, 1975).

3.1.1c. *Cellular Localization of GPDH Induction.* The close association of GPDH induction with myelination strongly suggested that the cellular localization of this phenomenon was in the oligodendrocyte; we attempted to verify this by *in situ* immunoperoxidase staining in purified cultures of oligodendrocytes and astrocytes. Cultures of purified astrocytes (Table I) did not have a significant induction of GPDH either in the presence of serum (McCarthy and de Vellis, 1980) or chemically defined medium (Morrison and de Vellis, 1982). In contrast, oligodendrocyte cultures (Table II) had a 16-fold induction of GPDH (McCarthy and de Vellis, 1980). In the original paper describing the isolation of astrocytes and oligodendrocytes, we indicated that astrocytes may be inducible (less than 2-fold) for GPDH by hydrocortisone. However, further studies showed that GPDH activity was not inducible nor was GPDH detectable by immunocytochemical staining techniques in purified astrocyte cultures (Leveille and de Vellis, 1982; de Vellis *et al.*, 1983). The most likely reason for our original finding of GPDH induction in astrocyte cultures was oligodendrocyte contamination. These data indicate that the inducibility of GPDH by hydrocortisone occurs in the oligodendrocyte.

Although specific markers for oligodendrocytes have been described (GPDH and lactate dehydrogenase inductions, CNPase activity, myelin

Table II. Regulation of Enzyme Activity[a]

Enzyme/treatment	Enzyme activity[b]	
	Astrocytes	Oligodendrocytes
CNPase[c]		
+ Bu$_2$cAMP	ND	178 ± 20.0
− Bu$_2$cAMP	ND	100 ± 7.0
GPDH		
+ hydrocortisone	2.82 ± 0.3	688.5 ± 5.1
− hydrocortisone	2.18 ± 0.7	43.0 ± 1.8
LDH		
+ Bu$_2$cAMP	2169.00 ± 69.0	2910.0 ± 112.0
− Bu$_2$cAMP	2060.00 ± 55.0	1147.0 ± 30.0

[a] The final concentration of hydrocortisone was 1.38 μM and Bu$_2$cAMP, 1 mM. Each value represents the mean of three cultures ± S.E.M. ND, nondetectable.
[b] Enzyme activity is expressed as nmoles substrate hydrolyzed per min per mg protein.
[c] Data from McMorris (1983).

basic protein, and galactocerebroside), the only unequivocal method for distinguishing glial cell types is histological characterization by electron microscopy. We found the localization of GPDH *in vivo* to be exclusively in the oligodendrocyte by this method (Leveille *et al.*, 1980). Immuno-peroxidase staining procedures at the light and electron microscopic levels have demonstrated the staining of only those cells that appeared to be oligodendrocytes by classical morphology (Fig. 8). Oligodendro-cytes found in perineuronal, interfascicular, and perivascular locations were stained positively while neuronal somas, synaptic profiles, den-drites, axons, and astrocytes were not stained. Thus, the *in vivo* and *in vitro* data conclusively prove that GPDH induction is an exclusive prop-erty of the oligodendrocyte. The lack of immunocytochemical staining of astrocytes found in tissue sections and the extremely low enzyme levels in isolated culture suggest that the constitutive levels of GPDH in astrocytes are extremely low (Morrison and de Vellis, 1981).

The question of whether the induced and uninduced enzymatic activities were in fact the same GPDH molecule was investigated bio-chemically and immunologically. We have shown by immunotitration, Ouchterlony double diffusion, and polyacrylamide gel electrophoresis that GPDH molecules isolated from the induced cells and uninduced cells are identical (McGinnis and de Vellis, 1977). These data demon-strate that in rat neural tissue, GPDH is a biochemical marker for oli-godendrocytes which are a target cell for glucocorticoid hormones.

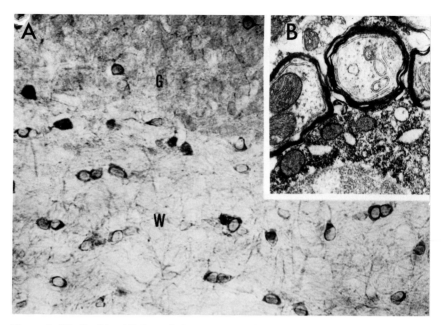

Figure 8. (A) Combined light and electron micrograph of GPDH in rat cerebellum. The light micrograph is a whole-mount section: rabbit anti-GPDH γ-globulins followed by peroxidase-labeled goat anti-rabbit γ-globulins. GPDH-positive oligodendrocytes, recognized by intense cytoplasmic staining, appear predominantly in white matter (W) and the granule cell layer (G). (B) Electron micrograph showing a GPDH-positive oligodendrocyte in relation to myelinated axons. Note the continuity between the myelin sheath and the stained process (arrow) of this oligodendrocyte.

Unlike dissociated and reaggregate neural cultures from rat, the induction of GPDH has not been found in mouse reaggregate cultures (Kozak, 1977). However, in SV40-transformed fetal mouse brain cultures, inducibility of GPDH was demonstrated (Benda *et al.*, 1977). Whether the lack of inducibility of GPDH is species specific requires further investigation. However, as found in rat brain, GPDH activity in mouse brain increases as development progresses, thereby suggesting the possible mediation of certain myelination events by GPDH. This increase in the activity of GPDH in the mouse brain results from the shift of the fetal gene product to the adult gene product (Kozak, 1977). Immunocytochemical methods indicate that the GPDH-positive cells in the mouse cerebral cortex are exclusively those defined morphologically as oligodendrocytes (Fisher *et al.*, 1981). However, some controversy exists as to whether other cell types are GPDH-positive in the mouse cerebellum. Although further studies are needed to settle this issue in the mouse cerebellum, immunological data indicate that GPDH is a reliable marker for oligodendrocytes in the mouse cerebrum.

3.1.2. Other Biochemical Events Influenced by Glucocorticoid Hormones. Glucocorticoid hormones are also implicated in regulating sulfolipid synthesis (Dawson and Kearns, 1978; Stephans and Pieringer, 1981). The glucocorticoid-sensitive enzyme, sulfotransferase, catalyzes the production of sulfogalactosylceramide. In a mouse glioma cell line, thought to be of oligodendrocyte origin, physiological concentrations of hydrocortisone induce a 36-fold increase in sulfotransferase (Dawson and Kearns, 1978). In addition, sulfotransferase is induced by hydrocortisone in dissociated embryonic mouse brain cultures (Stephans and Pieringer, 1981). Although cell specificity cannot be delineated from these experiments, the presence of sulfotransferase in bulk-isolated oligodendrocytes (Pleasure *et al.*, 1977) and its specific activity in dissociated mouse brain cultures, corresponding to the number of oligodendrocytes present (Herschkowitz *et al.*, 1982), further suggest the cellular location of this induction. However, there is no conclusive evidence that induction of this enzyme is oligodendrocyte-specific.

3.1.3. Peptide Hormones

3.1.3a. Hormones Not Linked to cAMP. Animal studies have indicated the importance of thyroid hormones for normal myelination. Thyroid deficiency in early life produces abnormal myelination with reduced amounts of several myelin components such as cholesterol, cerebrosides, sulfatides, and myelin-associated glycoproteins (Balazs *et al.*, 1969). Precocious myelination is observed in cultured cerebellar explants obtained from newborn rats following the administration of thyroid hormone (Hamburgh, 1966). Furthermore, in dissociated embryonic mouse brain cultures, the synthesis of myelin-associated glycolipid was dependent on the presence of thyroid hormones in the culture medium (Bhat *et al.*, 1979). These studies indicate that thyroid hormones may influence oligodendrocyte differentiation. However, further studies with purified cultures of oligodendrocytes are needed to characterize the specificity of thyroid hormone action.

3.1.3b. Hormones Directly Linked to cAMP. The use of mixed glial primary cultures and purified cultures indicates that the accumulation of intracellular cAMP via the stimulation of membrane receptors is regulated differently in the oligodendrocyte than in the astrocyte (Table III). The β-adrenergic agonists, norepinephrine, adenosine, and prostaglandin E_1, increase intracellular cAMP in both cell types (McCarthy and de Vellis, 1980). However, unlike astrocytes, α-adrenergic agonists do not modulate the cAMP response in oligodendrocytes (McCarthy and de

Table III. Regulation of cAMP[a]

Treatment	cAMP (pmoles/mg protein)	
	Astrocytes	Oligodendrocytes
Control	8.7 ± 0.2	8.9 ± 0.4
Norepinephrine	28.7 ± 2.9	50.1 ± 9.0
Norepinephrine + phentolamine[b]	180.6 ± 10.1	62.0 ± 4.4
Adenosine	44.3 ± 1.6	14.3 ± 0.7
Prostaglandin E_1	67.6 ± 8.8	187.4 ± 31.2

[a] The concentration of all drugs, except for adenosine, was 3 μM. Adenosine was used at 100 μM. All incubations were carried out for 5 min. Each value represents the mean of three cultures ± S.E.M.
[b] Phentolamine is a specific α-adrenergic antagonist.

Vellis, 1980). This indicates a difference in the regulation of intracellular cAMP accumulation in the two cell types. The importance of cAMP modulation remains to be elucidated, but the finding that the magnitude of the cAMP accumulation in response to β-adrenergic agonists increases during development (McCarthy and de Vellis, 1979) suggests that the control of cAMP regulation via membrane receptors may be important in glial differentiation.

Using the cAMP analog, $N^{6'}$, $O^{2'}$-dibutyryl cAMP (Bu_2cAMP), we have found that lactate dehydrogenase (LDH) (EC 1.1.1.27) induction occurs only in the oligodendrocyte (Kumar and de Vellis, 1981). LDH is a constitutive enzyme found in all cells and is composed of five isozymes. Its presence permits cells to maintain anaerobic glycolysis, thereby ensuring metabolic energy under anoxic conditions. Exposure to Bu_2cAMP for 9 hr induced a twofold increase in the rates of synthesis as well as a near doubling in the percent relative rates of synthesis of LDH-1, LDH-5, and total LDH in isolated cultures of oligodendrocytes (Kumar and de Vellis, 1981). Although not well understood, the greater tolerance to anoxia seen in young animals compared to adults may be partially explained by LDH induction (Nissen and Schousboe, 1979).

While Bu_2cAMP does not by itself induce GPDH, in combination with hydrocortisone the rate of GPDH synthesis is doubled (Breen and de Vellis, 1978). The mechanism of this enhancement of GPDH synthesis has not been elucidated.

Recently, McMorris (1983) (Table II) has demonstrated that Bu_2cAMP induces the myelin-associated enzyme 2′,3′-cyclic nucleotide-3-phosphohydrolase (CNPase) (EC 3.1.4.37). Increases in the activity of this enzyme correspond to myelination *in vivo* (Sprinkle *et al.*, 1978), *in vitro* (Fry *et al.*, 1973), and in bulk-isolated oligodendrocytes (Poduslo and Norton, 1972). Neither the actual substrate nor the function of this enzyme is known, although it has been shown to be identical or very similar to the Wolfgram proteins of myelin (Sprinkle *et al.*, 1980). Although CNPase hydrolyzes 2',3'-cyclic nucleotides, it has no activity toward the biologically important 3',5'-cyclic nucleotides (cAMP, cGMP). CNPase activity in oligodendrocytes from both mixed culture and isolated culture is induced by exposure to Bu_2cAMP (McMorris, 1983), and only occurs up to 13 days after explantation into culture. This narrow time frame of inducibility corresponds to the rise in CNPase activity *in vivo* (Sprinkle *et al.*, 1978). These data indicate that oligodendrocytes in culture may aid in the analysis of receptor–cAMP-mediated events involved in differentiation, especially myelination.

   3.1.4. Future Directions. Although far from being fully understood, myelination has been extensively studied. Specific events of the myelination process, such as the expression of enzymes (Snyder *et al.*, 1983) and specific myelin proteins (Schachner *et al.*, 1981), occur at different times during the formation of myelin. A few of the regulatory hormones and their modes of action have been defined. With the further use of purified cultures of oligodendrocytes, the entrance to or exit from a specific developmental stage within the myelination process will hopefully be characterized. Understanding of these events and their environmental and genetic controls may help in the treatment of myelin-related neurological disorders.

   The lack of proper markers remains a major obstacle in defining specific events of oligodendrocyte differentiation. These would be useful in analyzing gene expression during development and in the response to specific stimuli. Schachner *et al.* (1981) have demonstrated the usefulness of the monoclonal antibody approach and have described several surface antigens that are differentially expressed during development, although the functions of these antigens are not known. A recent study using immunocytochemical methods shows that CNPase appears prior to sulfatide on the oligodendrocyte membrane surface (Ranscht *et al.*, 1982). More studies such as those described above will help catalog specific events of oligodendrocyte differentiation.

   Immunocytochemical markers may also help in defining, isolating, and characterizing subpopulations of oligodendrocytes. Although much is known about myelination, other oligodendrocyte functions and interactions with other cell types are virtually unknown. Primary cultures may be useful in analyzing these phenomema.

3.2. Astrocytes

The description of astrocyte differentiation has centered around structural change, particularly the characteristic increase in 90-Å filaments and the decrease in microtubules (Peters and Vaughn, 1967). Recently, another structural component, vimentin, has been described as decreasing in amount during astrocyte differentiation (Schnitzer *et al.*, 1981). Although these structural changes are well defined, the regulatory agent(s) controlling their expression remains unknown. Use of purified astrocyte cultures has enabled the further description of their morphological and biochemical differentiation.

3.2.1. Chemically Defined Medium

3.2.1a. Morphological Differentiation. The highly controlled environment of cell culture allows the manipulation of the external milieu. However, as previously discussed, one of the uncontrollable parameters of cell culture is the presence of serum. To circumvent this, we have developed a chemically defined medium (CDM) that does not contain serum and allows purified astrocytes to proliferate at a rate comparable to those in serum-supplemented medium (Fig. 4 and 5) (Morrison and de Vellis, 1981). Astrocytes grown in CDM exhibit morphological and biochemical properties which appear to mimic a more differentiated state (Morrison and de Vellis, 1981, 1982).

Astrocytes grown in serum-supplemented medium are flat and polygonal, possess few processes, and contain 90-Å glial filaments or glial fibrillary acidic protein (GFA) (Fig. 6). In the presence of CDM (containing fibroblast growth factor, insulin, putrescine, hydrocortisone, and prostaglandin $F_{2\alpha}$) astrocytes exhibit a dramatic change in morphology (Fig. 9) (Morrison and de Vellis, 1981, 1982). They partially detach from the plastic surface, decrease in somal diameter, and extrude long branching processes. The soma of these cells exhibit many convoluted folds, but the surfaces of the processes are devoid of any distinguishable feature (Fig. 10). Greater than 95% of these cells stain positively for GFA and nearly 99% do not stain for fibronectin, suggesting that these cells are astrocytes. However, not all cells undergo induced morphological change in CDM; a small proportion of cells remain flat and polygonal. Furthermore, when the cultures are shifted back to serum-supplemented medium, most of the fibrous-like cells do not revert back to the flat, polygonal morphology (R. S. Morrison, personal communication). This suggests that CDM induces more than a transient morphological change. Which component or combination of components of CDM is involved in this phenomenon remains unknown. Although the morphological change is reminiscent of the morphology of differentiated astocytes *in*

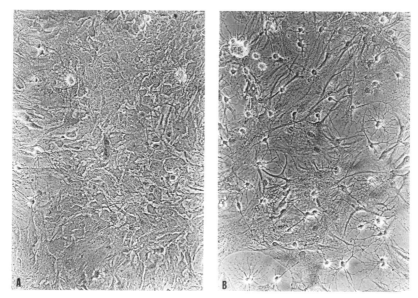

Figure 9. Phase-contrast micrographs of purified astrocyte cultures grown for 5 days in serum-supplemented medium (A) and chemically defined medium (B).

vivo, a more extensive examination of cultured astrocytes needs to be done before any conclusive statement can be made.

3.2.1b. Biochemical Differentiation. The components of CDM also produce a pronounced effect on the expression of a number of proteins in cultured astrocytes (Table I). Glutamine synthetase is a glia-specific marker (Norenberg and Martinez-Hernandez, 1979) and is inducible by hydrocortisone *in vitro* (Schousboe *et al.,* 1977). In the presence of CDM, glutamine synthesis is induced threefold by hydrocortisone (Table I). An increase in intracellular GFA represents the most prominent feature of astrocyte biochemical differentiation *in vivo* (Peters and Vaughn, 1967). CDM increases levels of intracellular GFA compared to control cultures (R. S. Morrison, personal communication). The content of S-100, a specific glial marker (Hyden and McEwen, 1966), increases during development *in vivo* (Herschman *et al.,* 1971). The cellular content of S-100 was demonstrated by microcomplement fixation to be significantly increased in astrocytes grown in CDM. The increase in GFA and S-100 suggests that CDM induces astrocytes to undergo a differentiation in culture similar to that seen *in vivo* (Morrison and de Vellis, 1983). Whether glutamine synthetase induction is a biochemical marker for astrocyte differentiation remains to be confirmed. Although more stud-

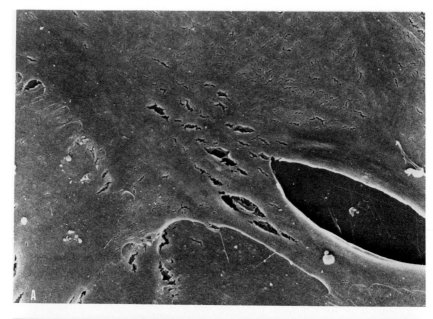

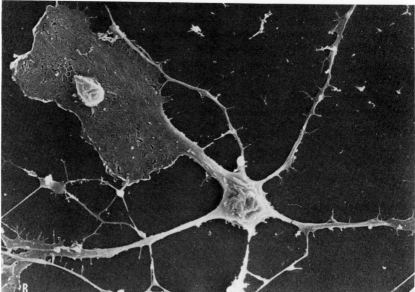

Figure 10. Scanning electron micrographs of astrocyte cultures raised in serum-supplemented medium (A) and chemically defined medium (B). Astrocytes were plated directly into serum-supplemented or chemically defined medium and maintained for 4 days before processing.

ies are needed, astrocytes in highly defined environments using CDM represent a good model system to study hormone-induced differentiation.

3.2.2. Peptide Hormones

3.2.2a. Hormones Directly Linked to cAMP. Exposure of purified astrocytes or oligodendrocytes to the β-adrenergic agonists, norepinephrine, adenosine, or prostaglandin E_1, increases intracellular levels of cAMP (McCarthy and de Vellis, 1980) (Table III). Adenosine elicited a greater response in astrocytes and norepinephrine and prostaglandin E_1 a greater response in oligodendrocytes. Astrocytes, but not oligodendrocytes, expressed α-adrenergic modulation of the cAMP response to β-adrenergic agonists (McCarthy and de Vellis, 1980). However, there are indications from studies in mixed cell cultures that the responsiveness of these receptors might change during development. The response to adenosine, norepinephrine, and prostaglandin E_1 significantly increases as the age of the tissue put into culture increases (McCarthy and de Vellis, 1979). With the differences in receptor response between oligodendrocytes and astrocytes and possible changes in the response during differentiation, it is tempting to speculate that receptor regulation of cAMP may be important in modulating some of the differentiation process.

Bu$_2$cAMP has been shown to induce morphological changes in a variety of cell types. In the presence of serum the majority of astrocytes remain flat and polygonal and are almost completely devoid of processes (Fig. 6). Within 2–3 hr after the addition of 1 mM Bu$_2$cAMP, a morphological transformation reminiscent of *in vivo* differentiation occurs. Cells partially detach from the plastic surface and send out long cytoplasmic processes with numerous microvilli and cytoplasmic blebs (Lim *et al.*, 1973; Moonen *et al.*, 1975; Hertz *et al.*, 1978; Kimelberg *et al.*, 1978). The observed morphological change is not a result of a generalized increase in levels of cAMP in that prostaglandin E_1 was not found to produce any morphological change corresponding to its induction of increased cAMP levels (Lim *et al.*, 1973). The continued presence of Bu$_2$cAMP is needed for the maintenance of fibrouslike morphology. When Bu$_2$cAMP is removed, the cells return to their flat and polygonal morphology.

Although the induced morphological change of astrocytes by Bu$_2$cAMP in serum-supplemented medium is similiar to that observed with these same cells grown in CDM, there are several observations suggesting that the induced change in cell shape may be distinct for each culture condition. The fibrouslike morphology in the presence of Bu$_2$cAMP occurs rapidly (2–3 hr) and nearly 100% of the cells are changed. While astrocytes grown in CDM take several days to achieve maximum morphological change, some remain flat and polygonal. The morphology of the fibrous-like cell also differs. There are blebs on the surface of cells grown in the presence of Bu_2cAMP that are not found on those grown in CDM. In addition, the reversal of the morphological change is virtually 100% after Bu_2cAMP removal (Haugen and Laerum, 1978), but only partial after CDM is replaced by serum-supplemented medium. These differences indicate that the switch in morphology induced by Bu_2cAMP may be distinct from that evident in CDM.

Bu_2cAMP also induces specific biochemical events, e.g., a significant increase in GFA content and glutamate uptake in cultured mouse astrocytes (Hertz et al., 1978). Activities of both carbonic anhydrase and Na^+,K^+-ATPase increase in the presence of Bu_2cAMP (Kimelberg et al., 1978). These enzyme activities increase with time in culture in the absence of Bu_2cAMP; the presence of Bu_2cAMP only served to enhance their expression. Furthermore, several other unidentified proteins appear to be induced by Bu_2cAMP as revealed by SDS gel electrophoresis (Hansson et al., 1980). These data indicate that Bu_2cAMP has pronounced effects on several biochemical parameters of astrocytes. The precocious enhancement of several enzyme activities both *in vivo* (Schousboe et al., 1975; Hertz et al., 1978) and *in vitro* and distinct changes in protein expression suggest that cultured astrocytes may be a good model system to study cAMP-mediated biochemical differentiation.

3.2.2b. Hormones Not Linked to cAMP. In addition to the influences of CDM and of Bu_2cAMP in serum-supplemented medium, extracts from brain tissue induce a morphological change in astrocytes (Fig. 11). Our laboratory has investigated the effect of extracts made from brains at different developmental times. Extracts from 16- to 18-day embryos, 1- to 2-day postnatal, and 60-day adult rats were all found to induce morphological changes in astrocytes, with the induction of fibrous-like morphology being greater as the age of the animal increased (Morrison et al., 1982). This is surprising since the vast majority of astrocyte differentiation occurs in the first postnatal month in the rat. We are currently investigating this puzzling finding.

The most studied and best characterized of the factors from brain extracts that induce morphological changes of cultured astrocytes is glial maturation factor (GMF) (Lim, 1980). Isolated from adult brain, this factor induces a morphological change very similar to that produced by Bu_2cAMP. The flat, polygonal, and epitheloidlike cell becomes more fibrous with extension of long cytoplasmic processes with numerous microvilli and cytoplasmic blebs in the presence of GMF (Athias et al., 1974; Sensenbrenner, 1977; Haugen and Laerum, 1978; Pettman et al.,

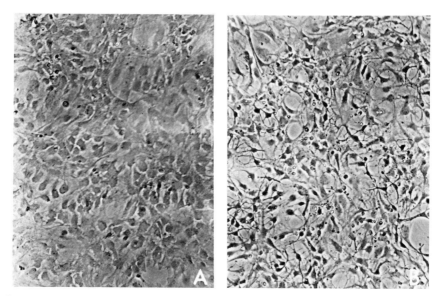

Figure 11. Phase-contrast micrographs of purified astrocytes grown for 5 days in serum-supplemented medium, without brain extract (A) and in the presence of 250 μg/ml adult brain extract for 24 hr (B).

1980b). Although exposure to GMF increased cAMP levels, it is very unlikely that the increase in cAMP is responsible for the morphological change (Lim *et al.*, 1973). The effect induced by Bu$_2$cAMP occurs within 2–3 hr whereas GMF needs 12 or more hr to induce a change in morphology. Furthermore, the increase in cAMP levels induced by GMF does not occur until approximately 4 days after treatment (Lim *et al.*, 1973). However, the expression of the morphological change, e.g., long cytoplasmic process with numerous microvilli and cytoplasmic blebs, along with the similar reversibility of the phenomenon upon removal of either compound, suggests that these two agents may act via the same pathway. The paucity of data makes this conclusion only speculative at present.

GMF has been shown to have pleiotypic effects on cellular physiology. During the first 3 days of exposure to GMF, levels of cGMP, DNA synthesis and cell division, RNA and protein synthesis, and morphological changes are enhanced. After these initial events, DNA synthesis and cell division are inhibited, elongation of cytoplasmic processes continues, and levels of cAMP and S-100 protein increase (Lim, 1980).

GMF has been highly purified from adult pig and beef brains and shown to be a protein (Pettman *et al.*, 1980b, Kato *et al.*, 1981). Kato *et al.* (1981) have shown that GMF can exist in at least two molecular weight forms of approximately 200,000 and 20,000. The smaller of these proteins has been highly purified from both pig and cow and shown to be acidic (isoelectric point ~ 4.8), resistant to trypsin, and heat-labile. Although both proteins have morphological and mitogenic activity, each differs in the concentration needed to elicit an effect. Whether this difference is species specific or reflects the purity of the preparation tested needs to be further elucidated.

There are several important questions about GMF that need to be addressed. Where is this molecule produced? What is the mechanism of action? How does the large molecule relate ontologically to the smaller molecule? How does this GMF correlate with the activity seen in trauma and pathological states? We have also found factors in embryonic brain extracts which induce morphological changes (Morrison *et al.*, 1982). Hence, are there multiple distinct GMF-like proteins during development, or is it the same molecule?

3.2.3. *Future Directions.* There are four major areas that need further study: (1) intra- and intercellular signaling during development, (2) elucidation of normal physiology, (3) identification of astrocyte subpopulations, and (4) characterization of regulatory agents involved in specific differentiation events.

The identification of specific molecules affecting differentiation would help in defining cell lineages. In addition, it would allow detection of developmental signals which control specific cellular functions, both in the normal and pathological state. Knowledge of these events would enable correlation of regulatory agents with specific developmental event during astrocyte differentiation.

Schachner and co-workers have used monoclonal antibodies to identify subpopulations of astrocytes in the mouse CNS and their developmental appearance both *in vivo* and *in vitro* (Lagenaur *et al.*, 1982). Other workers have described a monoclonal antibody that detected an antigen expressed during the astroblast stage of development (Cairncross *et al.*, 1982). Immunocytochemical techniques in combination with primary cell culture and other classical biochemical techniques will help in identifying the agents controlling differentiation and the specific events which mark different developmental windows. This will hopefully lead to further understanding of the normal physiology of the astrocyte *in vivo* and of the intra- and intercellular signaling during development.

4. CONCLUSION

Proliferation and differentiation of glial cells in the CNS involves the interaction of genetic and environmental factors, the regulation of which remains largely unknown. The theme of this chapter has been to describe how the orderly interaction of developmental events is controlled. There is ample evidence that hormones are an important part of this regulatory process.

In this chapter the hormonal influence on proliferation and differentiation was described in two distinct glial cell types, oligodendrocytes and astrocytes. Primary culture allows a simplified and controlled study of these cell types, while in the intact animal modulation of developmental events is complex and interwoven among cell types and their interactions with the environment. Herein lies cell culture's major problem—reduction of a highly complex organ with a hierarchy of tissue interactions to a model system that is homotypic and rigidly controlled. Although some events in primary culture are representative of *in vivo* events, some may not be; hence, every effort needs to be made to integrate findings in culture with those in the animal.

One of the obvious conclusions to be drawn from the data presented is how little we know of normal oligodendrocyte and astrocyte physiology. Through the use of primary culture and other cell culture methods, these functions will hopefully be further clarified. The interplay between CNS glia and neurons during development remains another area of limited understanding, and primary culture of specific tissues lends itself well to the study of such cellular interactions.

ACKNOWLEDGMENTS

The authors wish to thank Joyce Adler for preparation of the manuscript. This work was supported by NIH Grants HD-05615 and HD-06576 and DOE Contract DE-AMO3-76-SF-00012.

REFERENCES

Abney, E. R., Bartlett, P. P., and Raff, M. C., 1981, Astrocytes, ependymal cells, and oligodendrocytes develop on schedule in dissociated cell cultures of embryonic rat brain, *Develop. Biol.* **83**:301–310.

Arenander, A. T., and de Vellis, J., 1982, Glial-released proteins in neural intercellular communication: Molecular mapping, modulation and influence on neuronal differentiation, in: *Proteins in the Nervous System: Structure and Function* (B. Haber, J. R. Perez-Polo, and J. D. Coulter, eds.), Liss, New York, pp. 243–269.

Athias, P., Sensenbrenner, M., and Mandel, P., 1974, The behaviour of dissociated chick embryo brain cells in long-term cultures in presence and absence of brain extracts, *Differentiation* **2**:99–106.

Balazs, R., 1974, Influence of metabolic factors on brain development, *Br. Med. Bull.* **30**:126–134.

Balazs, R., Brookshank, B. W. L., Davison, A. L., Eayrs, J. T., and Wilson, D. A., 1969, The effect of neonatal thyroidectomy on myelination in the rat brain, *Brain Res.* **15**:219–232.

Balazs, R., Kovacs, S., Cocks, W. A., Johnson, A. L., and Eayrs, J. T., 1971, Effect of thyroid hormone on the biochemical maturation of rat brain: Postnatal cell formation, *Brain Res.* **25**:555–570.

Barkley, D. S., Rakic, L. L., Chaffee, J. K., and Wong, D. L., 1973, Cell separation by velocity sedimentation of postnatal mouse cerebellum, *J. Cell. Physiol.* **81**:271–280.

Benda, P., Illinger, D., Poindron, P., Fiszman, M., and Salimon, J. C., 1977, Passage through athymic nude mice of SV-40 virus-transformed mouse fetal brain cells, *Brain Res.* **122**:191–196.

Bhat, N. R., Sarlieve, L. L., Rao, G. S., and Pieringer, R., 1979, Investigations on myelination in vitro: Regulation by thyroid hormone in cultures of dissociated brain cells from embryonic mice, *J. Biol. Chem.* **254**:9342–9346.

Bhat, S., Barbarese, E., and Pfeiffer, S. E., 1981, Requirement for nonoligodendrocyte cell signals for enhanced myelinogenic gene expression in long-term cultures of purified rat oligodendrocytes, *Proc. Natl. Acad. Sci. USA* **78**:1283–1287.

Bock, E., Moller, M., Nissen, C., and Sensenbrenner, M., 1977, Glial fibrillary acidic protein in primary astroglial cell cultures derived from newborn rat brain, *FEBS Lett.* **83**:204–211.

Bologa, L., Bisconte, J.-C., Joubert, R., Marangos, P. J., Derbin, C., Rioux, F., and Herschkowitz, N., 1982a, Accelerated differentiation of oligodendrocytes in neuronal-rich embryonic mouse brain cell cultures, *Brain Res.* **252**:129–136.

Bologa, L., Z'Graggen, A., Rossi, E., and Herschkowitz, N., 1982b, Differentiation and proliferation: Two possible mechanisms for the regeneration of oligodendrocytes in culture, *J. Neurol. Sci.* **57**:419–434.

Bologa, L., Bisconte, J.-C., Joubert, R., Margules, S., and Herschkowitz, N., 1983, Proliferative activity and characteristics of immunocytochemically identified oligodendrocytes in embryonic mouse brain cell cultures, *Exp. Brain Res.* **50**:84–90.

Bologa, L., Z'Graggen, A., and Herschkowitz, N., 1984, Proliferation rate of oligodendrocytes in culture can be influenced by extrinsic factors, *Develop. Neurosci.* **6**:26–31.

Booher, J., and Sensenbrenner, M., 1972, Growth and cultivation of dissociated neurons and glial cells from embryonic chick, rat and human brain in flask cultures, *Neurobiology* **2**:29–105.

Breen, G. A. M., and de Vellis, J., 1974, Regulation of glycerol phosphate dehydrogenase by hydrocortisone in dissociated rat cerebral cell cultures, *Develop. Biol.* **41**:255–266.

Breen, G. A. M., and de Vellis, J., 1975, Regulation of glycerol phosphate dehydrogenase by hydrocortisone in rat brain explants, *Exp. Cell Res.* **91**:159–169.

Breen, G. A. M., and de Vellis, J., 1978, Regulation of glycerol phosphate dehydrogenase by N^6, O^2-dibutyryl cyclic AMP, norepinephrine and isobutyl methyl xanthine in rat brain cultures, *J. Biol. Chem.* **253**:2554–2562.

Bressler, J. P., Cole, R., and de Vellis, J., 1983, Neoplastic transformation of newborn rat oligodendrocytes in culture, *Cancer Res.* **43**:709–715.

Brockes, J. P., Lemke, G. E., and Balzer, D. R., 1980, Purification and preliminary characterization of a glial growth factor from the bovine pituitary, *J. Biol. Chem.* **255**:8374–8377.

Bunge, R., Moya, F., and Bunge, M., 1981, Observations on the role of cell secretion in Schwann cell–axon interactions, in: *Neurosecretion and Brain Peptides* (J. B. Martin, S. Reichlin, and K. L. Bick, eds.), Raven Press, New York, pp. 229–242.

Cairncross, J. G., Mattes, M. J., Beresford, H. R., Albino, A. P., Houghton, A. N., Lloyd, K. O., and Old, L. J., 1982, Cell surface antigens of human astrocytoma defined by mouse antibodies: Identification of astrocytoma subsets, *Proc. Natl. Acad. Sci. USA* **79**:5641–5645.

Campbell, G. L., Schachner, M., and Sharrow, S. O., 1977, Isolation of glial cell-enriched and depleted populations from mouse cerebellum by density gradient centrifugation and electronic cell sorting, *Brain Res.* **127**:69–86.

Carpenter, M. B., and Sutin, J., 1983, *Human Neuroanatomy*, eighth edition, Williams and Wilkins, Baltimore.

Casper, R., Vernadakis, A., and Timiras, P. S., 1967, Influence of estradiol and cortisol on lipids and cerebrosides in the developing brain and spinal cord of the rat, *Brain Res.* **5**:524–526.

Coceani, F., and Pace-Asciak, C. R., 1976, Prostaglandins: Physiological, pharmacological, and pathological aspects, in: *Advance in Prostaglandin Research* (S. M. Darim, ed.), University Park Press, Baltimore, 1–36.

Cohen, J., Balazs, R., Hajos, F., Currie, D. N., and Dutton, G. R., 1978, Separation of cell types from the developing cerebellum, *Brain Res.* **148**:313–331.

Curry, J. J., and Heim, L. M., 1966, Brain myelination after neonatal administration of oestradiol, *Nature* **209**:915–916.

Dalton, M., Hommes, O., and Leblond, C., 1968, Correlation of glial proliferation with age in the mouse brain, *J. Comp. neurol.* **134**:397–399.

Dawson, G., and Kearns, S. M., 1978, Mechanism of action of hydrocortisone potentiation of sulfogalactosylceramide synthesis in mouse olgodendroglioma cell lines, *J. Biol. Chem.* **254**:163–167.

del Cerro, M., and Swarz, J., 1976, Prenatal development of Bergmann glial fibers in rodent cerebellum, *J. Neurocytol.* **5**:669–676.

del Rio Hortega, P., 1919, El tercer elemento de los centros nervosos, *Bol. Soc. Esp. Biol.* **9**:68–83.

del Rio Hortega, P., 1928, Tercera apartacion al conosimanto morfologica interpretacion functional del la oligodendroglia, *Mem. R. Soc. Esp. Hist. Nat.* **14**:5–122.

de Vellis, J., and Brooker, G., 1973, Induction of enzymes by glucocorticoids in a rat glial cell line, in: *Tissue Culture of the Nervous System* (G. Sato, ed.), Plenum Press, New York, pp. 231–245.

de Vellis, J., and Inglish, D., 1968, Hormonal control of glycerolphosphate dehydrogenase in the rat brain, *J. Neurochem.* **15**:1061–1070.

de Vellis, J., and Inglish, D., 1973, Age-dependent changes in the regulation of glycerol phosphate dehydrogenase in the rat brain and in glial cell lines, *Prog. Brain Res.* **40**:321–330.

de Vellis, J., and Kukes, G., 1973, Regulation of glial cell functions by hormones and ions, *Tex. Rep. Biol. Med.* **31**:271–293.

de Vellis, J., Schjeide, O. A., and Clemente, C. D., 1967, Protein synthesis and enzymatic patterns in the development brain following head x-irradiation of newborn rats, *J. Neurochem.* **14**:499–511.

de Vellis, J., Inglish, D., Cole, R., and Molson, J., 1971, Effects of hormones on the differentiation of cloned lines of neurons and glial cells, in: *Influence of Hormones on the Central Nervous System* (D. Ford, ed.), Karger, Basel, pp. 25–39.

de Vellis, J., Breen, G. A. M., and McGinnis, J. F., 1975, Biochemical studies in various culture systems of neural tissues, in: *Brain Mechanisms in Mental Retardation* (N. A. Buchwald and M. A. B. Brazier, eds.), Academic Press, New York, pp. 115–122.

de Vellis, J., Peng, W. W., Pixley, S. K. R., and Tiffany-Castiglioni, E., 1983, Oligodendroglial, astroglial and glial tumor-associated antigens defined by monoclonal antibodies, in: *30th Annual Colloquium—Protides of the Biological Fluids* (H. Peeters, ed.), Pergamon Press, Elmsford, New York, pp. 99–102.

Dutrochet, H., 1824, Recherches anatomiques et physiologiques sur la structure interne des animaux et des vegetaux et sur leur motilite, Baillière, Paris.

Eayrs, J. T., 1964, Endocrine influences on cerebral development, *Arch. Biol.* **75**:529–565.

Ek, B., Westermark, B., Wasteson, A., and Heldin, C. H., 1982, Stimulation of tyrosine-specific phosphorylation by platelet-derived growth factor, *Nature* **295**:419–420.

Esber, H. J., Payne, I. J., and Bogden, A. E., 1973, Variability of hormone concentrations and ratios in commercial sera used for tissue culture, *J. Natl. Cancer Inst.* **50**:559–562.

Farooq, M., Cammer, W., Synder, D. S., Raine, C. S., and Norton, W. T., 1981, Properties of bovine oligodendroglia isolated by a new procedure using physiologic conditions, *J. Neurochem.* **36**:431–440.

Fewster, M. E., and Mead, J. F., 1968a, Fatty acid and fatty aldehyde composition of glial cell lipids isolated from bovine white matter, *J. Neurochem.* **15**:1303–1312.

Fewster, M. E., and Mead, J. F., 1968b, Lipid composition of glial cells isolated from bovine white matter, *J. Neurochem.* **15**:1041–1052.

Fewster, M. E., Blackstone, S. C., and Ihrig, T. J., 1973, The preparation and characterization of isolated oligodendroglia from bovine white matter, *Brain Res.* **63**:263–271.

Fisher, M., Gapp, D. A., and Kozak, L. P., 1981, Immunohistochemical localization of *sn*-glycerol-3-phosphate dehydrogenase in Bergmann glia and oligodendroglia in the mouse cerebellum, *Develop. Brain Res.* **1**:341–354.

Fry, J. M., Lehrer, G. M., and Bornstein, M. B., 1973, Experimental inhibition of myelination in spinal cord tissue cultures: Enzyme assays, *J. Neurobiol.* **4**:453–459.

Gebicke-Härter, P. J., Althaus, H. H., Schwartz, P., and Newhoff, V., 1981, Oligodendrocytes from postnatal cat brain in cell culture. I. Regeneration and maintenance, *Develop. Brain Res.* **1**:497–518.

Gospodarowicz, D., 1981, Epidermal and nerve growth factors in mammalian development, *Annu. Rev. Physiol.* **43**:251–263.

Hamburgh, M., 1966, Evidence for a direct effect of temperature and thyroid hormone on myelinogenesis in vitro, *Develop. Biol.* **13**:1253–1255.

Hanssen, E., Sellstrom, A., Persson, L. I., and Ronnback, L., 1980, Brain primary culture—A characterization, *Brain Res.* **188**:233–246.

Haugen, A., and Laerum, O. D., 1978, Induced glial differentiation of fetal rat brain cells in culture: An ultrastructural study, *Brain Res.* **150**:225–238.

Havranova, J., Roth, J., and Brownstein, M., 1978, Insulin receptors are widely distributed in the central nervous system of the rat, *Nature* **272**:827–829.

Heldin, C. H., Wasteson, A., and Estermark, B., 1977, Partial purification and characterization of platelet factors stimulating the multiplication of normal human glial cells, *Exptl. Cell Res.* **109**:429–438.

Herschkowitz, N., Bologa, L., and Siegrist, H. P., 1982, Characterization of mouse oligodendrocytes during development, *Trans. Am. Soc. Neurochem.* **13**:173.

Herschman, H. R., Levine, L., and de Vellis, J., 1971, Appearance of brain specific antigen (S-100 protein) in the developing rat brain, *J. Neurochem.* **18**:629–633.

Hertz, L., Bock, E., and Schousboe, A., 1978, GFA content, glutamate uptake and activity of glutamate metabolizing enzymes in differentiating mouse astrocytes in primary cultures, *Develop. Neurosci.* **1**:226–238.

His, W., 1889, Die Neuroblasten und Deren Entstehungen in Embryonalen Mark, *Arch. Anat. Physiol.* **5**:249–300.

Hyden, H., and McEwen, B., 1966, A glial protein specific for the nervous system, *Proc. Natl. Acad. Sci. USA* **35**:354–358.

Imamoto, K., Paterson, J., and Leblond, C., 1978, Radioautographic investigation of gliogenesis in the corpus callosum of young rats. I. Sequential changes in oligodendrocytes, *J. Comp. Neurol.* **180**:115–137.

Kaplan, M. S., and Hinds, J. W., 1980, Gliogenesis of astrocytes and oligodendrocytes in the neocortical grey and white matter of the adult rat: Electron microscopic analysis of light radioautographs, *J. Comp. Neurol.* **193**:711–727.

Kato, T., Fukui, Y., Turriff, D. E., Nakagawa, S., Lim, R., Arnason, B. G. W., and Tanaka, R., 1981, Glia maturation factor in bovine brain: Partial purification and physiochemical characterization, *Brain Res.* **212**:393–402.

Kershman, J., 1938, The medulloblast and the medulloblastoma, *Arch. Neurol. Psychiatry* **40**:937–967.

Kimelberg, H. K., Narumi, S., and Bourke, R. S., 1978, Enzymatic and morphological properties of primary rat brain astrocyte cultures, and enzymatic development in vivo, *Brain Res.* **153**:55–77.

Kozak, L. P., 1977, The transition from embryonic to adult isozyme expression in reaggregating cell cultures of mouse brain, *Develop. Biol.* **55**:160–169.

Kremzner, L. T., 1973, Polyamine metabolism in normal and neoplastic neural tissue, in: *Polyamines in Normal and Neoplastic Growth* (D. H. Russell, ed.), Raven Press, New York, pp. 27–40.

Kruger, L., and Maxwell, D. S., 1966, Electron microscopy of oligodendrocytes in normal rat cerebrum, *Am. J. Anat.* **118**:411–436.

Kumar, S., and de Vellis, J., 1981, Induction of lactate dehydrogenase by dibutyryl cAMP in primary cultures of central nervous tissue is an oligodendroglial marker, *Develop. Brain Res.* **1**:303–307.

Labourdette, G., Roussel, G., Ghandour, M. S., and Nussbaum, J. L., 1979, Cultures from rat brain hemispheres enriched in oligodendrocyte-like cells, *Brain Res.* **179**:199–203.

Labourdette, G., Roussel, G., and Nussbaum, J. L., 1980, Oligodendroglia content of glial cell primary cultures, from newborn rat brain hemispheres, depends on the initial plating density, *Neurosci. Lett.* **18**:203–209.

Lagenaur, C., Masters, C., and Schachner, M., 1982, Changes in expression of glial antigens M_1 and C_1 after cerebellar injury, *J. Neurosci.* **2**:470–476.

Leutz, A., and Schachner, M., 1981, Epidermal growth factor stimulates DNA synthesis of astrocytes in primary cerebellar cultures, *Cell Tissue Res.* **220**:393–404.

Leveille, P. J., and de Vellis, J., 1982, Studies of glycerol phosphate dehydrogenase and glucocorticoid receptors in glial cultures, *Trans. Am. Soc. Neurochem.* **13**:233.

Leveille, P. J., McGinnis, J. F., Maxwell, D. S., and de Vellis, J., 1980, Immunocytochemical localization of glycerol-3-phosphate dehydrogenase in rat oligodendroglia, *Brain Res.* **196**:287–305.

Levitt, P., and Rakic, P., 1980, Immunoperoxidase localization of glial fibrillary acidic protein in radial glial cells and astrocytes of the developing rhesus monkey brain, *J. Comp. Neurol.* **193**:815–840.

Lim, R., 1980, Glia maturation factor, *Curr. Top. Develop. Biol.* **16**:305–322.

Lim, R., Mitsunobu, K., and Li, W. K. P., 1973, Maturation-stimulated effect of brain extract and dibutyryl cyclic AMP on dissociated embryonic brain cells in culture, *Exp. Cell Res.* **79**:243–246.

McCarthy, K. D., and de Vellis, J., 1978, Alpha-adrenergic receptor modulation of beta-adrenergic 3'-5'-cyclic monophosphate levels in primary cultures of glia, *J. Cyclic Nucleotide Res.* **4**:15–26.

McCarthy, K. D., and de Vellis, J., 1979, The regulation of adenosine 3':5'-cyclic monophosphate accumulation in glia by alpha-adrenergic agonists, *Life Sci.* **24**:639–650.

McCarthy, K. D., and de Vellis, J., 1980, Preparation of separated astroglial and oligodendroglial cell cultures from rat cerebral tissue, *J. Cell Biol.* **85**:890–902.

McEwen, B. S., Davis, P. G., Parsons, B., and Pfaff, D. W., 1979, The brain as a target for steroid hormone action, *Annu. Rev. Neurosci.* **2**:65–112.

McGinnis, J. F., and de Vellis, J., 1974, Purification and characterization of rat brain glycerol phosphate dehydrogenase, *Biochim. Biophys. Acta* **364**:17–27.

McGinnis, J. F., and de Vellis, J., 1977, Differential hormonal regulation of L-glycerol-3-phosphate dehydrogenase in rat brain and skeletal muscle, *Arch. Biochem. Biophys.* **179**:682–691.

McMorris, F. A., 1983, Cyclic AMP induction of the myelin enzyme 2′,3′-cyclic nucleotide 3′-phosphohydrolase in rat oligodendrocytes, *J. Neurochem.* **41**:506–515.

Marchbanks, R. M., 1970, Ion transport and metabolism in brain, in: *Membrane and Ion Transport*, Volume 2 (E. E. Bittar, ed.), Wiley–Interscience, New York, pp. 145–184.

Massarelli, R., Sensenbrenner, M., Ebel, A., and Mandel, P., 1974, Kinetics of choline uptake in mixed neuronal-glial and exclusively glial cultures, *Neurobiology* **4**:414–418.

Meier, D., and Schachner, M., 1982, Immunoselection of oligodendrocytes by magnetic beads. II. *In vitro* maintenance of immunoselected oligodendrocytes, *J. Neurosci. Res.* **7**:135–145.

Meier, D. H., Lagenaur, C., and Schachner, M., 1982, Immunoselection of oligodendrocytes by magnetic beads. I. Determination of antibody coupling parameters and cell binding conditions, *J. Neurosci. Res.* **7**:119–134.

Moonen, G., Cam, Y., Sensenbrenner, M., and Mandel, P., 1975, Variability of the effects of serum-free medium, dibutyryl-cyclic AMP or theophylline on the morphology of cultured newborn rat astroblasts, *Cell Tissue Res.* **163**:365–372.

Mori, S., and Leblond, C. P., 1970, Electron microscopic identification of three classes of oligodendrocytes and a preliminary study of their proliferative activity in the corpus callosum of young rats, *J. Comp. Neurol.* **139**:1–30.

Morris, J. E., and Moscona, A. A. 1971, The induction of glutamine synthetase in cell aggregates of embryonic neural retina: Correlations with differentiation and multicellular organization, *Develop. Biol.* **25**:420–444.

Morrison, R. S., and de Vellis, J., 1981, Growth of purified astrocytes in a chemically defined medium, *Proc. Natl. Acad. Sci. USA* **78**:7205–7209.

Morrison, R. S., and de Vellis, J., 1982, Growth and differentiation of purified astrocytes in a chemically defined medium, in: *Growth of Cells in Hormonally Defined Media*, Volume 9, Cold Spring Harbor Laboratory, Cold Spring Harbor, N.Y., pp. 973–985.

Morrison, R. S., and de Vellis, J., 1983, Differentiation of purified astrocytes in a chemically defined medium, *Develop. Brain Res.* **9**:337–345.

Morrison, R. S., Saneto, R. P., and de Vellis, J., 1982, Developmental expression of rat brain mitogens for cultured astrocytes, *J. Neurosci. Res.* **8**:435–451.

Mugnaini, E., and Walberg, F., 1964, Ultrastructure of neuroglia, *Ergeb. Anat. Entwicklungsgesch.* **37**:194–236.

Nissen, C., and Schousboe, A., 1979, Activity and isozyme pattern of lactate dehydrogenase in astroblasts cultured from brains of newborn mice, *J. Neurochem.* **32**:1787–1792.

Norenberg, M. D., and Martinez-Hernandez, A., 1979, Fine structural localization of glutamine synthetase in astrocytes of rat brain, *Brain Res.* **161**:303–310.

Norton, W. T., and Poduslo, S. E., 1973, Myelination in rat brain: Changes in myelin composition during brain maturation, *J. Neurochem.* **21**:759–773.

Pacold, S. T., and Blackard, W. G., 1979, Central nervous system insulin receptors in normal and diabetic rats, *Endocrinology* **105**:1452–1457.

Palay, S. L., 1958, An electron microscopical study of neuroglia, in: *Biology of Neuroglia* (W. F. Windle, ed.) Thomas, Springfield, Illinois, pp. 24–38.

Paterson, J. A., Privat, A., Ling, E. A., and Leblond, C. P., 1973, Investigation of glial cells in semithin sections. III. Transformation of subependymal cells into glial cells as shown by radioautography after ³H-thymidine injection into the lateral ventricle of the brain of young rats, *J. Comp. Neurol.* **149**:83–102.

Penfield, W., 1932, Neuroglia: Normal and pathological, in: *Cytology and Cellular Pathology of the Nervous System* (W. Penfield, ed.), Harper & Row (Hoeber), New York, pp. 422–479.

Peters, A., and Vaughn, J. E., 1967, Microtubules and filaments in the axons and astrocytes of early postnatal rat optic nerves, *J. Cell Biol.* **32**:113–119.

Peters, A., Palay, S. L. and Webster, H. de F., 1976, *The Fine Structure of the Nervous System: The Neurons and Supporting Cells*, W. B. Saunders, Philadelphia.

Pettman, B., Delaunoy, J., Courageot, J., Devilliers, G., and Sensenbrenner, M., 1980a, Rat brain glial cells in culture: Effects of brain extracts on the development of oligodendroglia-like cells, *Develop. Biol.* **75**:278–287.

Pettman, B., Sensenbrenner, M., and Labourdette, G., 1980b, Isolation of a glial maturation factor from beef brain, *FEBS Lett.* **118**:195–199.

Pleasure, D., Abramsky, O., Silberberg, D., Quinn, B., and Parvis, J., 1977, Biochemical studies of oligodendrocytes from calf brain, *Trans. Am. Soc. Neurochem.* **8**:143.

Poduslo, S. E., and Norton, W. T., 1972, Isolation and some chemical properties of oligodendroglia from calf brain, *J. Neurochem.* **19**:727–736.

Prasad, K., 1977, Role of cyclic nucleotides in differentiation of nerve cells, in: *Cell, Tissue, and Organ Cultures in Neurobiology* (S. Federoff and L. Hertz, eds.), Academic Press, New York, pp. 447–484.

Pruss, R. M., Bartlett, P. F., Gavrilovic, J., Lisak, R. P., and Rattray, S., 1982, Mitogens for glial cells: A comparison of the response of cultured astrocytes, oligodendrocytes and Schwann cells, *Develop. Brain Res.* **2**:19–35.

Raff, M. C., Mirsky, R., Fields, K. L., Lisak, R. P., Dorfman, S. H., Silberberg, D. H., Gregson, N. A., Leibowitz, S., and Kennedy, M. C., 1978, Galactocerebroside is a specific marker for oligodendroglia in culture, *Nature* **274**:813–815.

Rakic, P., 1971, Neuron–glia relationship during granule cell migration in developing cerebellar cortex: A Golgi and electron microscopic study in macacus rhesus, *J. Comp. Neurol.* **141**:282–312.

Ramón y Cajal, S., 1909, *Histologie du Système Nerveux de l'Homme et des Vertébrœs*, Maloine, Paris.

Ramón y Cajal, S., 1913, Contribucion al conocimento de la neuroglia del cerebro humano, *Trab. Lab. Invest. Biol. Univ. Madrid* **11**:255–315.

Ranscht, B., Clapshaw, P. A., Price, J., Noble, M., and Seifert, W., 1982, Development of oligodendrocytes and Schwann cells studied with a monoclonal antibody against galactocerebroside, *Proc. Natl. Acad. Sci. USA* **79**:2709–2713.

Saneto, R. P., Morrison, R. S., and de Vellis, J., 1982, Isolation and characterization of an astroglial mitogenic factor, *Soc. Neurosci. Abstr.* **8**:401.

Schachner, M., Schoonmaker, G., and Hynes, R. O., 1978, Cellular and subcellular localization of LETS protein in the nervous system, *Brain Res.* **158**:149–158.

Schachner, M., Kim, S. K., and Zehule, R., 1981, Developmental expression in central and peripheral nervous system of oligodendrocyte cell surface antigen (O antigens) recognized by monoclonal antibodies, *Develop. Biol.* **83**:328–338.

Schnitzer, J., Franke, W. W., and Schachner, M., 1981, Immunocytochemical demonstration of vimentin in astrocytes and ependymal cells of developing and adult mouse nervous system, *J. Cell Biol.* **90**:435–447.

Schousboe, A., Fosmark, H., and Hertz, L., 1975, High content of glutamate and of ATP in astrocytes cultured from rat brain hemispheres; effect of serum withdrawal and of cAMP, *J. Neurochem.* **25**:909–911.

Schousboe, A., Bock, E., and Hertz, L., 1977, Effect of Bt₂ cAMP and serum withdrawal on morphological and biochemical differentiation of normal astrocytes in culture, *Proc. Int. Soc. Neurochem.* **6**:435.

Schwartz, H. L., and Oppenheimer, J. H., 1978, Physiologic and biochemical actions of thyroid hormones, *Pharmacol. Ther. B.* **3**:349–376.

Sensenbrenner, M., 1977, Dissociated brain cells in primary culture, in: *Cell, Tissue, and Organ Cultures in Neurobiology* (S. Fedoroff and L. Hertz, eds.) pp. 191–213, Academic Press, New York.

Shein, H. M., 1965, Propagation of human fetal spongioblasts and astrocytes in dispersed cell cultures, *Exp. Cell Res.* **40**:554–569.

Simpson, D. L., Morrison, R., de Vellis, J., and Herschman, H. R., 1982, Epidermal growth factor binding and mitogenic activity on purified populations of cells from the central nervous system, *J. Neurochem. Res.* **8**:453–462.

Skoff, R., Price, D., and Stocks, A., 1976, Electron microscopic autoradiographic studies of gliogenesis in rat optic nerve. I. Cell proliferation, *J. Comp. neurol.* **169**:291–312.

Snyder, D. S., Zimmerman, T. R., Farooq, M., Norton, W. T., and Cammer, W., 1983, Carbonic anhydrase, 5'-nucleotidase, and 2',3'-cyclic nucleotide-3-phosphodiesterase activities in oligodendrocytes, astrocytes and neurons isolated from the brain of developing rats, *J. Neurochem.* **40**:120–127.

Sprinkle, T. J., Zaruba, M. E., and McKhann, G. M., 1978, Activity of 2',3'-cyclic nucleotide 3'-phosphodiesterase in regions of rat brain during development: Quantitative relationship to myelin basic protein, *J. Neurochem.* **30**:309–314.

Sprinkle, T. J., Wells, M. R., Garver, F. A., and Smith, D. B., 1980, Studies on the Wolfgram high molecular weight CNS myelin proteins: Relationships to 2',3'-cyclic nucleotide 3'-phosphodiesterase, *J. Neurochem.* **35**:1200–1208.

Stephans, J., and Pieringer, R. A., 1981, Hydrocortisone stimulates myelination *in vitro* in defined media, *Trans. Am. Soc. Neurochem.* **12**:226.

Szuchet, S., and Stefansson, K., 1980, *In vitro* behavior of isolated oligodendrocytes, *Adv. Cell. Neurobiol.* **1**:313–345.

Szuchet, S., Stefansson, K., Wollman, R. L., Dawson, G., and Arnason, B. G. W., 1980, Maintenance of isolated oligodendrocytes in long-term culture, *Brain Res.* **200**:151–164.

Tabor, C. W., and Tabor, H., 1976, 1,4-Diaminobutane (putrescine), spermidine, and spermine, *Annu. Rev. Biochem.* **45**:285–306.

Tata, J. R., Ernster, L., Lindberg, O., Arrhenius, E., Pedersen, S., and Hedman, R., 1963, The action of thyroid hormones at the cell level, *Biochem. J.* **86**:408–428.

Vaughn, J., 1969, An electron microscopic analysis of gliogenesis in rat optic nerves, *Z. Zellforsch. Mikrosk. Anat.* **94**:293–324.

Vernadakis, A., 1971, Hormonal factors in the proliferation of glial cells in culture, in: *Influence of Hormones on the Nervous System* (D. H. Ford, ed.), Karger, Basel, pp. 42–55.

Viarengo, A., Zoricheddu, A., Taningher, M., and Orunesu, M., 1975, Sequential stimulation of nuclear RNA polymerase activities in livers from thyroidectomized rats treated with triiodothyronine, *Endocrinology* **97**:955–961.

Virchow, R., 1860, *Cellular Pathology as Based upon Physiological and Pathological Histology* (edited and translated by F. Chance), Churchill, London.

Westermark, B., and Wasteson, A., 1975, The response of cultured human normal glial cells to growth factors, *Adv. Metab. Disord.* **8**:85–100.

Witter, B., and Debuch, H., 1982, On the phospholipid metabolism of glial cell primary cultures: Cell characterization and their utilization of 1-alkyl-glycerophosphoethanolamine, *J. Neurochem.* **38:**1029–1037.

Yamamoto, K. R., and Alberts, B. M., 1976, Steroid receptor elements for modulation of eukaryotic transcription, *Annu. Rev. Biochem.* **45:**721–746.

5

Environmental Influences on the Development of Sympathetic Neurons

STORY C. LANDIS

Peripheral autonomic ganglia provide an excellent source of neurons for tissue culture. The ganglia represent, in most cases, discrete and easily dissected packets of neurons. These packets contain relatively homogeneous populations of neurons whose neurotransmitter properties are largely known and for which a number of assays, cytochemical, biochemical, and eletrophysiological, are readily available. In the case of sympathetic ganglia, the neurons are still relatively immature at birth and therefore amenable to dissociation and culturing. Further, the trophic factor, nerve growth factor (NGF), for these cells is not only known but can readily be purified in reasonable quantities from a relatively accessible source. All of these advantages have in aggregate allowed the exploitation of a cell culture system for dissociated neurons from the superior cervical ganglion (SCG) of the newborn rat. This system has yielded a number of new insights into neurotransmitter plasticity and stability, multiple neurotransmitter function, and environmental influences on development. The purpose of this review is to summarize what has been learned from this culture system and to briefly

STORY C. LANDIS • Department of Neurobiology, Harvard Medical School, Boston, Massachusetts 02115.

describe recent studies aimed at establishing the relevance of these findings to normal development in the intact animal.

1. DEVELOPMENT OF SYMPATHETIC NEURONS IN CULTURE

1.1. Early Noradrenergic Phenotype

Neurons can be dissociated from the SCG of newborn rats and grown in culture (Fig. 1 and 2). Initially, all of the neurons appear to synthesize and store catecholamines. Following permanganate fixation, which reveals vesicular stores of norepinephrine (NE) as small granular vesicles (SGV) (Richardson, 1966), the growth cones of these neurons contain numerous SGV (Landis, 1978), and all of the synapses and varicosities which form during the first week after plating contain SGV when endogenous stores of catecholamine are localized (Landis, 1980) (see Fig. 5) or when exogenously supplied catecholamines are examined (Johnson et al., 1976, 1980b). Further, only catecholamine synthesis can be detected when transmitter synthesis is assayed biochemically during the first week after plating (Mains and Patterson, 1973; Patterson and Chun, 1977b). The early expression of noradrenergic properties by dissociated sympathetic neurons is not surprising. The neural crest cells that will give rise to sympathetic neurons appear to receive an adrenergic signal from their environment during migration (Cohen, 1972; Norr, 1974; Teillet et al., 1978). As soon as sympathetic ganglia can be discerned, immature neurons are seen which exhibit formaldehyde-induced catecholamine histofluorescence and tyrosine- and dopamine-β-hydroxylase-like immunoreactivities (DeChamplain et al., 1970; Cochard et al., 1978, 1979; Teitelman et al., 1978, 1979). By birth in the rat, virtually all of the neurons in the SCG contain catecholamine fluorescence (Eranko, 1972). At present, there is no evidence for comparably early expression of cholinergic function in rat sympathetic neurons or their precursors in vivo or in culture of their precursors. This is in contrast to avian development: acetylcholine (ACh) synthesis has been detected in populations of migrating neural crest cells from both mesencephalic and trunk levels (Smith et al., 1979).

1.2. Conditions That Promote Noradrenergic Development

Under certain culture conditions, the dissociated sympathetic neurons continue to differentiate noradrenergically and develop many of the properties characteristic of mature sympathetic neurons in vivo. One

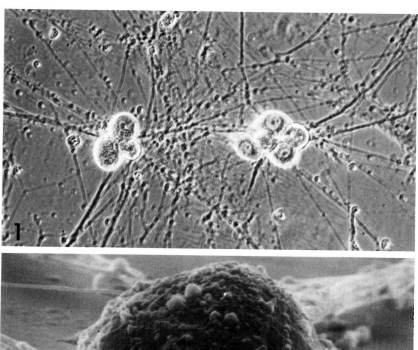

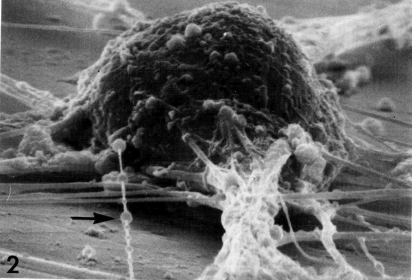

Figure 1. Phase micrograph of dissociated sympathetic neurons in culture. After 2 weeks in culture, the neuron cell bodies are reasonably large and interconnected by a still sparse plexus of axons. These neurons were enzymatically dissociated from the superior cervical ganglia of newborn rats. The debris results from nonneuronal cells dying after treatment with antimitotic agents. Two nonneuronal cells still remain in this field. × 250.

Figure 2. Scanning electron micrograh of a cultured sympathetic neuron. This micrograph was taken at high tilt so that the observer has the sense of standing on the dish next to the neuron. Note that the neuron cell body does not rest directly on the dish next to the neuron. Bundles of processes join this neuron with others in the culture. The core of the process bundle coming directly out from the cell is likely to be a dendrite along which a number of axons course. The arrow indicates a single·axon with several varicosities along its length. × 2500.

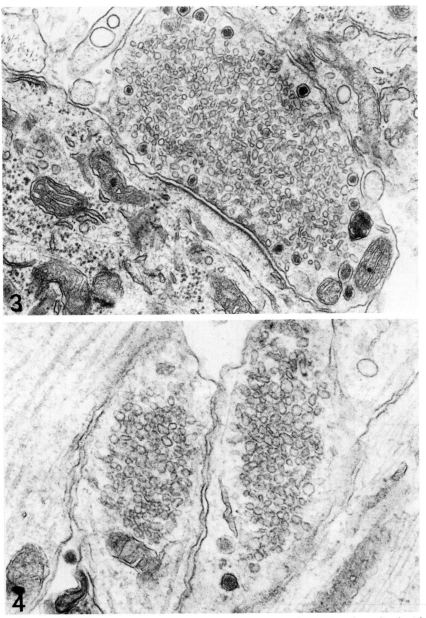

Figure 3. Electron micrograph of a synapse from a mature adrenergic culture fixed with aldehyde–osmium. The presynaptic ending contains numerous pleiomorphic synaptic vesicles, mitochondria, and large dense-core vesicles. Discontinuous dense material lines the presynaptic membrane and contrasts with the more uniform postsynaptic density. These

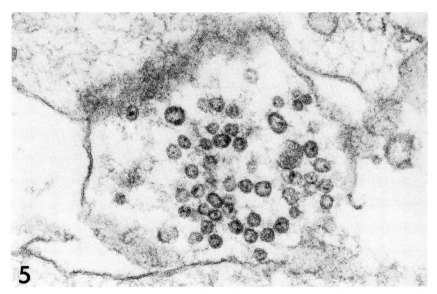

Figure 5. Electron micrograph of a varicosity from a very young culture grown under cholinergic-promoting conditions and fixed with permanganate. The first synapses and varicosities that form in the cultures of dissociated sympathetic neurons contain numerous small granular vesicles indicating their content of endogenous catecholamines. This is true whether the cultures are grown under adrenergic- or cholinergic-promoting conditions. × 40,000.

such culture condition involves maintaining the dissociated sympathetic neurons in the virtual absence of nonneuronal cells (Figs. 1 and 2). This can be accomplished in several ways: growth in medium that lacks bicarbonate ions (Mains and Patterson, 1973), several treatments with an antimitotic agent such as cytosine arabinoside (Hawrot and Patterson, 1979) or 5-fluorodeoxyuridine (Wakshull *et al.*, 1978). In general, it has proven easier to obtain pure cultures of neurons if the sympathetic ganglia are mechanically rather than enzymatically dissociated. Even more effective in promoting exclusively noradrenergic differentiation is growth under depolarizing conditions such as the presence of elevated

---

membrane specializations are identical under all growth conditions including in defined medium. × 40,000.

Figure 4. Electron micrograph of a varicosity from a mature adrenergic culture fixed with aldehyde–osmium. As at synapses, the axonal varicosity contains many synaptic vesicles. However, no postsynaptic target is evident and no membrane specializations can be discerned in the terminal. These varicosities are seen frequently in the axon bundles and adjacent to but not directly apposed to cell bodies. × 40,000.

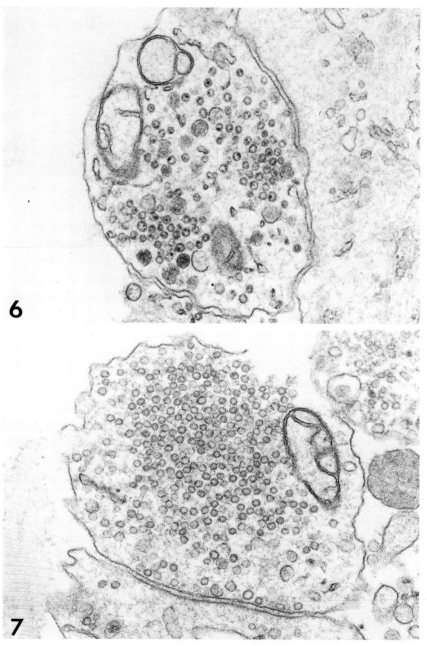

Figure 6. Electron micrograph of a synapse from a mature adrenergic culture fixed with permanganate. After several weeks in culture, all of the synapses and varicosities present

potassium levels (20 mM instead of 5 mM) or veratridine (Walicke *et al.*, 1977).

Mature cultures of neurons grown under these adrenergic-promoting conditions synthesize and store primarily the catecholamines dopamine and NE (Mains and Patterson, 1973; Patterson and Chun, 1977a). They can take up and store exogenous catecholamines and release them in a calcium-dependent manner (Burton and Bunge, 1975; Patterson *et al.*, 1975). *In vitro* as *in vivo*, these sympathetic neurons possess many axonal varicosities containing numerous synaptic vesicles (Figs. 2–4). Some varicosities form morphologically specialized synapses on neuronal cell bodies and dendrites (Rees and Bunge, 1974; Buckley and Landis, 1983a) with pre- and postsynaptic membrane specializations characteristic of asymmetric synapses like those which these neurons receive from preganglionic axons *in vivo* (Figs. 3 and 4). The synaptic terminals and varicosities in culture contain predominantly SGV after permanganate fixation (Rees and Bunge, 1974; Landis, 1980) (Fig. 6) and appear similar to those that the neurons would have formed in the SCG itself (Grillo, 1966; Matthews, 1974) and in target tissues such as the iris and salivary gland (Hokfelt, 1969). Morphological examination of depolarized and recovering terminals suggests that transmitter release occurs from both morphologically specialized synapses and unspecialized vesicle-containing varicosities with approximately equal frequencies by an exocytotic mechanism (Buckley and Landis, 1983b). In culture, sympathetic neurons are relatively insensitive to catecholamines (O'Lague *et al.*, 1978a,b; Wakshull *et al.*, 1979), and synaptic interactions have not been detected between noradrenergic neurons (O'Lague *et al.*, 1978b). Thus, the numerous morphologically specialized synapses present appear to be electrophysiologically silent.

1.3. Conditions That Promote Cholinergic Development

It has also proven possible to grow cultures of dissociated sympathetic neurons under conditions such that the cultures develop cholinergic as well as noradrenergic properties. One condition which fosters the induction of cholinergic properties is the presence of certain nonneuronal cells (Patterson and Chun, 1974, 1979a). A number of kinds

---

in cultures grown under adrenergic-promoting conditions contain almost exclusively small granular vesicles. × 40,000.

Figure 7. Electron micrograph of a synapse from a mature cholinergic culture fixed with permanganate. After several weeks in culture, many of the synapses and varicosities present in cultures grown under cholinergic-promoting conditions contain no small granular vesicles, but only clear ones, × 40,000.

of rat nonneuronal cells have proven effective: ganglionic nonneuronal cells; heart cells, both myocytes and fibroblasts; and skeletal myotubes among others. In general, all tissues that receive a cholinergic innervation, sympathetic or otherwise, seem able to induce cholinergic function while tissues such as liver which do not receive any cholinergic innervation appear incapable of inducing cholinergic properties. The effect also is species-specific in that chick and mouse nonneuronal cells have no effect. Under these growth conditions, significant amounts of ACh as well as catecholamines are synthesized (Patterson and Chun, 1974, 1977a); choline acetyltransferase (CAT) activity increases (Johnson et al., 1976, 1980a; Patterson and Chun, 1977a) and the neurons form excitatory cholinergic synapses with each other (O'Lague et al., 1974, 1978a,b; Ko et al., 1976; Wakshull et al., 1979) and cholinergic junctions with heart myocytes (Furshpan et al., 1976) as well as skeletal myotubes (Nurse and O'Lague, 1975; Nurse, 1982). As under adrenergic-promoting growth conditions, many axonal varicosities are evident along the neuronal processes and some of these also participate in morphologically specialized junctions (Buckley and Landis, 1983a). The membrane specializations at these synapses are indistinguishable in both thin section and freeze-fracture from those present in adrenergic cultures. The synapses and varicosities contain almost exclusively clear synaptic vesicles after permanganate fixation, which is consistent with but not proof of cholinergic function (Johnson et al., 1976, 1980b; Landis, 1976, 1980) (Fig. 7).

1.4. Effects of "Cholinergic Factor"

The induction of cholinergic properties by appropriate rat nonneuronal cells can occur through growth in medium conditioned (CM) by the nonneuronal cells, since they release a soluble cholinergic factor into the medium (Patterson et al., 1975; Landis et al., 1976; Patterson and Chun, 1977a). This effect has been examined most thoroughly in the case of medium conditioned by heart cells. Induction can also occur through direct contact with heart cell surfaces, since growth on heart cell monolayers killed by paraformaldehyde fixation induces ACh synthesis in the sympathetic neurons (Hawrot, 1980). At present, it is not clear whether the surface factor is identical to or different from the soluble factor. Growth in high concentrations of heart cell CM not only induces cholinergic properties but also causes a simultaneous decline in catecholamine synthesis (Patterson and Chun, 1977a; Reichardt and Patterson, 1977; Fukada, 1980). More recently, the effect of CM on the catecholamine synthetic enzymes has been examined directly; tyrosine hydroxylase activity and immunoreactivity is decreased under strongly cholinergic-promoting growth conditions as is dopamine-β-hydroxylase activity (Wolinsky and Patterson, 1983; Swerts et al., 1983). Bunge and his colleagues have found that cholinergic function can be induced by growth in high concentrations of human placental serum and chick embryo extract in the absence of nonneuronal cells (Wakshull et al., 1978). These agents do not, however, appear to lead to a simultaneous fall in catecholamine synthetic enzymes as does a high concentration of CM (Higgins et al., 1981; Iacovitti et al., 1981). The potential of medium additives such as serum for influencing neuronal phenotypic properties has been underscored by comparison of sympathetic cultures grown in the presence or absence of such complex medium additives. Iacovitti et al. (1982) reported that sympathetic neurons grown in N2 defined medium (Bottenstein and Sato, 1979) synthesized no ACh and surprisingly stored little NE. The addition of adult rat serum to cultures grown under similar but not identical serum-free conditions results in a dose-dependent induction of ACh synthesis (Wolinsky et al., 1983).

Several of the properties of the diffusible cholinergic factor secreted by heart cells have been described and work is in progress to purify and characterize it. The cholinergic factor has been partially purified from serum-containing CM and has an approximate molecular weight of 50,000. It is highly sensitive to periodate but relatively stable to heat, urea, guanidine, and mercaptoethanol (Weber, 1981). Heart cells can also condition serum-free medium. The production or release of the cholinergic factor in serum-free medium is influenced by certain hormones and growth factors; epidermal growth factor (EGF) increases its release whereas glucocorticoids decrease its release (Fukada, 1980) and therefore the cholinergic induction (McLennan et al., 1980). Additional purification has been achieved from this defined medium with an increase in specific activity of more than 10,000-fold. The most purified activity is sensitive to trypsin and both induces cholinergic function and inhibits the development of adrenergic properties in sympathetic cultures (Fukada, 1983). It is clear that the cholinergic factor is different from nerve growth factor (NGF) since NGF is required for survival and stimulates the growth and differentiation of both noradrenergic and cholinergic neurons while CM has no effect on survival or growth but selectively increases cholinergic differentiation (Chun and Patterson, 1977a,b).

CM not only affects the neurotransmitter phenotype of dissociated sympathetic neurons developing in culture but also influences a number of other properties. Soybean agglutinin binding sites are decreased fourfold when cultures are grown under cholinergic- as opposed to adrenergic-promoting conditions (Schwab and Landis, 1981); these binding sites appear to be glycolipids, globoside and lesser amounts of two others (Zurn, 1982). In contrast, there is an increase in cholera toxin binding sites under cholinergic-promoting conditions, but no change in tetanus toxin binding (Schwab and Landis, 1981). In addition, there are changes in the expression of monoamine oxidase (Pintar *et al.*, 1981) and of certain membrane proteins as well as secreted and substrate-attached proteins (Braun *et al.*, 1981; Sweadner, 1981). The changes in cell surface properties and in the nature of the secreted proteins could play an important role in selective synaptogenesis or in trophic interactions during normal development *in vivo*.

The cholinergic factor produced by nonneuronal cells induces neurons to become cholinergic that have alredy begun to differentiate along a noradrenergic pathway. As described above, shortly after plating all the dissociated neurons exhibit noradrenergic properties, and cholinergic ones appear only later (Johnson *et al.*, 1976, 1980b; Patterson and Chun, 1977b; Landis, 1980). Further, under the most cholinergic-promoting conditions, reciprocity is evident between adrenergic and cholinergic functions (Patterson and Chun, 1977a; Reichardt and Patterson, 1977; Fukada, 1980; Wolinsky and Patterson, 1983; Swerts *et al.*, 1983), while neuronal number remains constant.

Physiological and morphological studies of microcultures have provided direct evidence for a transition from noradrenergic to cholinergic function during development in culture. The microcultures used in these studies consist of one to several neurons growing on a small island of heart myocytes and fibroblasts approximately 300 to 500 μ in diameter (Fig. 8). Usually 25 to 30 of these microcultures will be grown in the center of a 35-mm culture dish. The myocytes are sensitive to both NE and ACh and serve as a bioassay for these two neurotransmitters in physiological studies; the use of appropriate antagonists permits further dissection of neuronal action on the heart. After the neurotransmitter phenotype of the neuron has been characterized physiologically and pharmacologically, then the microculture can be prepared for electron microscopy and its fine structure examined. Such studies allow an unambiguous correlation of structure and function at the single-cell level. Some neurons have been identified which appear to only excite the heart myocytes; this effect can be blocked by propranolol or atenolol, and the terminals of these neurons contain many SGV after permanganate fixation (Furshpan *et al.*, 1976, 1982; Landis, 1976; Potter *et al.*, 1981a,b). Other neurons appear to have only an inhibitory effect on the heart cells which could be blocked by atropine. The terminals of these neurons contained only clear synaptic vesicles after permanganate fixation and

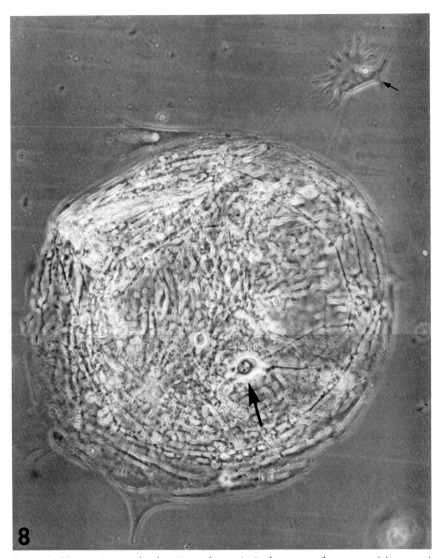

Figure 8. Phase micrograph of a microculture. A single neuron (large arrow) is present on an island of heart myocytes and fibroblasts. The neuron is still relatively young so that the individual processes can be distinguished on the heart monolayer. In the upper right is a fibroblast (small arrow). A single neurite from the neurons has been carried with this nonneuronal cell and appears out of focus. ×200.

have thus been identified as functionally purely cholinergic. In addition, many neurons have now been identified that are bifunctional and release both ACh and NE. The terminals of these neurons contain both small granular and clear synaptic vesicles and therefore appear intermediate in function (Furshpan et al., 1976, 1982; Landis, 1976; Potter et al., 1980, 1981a,b). Among these single neurons, the relative balance of noradrenergic and cholinergic function, assayed both physiologically and morphologically, varies. This variation is consistent with a shift in neurotransmitter function. Further, repeated physiological assays of single neurons over time have disclosed transitions from noradrenergic to bifunctional and from bifunctional to cholinergic. Most significantly, in several instances a complete transition from noradrenergic to bifunctional to cholinergic has been demonstrated in a single neuron (Potter et al., 1981b).

Most recently, the release of an additional neurotransmitter candidate has been detected in the microculture system. Some neurons cause an atropine-resistant hyperpolarization in the myocytes. This effect can be mimicked by puffing adenosine onto the heart cells. It can be blocked by adenosine deaminase, which deaminates adenosine to form inosine, and by the adenosine antagonist 8-phenyltheophylline (Furshpan et al., 1982). These observations suggest that the dissociated sympathetic neurons may release a purine, adenosine, as well as ACh and NE (for reviews of purinergic transmission see Burnstock, 1972, 1976). Neurons have been observed in microcultures which appear to release adenosine only, as well as in combination with either or both ACh and NE. Preliminary ultrasturctural observations on the terminals of neurons physiologically characterized as strongly purinergic have disclosed the presence of synaptic-size vesicles with a dense core after glutaraldehyde–osmium but not permanganate fixation (S. Landis, unpublished observations); similar vesicles have been described previously in vivo in regions where nonadrenergic, noncholinergic (and therefore possibly purinergic) transmission occurs (Wilson et al., 1979; Iijima, 1981; Gibbons, 1982). Additional studies are in progress to confirm this association of vesicle morphology and purinergic transmission.

The effect of the cholinergic factor on neurotransmitter choice appears to be dose-dependent. In mass cultures containing several thousand neurons, the higher the proportion of CM in the growth medium, the more ACh is synthesized, the more cholinergic interactions are observed physiologically, and the more apparently cholinergic synapses are identified morphologically (Landis et al., 1976; Patterson and Chun, 1977a; Landis, 1980). Although at low concentrations of CM, or in the presence of other weakly inducing agents such as chick embryo extract or rat serum, catecholamine production and the activities of the catecholamine synthetic enzymes are not reduced, at high concentrations of CM, these noradrenergic functions are significantly suppressed (Patterson and Chun, 1977; Iacovitti *et al.*, 1981; Wolinsky and Patterson, 1983; Swerts *et al.*, 1983). Biochemical studies of single neurons indicate that the proportion of neurons that undergo transition is dependent upon the strength of the cholinergic stimulus (Reichardt and Patterson, 1977). In addition, physiological studies of individual neurons in microcultures make it clear that the rate of transition varies from neuron to neuron and suggest that the strength of the cholinergic stimulus is one of the factors that affect the rate (Potter *et al.*, 1980, 1981b). Thus, in general, transitions appear to occur more slowly in microcultures where relatively few heart cells are present than in mass cultures or single-neuron microcultures treated with high concentrations of CM (Patterson and Chun, 1977a,b; Reichardt and Patterson, 1977; Potter *et al.*, 1980, 1981a,b).

The induction of ACh synthesis need not result in the immediate turnoff of noradrenergic functions. In the microcultures, neurons have been observed to secrete both NE and ACh for several weeks (Potter *et al.*, 1980, 1981a,b). Under culture conditions that apparently provide a relatively weak cholinergic stimulus, mass cultures can show coordinate increases in both noradrenergic and cholinergic synthetic enzyme activities (Iacovitti *et al.*, 1981) and 90% of the neurons may exhibit tyrosine hydroxylase-like immunoreactivity in cultures where 85% of the cells interact cholinergically (Higgins *et al.*, 1981). Further, not all noradrenergic properties are lost at the same rate and it is possible that some noradrenergic properties may only be reduced and not completely eliminated even when the transition is complete. For example, biochemical and correlated physiological and morphological studies of single neurons (Furshpan *et al.*, 1976; Landis, 1976; Potter *et al.*, 1980, 1981b) have demonstrated that neurons that no longer synthesize and store or secrete detectable quantities of catecholamines can still take up and store some exogenous catecholamine.

The ability of sympathetic neurons to respond to cholinergic factors appears to decrease with age under some experimental conditions. When neurons are dissociated from the SCG of newborn rats, they are more responsive to CM added during the first or second week than during the third or fourth (Patterson and Chun, 1977b). Cholinergic induction which is age-dependent has also been described in explant cultures. If explants of SCG are taken from neonatal rats, the neurons in these cultures will develop cholinergic properties, CAT activity, and the number of apparently cholinergic endings increase with time in culture; and coculture with heart muscle or growth in a cardiac extract causes greater cholinergic induction (Hill and Hendry, 1977; Ross et al., 1977; Hill et al., 1980; Johnson et al., 1980a). If instead of explant cultures, neurons from adult animals are dissociated and then grown in culture, at least some of these cells are able to form cholinergic synapses with each other and with skeletal myotubes (Wakshull et al., 1979). It is unlikely that the dissociation procedure somehow selects for the small population of cholinergic sympathetic neurons thought to be present in the adult SCG, since preliminary examination of dissociated adult neurons in microcultures of cardiac myocytes has shown that many of these neurons initially release only NE and become bifunctional with time, secreting both NE and ACh (Potter et al., 1981b). Several explanations exist for the observed difference in plasticity between mature neurons in explants and after dissociation; for example, the organotypic environment of the explant may protect the neurons from cholinergic influences or the dissociation procedure may be more traumatic than explantation and case the neurons to "dedifferentiate" and become susceptible again to cholinergic influences.

Neuronal activity has also been shown to play a role in influencing neurotransmitter choice in this culture system. The noradrenergic differentiation in vitro is stabilized and enhanced by growing the neurons under depolarizing conditions or by stimulating the neurons to fire electrophysiologically (Walicke et al., 1977). Such conditions both increase catecholamine synthesis and tyrosine hydroxylase activity and can largely prevent the neurons from responding to the cholinergic factor in CM. The effect of depolarization appears to be mediated by calcium ions (Walicke and Patterson, 1981). However, evidence for the control of neurotransmitter choice by activity in vivo is lacking (Hill and Hendry, 1979).

The multidisciplinary examination of the development of dissociated newborn rat sympathetic neurons in mass cultures and in microcultures has disclosed a number of surprising observations. First these neurons are plastic with regard to their neurotransmitter phenotype, even after they have begun to express one set of differentiated neurotransmitter properties. Second, the environment in which these neurons develop can have a profound influence on their phenotype, both with respect to neurotransmitter function as well as other biochemical properties. Finally, a single neuron can release at least two traditional neurotransmitters, NE and ACh, and the neurotransmitter repertoire of individual neurons may include purines and peptides as well. An obvious question that arises from these studies concerns the relationship of these cell culture properties to those of analogous neurons in vivo. In short, are these cell culture artifacts? In one sense, these properties can never be artifacts of cell culture since they represent the biological potential of these neurons. However, the neurotransmitter plasticity and environmental control of phenotype need not necessarily mirror normal developmental processes in the intact animal. In order to examine this issue, we have begun to study the development of cholinergic sympathetic neurons *in vivo* to determine how closely their developmental history parallels that observed in culture.

2. COMPARISONS WITH THE DEVELOPMENT OF CHOLINERGIC SYMPATHETIC NEURONS *IN VIVO*

2.1. Cholinergic Sympathetic Innervation of Sweat Glands

The first task in these studies has been to choose and characterize an appropriate cholinergic sympathetic system for analysis. The best characterized cholinergic sympathetic neurons are those which innervate eccrine sweat glands. Langley (1891, 1894) demonstrated that stimulation of the sympathetic outflow from the stellate and certain lumbar ganglia caused sweating in the cat and that the pharmacology of this response was cholinergic rather than adrenergic, as in most other sympathetic targets (Langley, 1922). In 1934, Dale and Feldberg demonstrated the presence of ACh in the venous effluent from gland-containing regions of the paw after nerve stimulation. In addition, AChE staining is pronounced around the sweat glands and in a small proportion of ganglionic neurons that are concentrated in those cat sympathetic ganglia that yielded the greatest sweating with nerve stimulation (Sjoqvist, 1963a,b). Recently, Lundberg et al. (1979) described the presence of vasoactive intestinal polypeptide (VIP)-like immunoreactivity in the fibers that innervate sweat glands and in strongly AChE-positive neurons in the cat.

Rats, like cats, have sweat glands concentrated in their footpads (Ring and Randall, 1946). Each gland contains a single, unbranched but tightly coiled secretory tubule which is ensheathed by a thick connective tissue capsule. As in the cat, sweating can be induced by muscarinic agonists (Weschler and Fisher, 1968; Quatrale and Laden, 1968; Sato and Sato, 1978; L. Stevens and S. Landis, unpublished observations) as well as by nerve stimulation (Ring and Randall, 1946); nerve-evoked sweating can be blocked by muscarinic antagonists (L. Stevens and S. Landis, unpublished observations). The glands possess an AChE- and VIP-positive nerve plexus (Winkelman and Schmit, 1959; Siegel et al.,

1982; Landis and Keefe, 1983). In thin sections, the AChE-stained fibers are seen as bundles of 8–12 axons that course throughout the gland. Varicosities containing the usual complement of small clear synaptic and large dense-core vesicles are numerous but they do not form close or specialized junctions (Landis and Keefe, 1983). The pattern of innervation is very similar to that described previously in the primate (Uno and Montagna, 1975). In adult rats, there is no evidence for the presence of endogenous catecholamines in the axons that innervate the sweat glands; no fluorescent fibers are present in Falck–Hillarp or glyoxylic acid preparations and no SGV are seen after permanganate fixation (Landis and Keefe, 1983). In contrast, in primates occasional fluorescent fibers and SGV-containing terminals are seen (Uno and Montagna, 1975).

2.2. Developmental Changes in the Transmitter-Related Phenotype of Sweat Gland Innervation

The hind footpads and the sweat glands which they contain develop during the first 3 weeks of life in the rat (Landis and Keefe, 1983). The arrival of innervating axons can first be detected with catecholamine fluorescent techniques. At 4 days, noradrenergic fibers are associated with both the forming glands and adjacent blood vessels. Endogenous catecholamines persist in the developing innervation until 21 to 25 days; although from 14 days on, the fibers associated with the developing glands are increasingly less fluorescent than those innervating adjacent blood vessels. Permanganate fixation and ultrastructural examination of the developing innervation have shown that all of the axon profiles at 7 and 10 days contain SGV, indicating the synthesis and storage of catecholamine (Fig. 9). Relatively few SGV are present at 14 days and by 21 days the SGV have disappeared (Fig. 10). At no time have we observed axonal degeneration in the developing plexus. These observations indicate that the developing sweat glands were innervated by noradrenergic axons which lost their stores of endogenous catecholamines as they formed an axonal plexus in the maturing gland.

The mature sweat gland innervation is characterized by AChE staining and immunoreactivity for VIP (Siegel et al., 1982; Landis and Keefe, 1983). In contrast to the early appearance of noradrenergic function, AChE staining is first observed around a few glands at 7 days. It is present in all of the glands at 10 days and reaches adult levels by 21 days. VIP-like immunoreactivity appears slightly later than AChE. Thus, the developing innervation initially contains catecholamines, while AChE and VIP-like immunoreactivity appear later but before the catecholamine histofluorescence and SGV have disappeared. Although

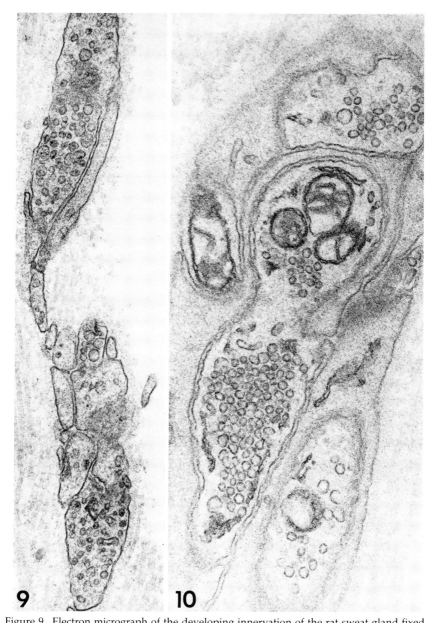

Figure 9. Electron micrograph of the developing innervation of the rat sweat gland fixed with permanganate. Numerous small granular vesicles are present in the axonal varicosities of the developing cholinergic sympathetic innervation of this target. × 35,000.

Figure 10. Electron micrograph of the mature innervation of the rat sweat gland fixed with permanganate. No small granular vesicles are present in the axonal varicosities of the adult innervation. This is similar to the changes described during the development of cholinergic sympathetic neurons in culture. × 45,000.

AChE and VIP staining are present in the mature innervation, they represent at best indirect assays for the appearance of cholinergic function and it will be important to examine cholinergic properties directly.

This descriptive analysis of the developing innervation is consistent with a transition from noradrenergic function to cholinergic *in vivo* as in culture. Two additional lines of evidence provide further support for such a transition. The first comes from the observation that the mature innervation, although functionally cholinergic, retains some noradrenergic properties. If adult rats or footpad slices are exposed to exogenous catecholamine, a plexus of fluorescent fibers appears in the sweat glands and each axonal varicosity contains a small proportion of SGV (Landis and Keefe, 1983). The uptake and storage exhibit characteristic adrenergic pharmacology and appear to be restricted to peripheral cholinergic neurons that are sympathetic. Not only do these cholinergic sympathetic neurons retain a catecholamine uptake and storage system, but they also possess some immunoreactivity for the catecholamine synthetic enzymes, tyrosine hydroxylase and dopamine-β-hydroxylase (Siegel *et al.*, 1982). Although these noradrenergic characteristics are detectable, they are reduced in extent from the same properties in adrenergic sympathetic neurons. The second line of evidence comes from studies on the effect of 6-hydroxydopamine (6-OHDA) (Yodlowski *et al.*, 1984), which is a toxic congener of NE that accumulates in and selectively destroys adrenergic terminals. If neonatal rats are treated with 6-OHDA during the first postnatal week, not only do the axons degenerate, but also the neuronal cell bodies, resulting in a virtually complete sympathectomy (Angeletti and Levi-Montalcini, 1970; Angeletti, 1971; Finch *et al.*, 1973). We have found that neonatal treatment with 6-OHDA causes not only the loss of the adrenergic sympathetic plexus but also the loss of the cholinergic sympathetic innervation of sweat glands. Although the sweat glands appear to develop normally, AChE and VIP staining and the characteristic axonal varicosities are absent from the glands. In contrast, if adult rats are treated with identical doses of 6-OHDA, only the adrenergic sympathetic plexus is affected. Thus, cholinergic sympathetic axons only appear to be sensitive to 6-OHDA treatment early in development.

The studies summarized above have demonstrated a number of similarities between the development of cholinergic sympathetic neurons in cell culture and *in vivo*. In both instances, there is evidence for early noradrenergic function which is then lost and for the continued presence of at least some noradrenergic properties, although at a reduced level, in neurons that are functionally cholinergic. Moreover, the neurotransmitter plasticity exhibited by cholinergic sympathetic neurons during development does not appear to be unique. Previous studies of the embryonic gut have described the presence of cells that transiently express noradrenergic properties (Cochard *et al.*, 1978, 1979; Teitelman *et al.*, 1979). Although the differentiated fate of these cells is, with one exception, unknown, it has been generally assumed that they develop into nonadrenergic enteric neurons. In one instance, the transient catecholaminergic cells that lie in the developing pancreas have been shown to become glucagon-containing cells of the pancreatic islets (Teitelman *et al.*, 1981). In the sympathetic neuron culture system, which permitted the first and most convincing demonstration of transmitter plasticity in single neurons, it has been possible to elucidate partially the developmental signals that affect neurotransmitter choice and plasticity. Having obtained evidence for a similar plasticity during the development of analogous neurons *in vivo*, it will be important to determine if these same signals play a role during normal development.

REFERENCES

Angeletti, P. U., 1971, Chemical sympathectomy in newborn animals, *Neuropharmacology* **10:**55–59.

Angeletti, P. U., and Levi-Montalcini, R., 1970, Sympathetic nerve cell destruction in newborn mammals by 6-hydroxydopamine, *Proc. Natl. Acad. Sci. USA* **65:**114–121.

Bottenstein, J., and Sato, G., 1979, Growth of a rat neuroblastoma cell line in serum-free supplemented medium, *Proc. Natl. Acad. Sci. USA* **76:**514–517.

Braun, S. J., Sweadner, K., and Patterson, P. H., 1981, Neuronal cells surfaces: Distinctive glycoproteins of cultured adrenergic and cholinergic sympathetic neurons, *J. Neurosci.* **1:**1397–1406.

Buckley, K. B., and Landis, S. C., 1983a, Morphological studies of synapses and varicosities in dissociated cell cultures of sympathetic neurons, *J. Neurocytol.* **12:**67–92.

Buckley, K. B., and Landis, S. C., 1983b, Morphological studies of neurotransmitter release and membrane recycling in sympathetic nerve terminals in culture, *J. Neurocytol.* **12:**93–116.

Burnstock, G., 1972, Purinergic nerves, *Pharmac. Rev.* **24:**509–581.

Burnstock, G., 1976, Purine nucleotides, *Adv. Biochem. Psychopharmacol.* **15:**225–235.

Burton, H., and Bunge, R. P., 1975, A comparison of the uptake and release of [^{3}H]-norepinephrine in rat autonomic and sensory ganglia in tissue culture, *Brain Res.* **97:**157–162.

Chun, L. L. Y., and Patterson, P. H., 1977a, Role of nerve growth factor in the development of rat sympathetic neurons in vitro. I. Survival, growth and differentiation of catecholamine production, *J. Cell Biol.* **75:**694–704.

Chun, L. L. Y., and Patterson, P. H., 1977b, Role of nerve growth factor in the development of rat sympathetic neurons in vitro. III. Effect on acetylcholine production. *J. Cell Biol.* **75:**712–718.

Cochard, P., Goldstein, M., and Black, I. B., 1978, Ontogenetic appearance and disappearance of tyrosine hydroxylase and catecholamines in the rat embryo, *Proc. Natl. Acad. Sci. USA* **75:**2986–2990.

Cochard, P., Goldstein, M., and Black, I. B., 1979, Initial development of the noradrenergic phenotype in autonomic neuroblasts of the rat embryo in vivo, *Develop. Biol.* **71:**100–114.

Cohen, A. M., 1972, Factors directing the expression of sympathetic nerve traits in cells of neural crest origin, *J. Exp. Biol.* **97:**167–182.

Dale, H. H., and Feldberg, W., 1934, The chemical transmission of secretory impulses to the sweat glands of the cat, *J. Physiol.* **82:**121–128.

DeChamplain, J., Malmfors, T., Olson, L., and Sachs, C., 1970, Ontogenesis of peripheral adrenergic neurons in the rat: Pre- and postnatal observations, *Acta Physiol. Scand.* **80:**276–288.

Eranko, L., 1972, Ultrastructure of the developing sympathetic nerve cell and the storage of catecholamines, *Brain Res.* **46:**159–172.

Finch, L., Haeusler, G., and Thoenen, H., 1973, A comparison of the effects of chemical sympathectomy by 6-hydroxydopamine in newborn and adult rats, *Br. J. Pharmacol.* **47:**249–260.

Fukada, K., 1980, Hormonal control of neurotransmitter choice in sympathetic neurone cultures, *Nature* **287:**553–555.

Fukada, K., 1983, Studies on the cholinergic differentiation factor for sympathetic neurons, *Soc. Neurosci. Abstr.* **9:**182.5.

Furshpan, E. J., MacLeish, P. R., O'Lague, P. H., and Potter, D. D., 1976, Chemical transmission between rat sympathetic neurons and cardiac myocytes developing in microcultures: Evidence for cholinergic, adrenergic and dual-function neurons, *Proc. Natl. Acad. Sci. USA* **73:**4225–4229.

Furshpan, E. J., Potter, D. D., and Landis, S. C., 1982, On the transmitter repertoire of sympathetic neurons in culture, *Harvey Lect.* **76:**149–191.

Gibbons, I. L., 1982, Lack of correlation between ultrastructural and pharmacological types of non-adrenergic autonomic nerves, *Cell Tissue Res.* **221:**551–581.

Grillo, M. A., 1966, Electron microscopy of sympathetic tissues, *Pharmacol. Rev.* **18:**387–399.

Hawrot, E., 1980, Cultured sympathetic neurons: Effects of cell-derived and synthetic substrata on survival and development, *Develop. Biol.* **74:**136–151.

Hawrot, E., and Patterson, P. H., 1979, Long term culture of dissociated sympathetic neurons, *Methods Enzymol.* **58:**574–584.

Higgins, D., Iacovitti, L., Joh, T. H., and Burton, H., 1981, The immunocytochemical localization of tyrosine hydroxylase within rat sympathetic neurons that release acetylcholine in culture, *J. Neurosci.* **1:**126–131.

Hill, C. E., and Hendry, I. E., 1977, Development of neurons synthesizing noradrenaline and acetylcholine in the superior cervical ganglion of the rat in vivo and in vitro, *Neuroscience* **2:**741–749.

Hill, C. E., and Hendry, I. E., 1979, The influence of preganglionic nerves on the superior cervical ganglion of the rat, *Neurosci. Lett.* **13:**133–139.

Hill, C. E., Hendry, I. A., and McLennan, I. S., 1980, Development of cholinergic neurons in cultures of rat superior cervical ganglia. Role of calcium and macromolecules, *Neuroscience* **5:**1027–1032.

Hokfelt, T., 1969, Distribution of noradrenaline storing particles in peripheral adrenergic neurons as revealed by electron microscopy, *Acta Physiol. Scand.* **76:**427–440.

Iacovitti, L., Joh, T. H., Park, D. H., and Bunge, R. P., 1981, Dual expression of neurotransmitter synthesis in cultured neurons, *J. Neurosci.* **1:**685–690.

Iacovitti, L., Johnson, M. I., Joh, T. H., and Bunge, R. P., 1982, Biochemical and morphological characterization of sympathetic neurons grown in a chemically-defined medium, *Neuroscience* **7:**2225–2239.

Iijima, T., 1981, Occurrence of uranaffin-positive synaptic vesicles in both adrenergic and non-adrenergic nerves of the rat anococcygeus muscle, *Cell Tissue Res.* **220**:427–433.

Johnson, M. I., 1978, Adult rat dissociated sympathetic neurons in culture: Morphological and cytochemical studies, *Soc. Neurosci. Abstr.* **8**:343.

Johnson, M., Ross, C. D., Meyers, M., Rees, R., Bunge, R., Wakshull, E., and Burton, H., 1976, Synaptic vesicle cytochemistry changes when cultured sympathetic neurones develop cholinergic interactions, *Nature* **262**:308–310.

Johnson, M. I., Ross, C. D., and Bunge, R. P., 1980a, Morphological and biochemical studies on the development of cholinergic properties in cultured sympathetic neurons. II. Dependence on postnatal age, *J. Cell Biol.* **84**:692–704.

Johnson, M. I., Ross, C. D., Meyers, M., Spitznagel, E. L., and Bunge, R. P., 1980b, Morphological and biochemical studies of the development of cholinergic properties in cultured sympathetic neurons. I. Correlative changes in choline acetyltransferase and synaptic vesicle cytochemistry, *J. Cell Biol.* **84**:680–691.

Ko, C. P., Burton, H., Johnson, M. I., and Bunge, R. P., 1976, Synaptic transmission between rat superior cervical ganglion neurons in dissociated cell cultures, *Brain Res.* **117**:461–485.

Landis, S. C., 1976, Rat sympathetic neurons and cardiac myocytes developing in microcultures: Correlation of the fine structure of endings with neurotransmitter function in single neurons, *Proc. Natl. Acad. Sci. USA* **73**:4220–4224.

Landis, S. C., 1978, Growth cones of cultured sympathetic neurons contain adrenergic vesicles, *J. Cell Biol.* **78**:R8–14.

Landis, S. C., 1980, Developmental changes in the neurotransmitter properties of dissociated sympathetic neurons: A cytochemical study of the effects of medium, *Develop. Biol.* **77**:349–361.

Landis, S. C., and Keefe, D., 1983, Evidence for neurotransmitter plasticity in vivo: Developmental changes in the properties of cholinergic sympathetic neurons, *Develop. Biol.* **98**:349–372.

Landis, S. C., MacLeish, P. R., Potter, D. D., Furshpan, E. J., and Patterson, P. H., 1976, Synapses formed between dissociated sympathetic neurons: The influence of conditioned medium, *6th Annu. Meet. Soc. Neurosci. Abstr.* 280.

Langley, J. N., 1891, On the course and connections of the secretory fibers supplying the sweat glands of the feet of the cat, *J. Physiol.* **12**:347–374.

Langley, J. N., 1894, Further observations on the secretory and vaso-motor fibres of the foot of the cat, with notes on other sympathetic nerve fibres, *J. Physiol.* **17**:296–314.

Langley, J. N., 1922, The secretion of sweat. Part I. Supposed inhibitory nerve fibres on the posterior nerve roots. Secretion after denervation, *J. Physiol.* **56**:110–119.

Lundberg, J. M., Hokfelt, T., Schultzberg, M., Uvnas-Wallenstein, K., Kohler, C., and Said, S. I., 1979, Occurrence of vasoactive intestinal polypeptide (VIP)-like immunoreactivity in certain cholinergic neurons of the cat: Evidence from combined immunohistochemistry and acetylcholinesterase staining, *Neuroscience* **4**:1539–1559.

MacLennan, I.S., Hill, C. E., and Hendry, I. A., 1980, Glucocorticosteroids modulate transmitter choice in developing superior cervical ganglion, *Nature* **283**:206–207.

Mains, R. E., and Patterson, P. H., 1973, Primary cultures of dissociated sympathetic neurons. I. Establishment of long-term growth in culture and studies of differentiated properties, *J. Cell Biol.* **59**:329–345.

Matthews, M. R., 1974, Ultrastructure of ganglionic junctions, in: *The Peripheral Nervous System* (J. I. Hubbard, ed.) Plenum Press, New York, pp. 111–149.

Norr, S., 1974, In vitro analysis of sympathetic neuron differentiation from chick neural crest cells, *Develop. Biol.* **34**:16–38.

Nurse, C. A., 1982, Interactions between dissociated rat sympathetic neurons and skeletal muscle cells developing in cell culture, *Develop. Biol.* **88**:55–70.

Nurse, C. A., and O'Lague, P. H., 1975, Formation of cholinergic synapses between dissociated sympathetic neurons and skeletal myotubes of the rat in cell culture, *Proc. Natl. Acad. Sci. USA* **72**:1955–1959.

O'Lague, P. H., Obata, K., Claude, P., Furshpan, E. J., and Potter, D. D., 1974, Evidence for cholinergic synapses between dissociated rat sympathetic neurons in cell culture, *Proc. Natl. Acad. Sci. USA* **71**:3602–3606.

O'Lague, P. H., Furshpan, E. J., and Potter, D. D., 1978a, Studies on rat sympathetic neurons developing in cell culture. II. Synaptic mechanisms, *Develop. Biol.* **67**:404–423.

O'Lague, P. H., Potter, D. D., and Furshpan, E. J., 1978b, Studies on rat sympathetic neuron developing in cell culture. III. Cholinergic transmission, *Develop. Biol.* **67**:424–443.

Patterson, P. H., and Chun, L. L. Y., 1974, The influence of non-neuronal cells on catecholamine and acetylcholine synthesis and accumulation in cultures of dissociated sympathetic neurons, *Proc. Natl. Acad. Sci. USA* **71**:3607–3610.

Patterson, P. H., and Chun, L. L. Y., 1977a, Induction of acetylcholine synthesis in primary cultures of dissociated rat sympathetic neurons. I. Effects of conditioned medium, *Develop. Biol.* **56**:263–280.

Patterson, P. H., and Chun, L. L. Y., 1977b, Induction of acetylcholine synthesis in primary cultures of dissociated rat sympathetic neurons. II. Developmental aspects, *Develop. Biol.* **60**:473–481.

Patterson, P. H., Reichardt, L. F., and Chun, L. L. Y., 1975, Biochemical studies on the development of primary sympathetic neurons in cell culture, *Cold Spring Harbor Symp. Quant. Biol.* **40**:389–397.

Pintar, J. E., Maxwell, G. D., Sweadner, K. J., Patterson, P. H., and Breakefield, X., 1981, Monoamine oxidase activity in early quail embryos and rat neuron cultures with different transmitter phenotypes, *Soc. Neurosci. Abstr.* **7**:848.

Potter, D. D., Landis, S. C., and Furshpan, E. J., 1980, Dual function during the development of rat sympathetic neurons in culture, *J. Exp. Biol.* **89**:57–71.

Potter, D. D., Landis, S. C., and Furshpan, E. J., 1981a, Adrenergic–cholinergic dual function in cultured sympathetic neurons of the rat, *Ciba Symp.* **83**:123–138.

Potter, D. D., Landis, S. C., and Furshpan, E. J., 1981b, Chemical differentiation of sympathetic neurons, in: *Neurosecretion and Brain Peptides: Implications for Brain Function and Neurological Disease* (J. Martin, S. Reichlin, and K. L. Bick, eds.), Raven Press, New York, pp. 275–285.

Quatrale, R. P., and Laden, K., 1968, Solute and water secretion by the eccrine sweat glands of the rat, *J. Invest. Dermatol.* **51**:502–504.

Rees, R., and Bunge, R. P., 1974, Morphological and cytochemical studies of synapses formed in culture between isolated rat superior cervical ganglion neurons, *J. Comp. Neurol.* **157**:1–12.

Reichardt, L. F., and Patterson, P. H., 1977, Neurotransmitter synthesis and uptake by isolated sympathetic neurons in microcultures, *Nature* **270**:147–151.

Richardson, K. C., 1966, Electron microscopic identification of autonomic nerve endings, *Nature* **210**:756.

Ring, J. R., and Randall, W. C., 1946, The distribution and histological structure of sweat glands in the albino rat and their response to prolonged nervous stimulation, *Anat. Rec.* **99**:7–16.

Ross, D., Johnson, M., and Bunge, R. P., 1977, Development of cholinergic characteristics in adrenergic neurones is age dependent, *Nature* **267**:536–539.

Sato, F., and Sato, K., 1978, Secretion of a potassium-rich fluid by the secretory coil of the rat paw eccrine sweat gland, *J. Physiol.* **274**:37–50.

Schwab, M., and Landis, S. C., 1981, Membrane properties of cultured rat sympathetic neurons: Morphological studies of adrenergic and cholinergic differentiation, *Develop. Biol.* **84**:67–78.

Siegel, R. E., Schwab, M., and Landis, S. C., 1982, Developmental changes in the neurotransmitter properties of cholinergic sympathetic neurons in vivo, *Soc. Neurosci. Abstr.* **8**:7.

Sjoqvist, F., 1963a, The correlation between the occurrence and localization of acetylcholinesterase-rich cell bodies in the stellate ganglion and the outflow of cholinergic sweat secretory fibers to the fore paw of the cat, *Acta Physiol. Scand.* **57**:339–352.

Sjoqvist, F., 1963b, Pharmacological analysis of acetylcholinesterase-rich ganglion cells in the lumbo-sacral sympathetic system of the cat, *Acta Physiol. Scand.* **57**:353–362.

Smith, J., Fauquet, M., Ziller, C., and LeDouarin, N. M., 1979, Acetylcholine synthesis by mesencephalic neural crest cells in the process of migration in vivo, *Nature* **282**:853–855.

Sweadner, K. J., 1981, Environmentally regulated expression of soluble extracellular proteins of sympathetic neurons, *J. Biol. Chem.* **256**:4063–4070.

Swerts, J.-P., Le Van Thai, A., and Weber, M. J., 1983, Regulation of enzymes responsible for transmitter synthesis and degradation in cultured rat sympathetic neurons. I. Effect of muscle conditioned medium, *Develop. Biol.* **100**:1–11.

Teillet, M. A., Cochard, P., and LeDouarin, N. M., 1978, Relative roles of the mesenchymal tissues and of the complex neural tube-notochord on the expression of adrenergic metabolism in neural crest cells, *Zoon* **6**:115–122.

Teitelman, G., Joh, T. H., and Reis, D. J., 1981, Transformation of catecholaminergic precursors into glucagon (A) cells in mouse embryonic pancreas, *Proc. Natl. Acad. Sci.* **78**:5225–5229.

Teitelman, G., Joh, T. H., and Reis, D. J., 1978, Transient expression of a noradrenergic phenotype in cells of the rat embryonic gut, *Brain Res.* **158**:229–234.

Teitelman, G., Baker, H., Joh, T. H., and Reis, D. J., 1979, Appearance of catecholamine-synthesizing enzymes during development of the rat sympathetic nervous system: Possible role of tissue environment, *Proc. Natl. Acad. Sci. USA* **76**:509–513.

Uno, H., and Montagna, W., 1975, Catecholamine-containing nerve terminals of the eccrine sweat glands of macaques, *Cell Tissue Res.* **155**:1–13.

Wakshull, E., Johnson, M. I., and Burton, H., 1978, Persistence of an amine uptake system in cultured rat sympathetic neurons which use acetylcholine as their transmitter, *J. Cell Biol.* **79**:121–131.

Wakshull, E., Johnson, M. I., and Burton, H., 1979, Postnatal rat sympathetic neurons in culture. I. A comparison with embryonic neurons, *J. Neurophysiol.* **42**:1410–1425.

Walicke, P. A., and Patterson, P. H., 1981, On the role of CA^{++} in the transmitter choice made by cultured sympathetic neurons, *J. Neurosci.* **1**:343–350.

Walicke, P. A., Campenot, R. B., and Patterson, P. H., 1977, Determination of transmitter function by neuronal activity, *Proc. Natl. Acad. Sci. USA* **74**:5767–5771.

Weber, M., 1981, A diffusible factor responsible for the determination of cholinergic functions in cultured sympathetic neurons: Partial purification and characterization, *J. Biol. Chem.* **256**:3447–3453.

Weschler, H. L., and Fisher, E. R., 1968, Eccrine glands of the rat, *Arch. Dermatol.* **97**:189–201.

Wilson, A. J., Furness, J. B., and Costa, M., 1979, A unique population of uranaffin-positive intrinsic nerve endings in the small intestine, *Neurosci. Lett.* **14**:303–308.

Winkelman, R. K., and Schmit, R. W., 1959, Cholinesterase in the skin of the rat, dog, cat, guinea pig and rabbit, *J. Invest. Dermatol.* **33**:185–190.

Wolinsky, E., and Patterson, P. H., 1983, Tyrosine hydroxylase activity decreases with induction of cholinergic properties in cultured sympathetic neurons, *J. Neurosci.* **3**:1495–1500.

Wolinsky, E., Patterson, P. H., and Landis, S. C., 1983, The influence of serum on the development of sympathetic neurons in culture, *Soc. Neurosci. Abstr.* **9**:5.2.

Yodlowski, M., Fredieu, J. R., and Landis, S. C., 1984, Treatment of neonatal rats with 6-hydroxydopamine prevents the development of cholinergic sympathetic innervation of sweat glands and permits sensory sprouting, *J. Neurosci.*, **4**:1535–1548.

Zurn, A. D., 1982, Identification of glycolipid binding sites for soybean agglutinin and differences in the surface glycolipid of cultured adrenergic and cholinergic sympathetic neurons, *Develop. Biol.* **94**:483–498.

6

In Vitro Analysis of Quail Neural Crest Cell Differentiation

MAYA SIEBER-BLUM and FRITZ SIEBER

1. DERIVATIVES OF THE NEURAL CREST

Many organs and tissues of the adult vertebrate organism are derived from a common embryonic structure, the neural crest. Neural crest cells are of neuroectodermal origin and are initially localized in a midline position along the entire neuraxis. Later in development, they migrate into the embryo, home into various locations, and differentiate. They contribute to the cranial nerves V, VII, IX, and X, and they give rise to autonomic ganglia, nerve-supporting cells of the PNS, pigment cells of the dermis, the epidermis, the mesenteries, and internal organs, sensory ganglia, and certain endocrine cells, e.g., adrenal medulla and calcitonin-producing cells in the ultimobranchial bodies. In the head region, neural crest cells also form bones and cartilage of the facial and visceral skeleton, dermis of the face and the ventral part of the neck, connective tissue, ciliary muscles, and the musculoconnective wall of the arteries derived from aortic arches, and they contribute to striated muscles in the face, jaw, and tongue (Weston, 1970; Noden, 1980; Le Douarin, 1980; Ayer-LeLièvre and Fontaine-Perus, 1982).

MAYA SIEBER-BLUM • Department of Cell Biology and Anatomy, The Johns Hopkins University School of Medicine, Baltimore, Maryland 21205. FRITZ SIEBER • Department of Medicine, The Johns Hopkins University School of Medicine, Baltimore, Maryland 21205.

The diversity of its progeny, the various dysgenetic and neoplastic disorders, and a series of technical advances in *in vivo* and *in vitro* analyses of neural crest cell development make the neural crest an attractive experimental system to study cell differentiation.

2. ORIGIN AND MIGRATION OF NEURAL CREST CELLS

The neural crest first appears as a thickening of the neural folds along the entire neuraxis. As the neural folds fuse, crest cells leave the midline bilaterally, starting at the fourth somite and proceeding progressively rostrad and caudad. Emigration of the neural crest cells is preceded by the formation of discontinuities in the basal lamina of the dorsal neural tube. As the neural crest cells are released, they initially migrate tangentially to the neural tube. They then diverge into two streams, a dorsolateral branch in close proximity to the ectoderm and a dorsoventral branch between neural tube and somites. The crest cells first encounter a large cell-free space filled with a three-dimensional network of extracellular matrix fibrils which serve as a substratum for the migrating cells (Johnston, 1966; Johnston and Listgarten, 1972; Tosney, 1978). This extracellular matrix consists of glycosaminoglycans, i.e., mainly hyaluronic acid and to a lesser extent chondroitin and sulfated glycosaminoglycans (Pratt *et al.*, 1975; Derby, 1978; Pintar, 1978; Bolender *et al.*, 1980). By contrast, after completion of migration, the differentiating neural crest cells (e.g., the nascent dorsal root ganglia) are in an environment that is poor in extracellular glycosaminoglycans (Derby, 1978). Toole and collaborators (Toole and Gross, 1971; Toole, 1973, 1976) have hypothesized that hyaluronate-rich extracellular matrix supports cell migration and proliferation and prevents precocious differentiation.

In addition to glycosaminoglycans, migrating crest cells also encounter collagen (Cohen and Hay, 1971; Hay, 1981) and fibronectin (Linder *et al.*, 1975; Wartiovaara *et al.*, 1979; Newgreen and Thiery, 1980; Mayer *et al.*, 1981). Antifibronectin staining is not only associated with fibrils but also with interstitial bodies, a characteristic component of embryonic matrices with which the migrating neural crest cells are in close contact (Mayer *et al.*, 1981; Tosney, 1982).

Neural crest cells are highly motile and invasive. However, dissemination along the "neural crest cell pathways" in the embryo is not unique to neural crest cells. Injected sarcoma 180 cells (Erickson *et al.*, 1980) and retinal epithelium cells translocate along the same routes, as do latex beads (Bronner-Fraser, 1982). The latter observation illustrates the importance of mechanisms other than active cell migration for neural crest cell translocation. Physical changes such as the degree of hydration (swelling) of the hyaluronate matrix may also affect cell translocation. Displacement of neural crest cells, as well as of mesenchymal cells in the chick cornea (Toole and Trelstad, 1971), cardiac cushion cells (Markwald et al., 1978), sclerotomal cells (Toole, 1972; Solursh et al., 1979), and primary mesenchyme (Fisher and Solursh, 1977; Solursh and Morris, 1977), occurs within highly hydrated hyaluronate-rich matrices. Loss of water is concomitant with termination of migration. Simultaneous morphogenetic movements of adjacent cell populations, such as sclerotomal cells, may crowd the available space and thus affect neural crest cell migration. Finally, neural crest cells that are in close proximity with the ectoderm or the neural tube may be displaced because these tissues grow and expand very rapidly.

3. ANALYSIS OF NEURAL CREST CELL DIFFERENTIATION *IN VIVO*

The heterospecific quail–chick transplantation method was instrumental in linking certain levels of the neuraxis with particular neural crest-derived tissues in the mature organism (Le Douarin and Teillet, 1973; Le Douarin, 1977, 1980). Vagal neural crest (level of somites 1–7) gives rise to all the enteric ganglia of the preumbilical gut and contributes to the innervation of the postumbilical gut. The lumbosacral region of the neural crest (posterior to somite 28) gives rise to the ganglion of Remak (in birds), to most of the ganglia of the postumbilical gut, and to the orthosympathetic chain at the lumbosacral level. The orthosympathetic chain derives from neural crest posterior to somite 5 and adrenomedullary cells originate from somitic levels 18–24. Crest cells derived from somitic levels 7–28 do not participate in the formation of the enteric ganglia.

Heterotopic transplantations have been used to investigate the differentiative potential of neural crest cells. Such experiments have shown that quail neural crest of the adrenomedullary level (presumptive adrenergic neurons) can colonize the gut and form functional (cholinergic) enteric ganglia when grafted to the vagal level of chick hosts. Alternatively, when rhombencephalic or vagal neural crest cells (presumptive cholinergic neurons) are transplanted to the adrenomedullary region, they populate predominantly the adrenal gland, and develop into adrenergic cells. From these results, it was concluded that the commitment of neural crest cells to different neuronal lineages is largely under the control of the postmigratory environment (Le Douarin and Teillet, 1974; Le Douarin *et al.*, 1975). By contrast, heterotopic grafting experiments in the head region showed that the pharynx and the pharyngeal pouches, which surround postmigratory head crest cells, do not influence the patterning of the skeletal and connective tissue of the branchial arches. When presumptive second or third arch neural crest cells were excised from chick hosts and replaced with presumptive first arch crest cells, the grafted cells migrated along the usual, second and third arch pathways, but formed a complete duplication of the first arch skeletal system and first arch-type muscles (Noden, 1983). *In vitro* clonal studies (Sieber-Blum and Cohen, 1980) with quail neural crest cells from the trunk region also indicate that commitment is largely preprogrammed in the early neural crest and not dependent on close contacts with surrounding tissues.

There is increasing evidence that at least some future cholinergic neurons undergo a transient developmental stage during which they store catecholamines before they assume their definitive cholinergic function (Jonakait *et al.*, 1979; Potter *et al.*, 1980; Landis and Keefe, 1983). This may explain some of the conflicting conclusions drawn from heterotopic grafting experiments of head and trunk neural crest. Furthermore, since the transplantation of neural crest segments involves the transfer of rather large cell populations, it is impossible to account for every single transplanted cell, and it is therefore difficult to distinguish unambiguously between an effect of the postmigratory microenvironment on the determination of neural crest cells and a growth advantage for certain subpopulations of committed cells. Methods for the *in vitro* clonal culture of neural crest cells, however, hold promise for a detailed and quantitative analysis of some aspects of neural crest cell development under well-controlled conditions.

4. *IN VITRO* ANALYSIS OF NEURAL CREST CELL DIFFERENTIATION

4.1. Primary Cultures

During embryonic development, neural crest cells of the trunk region leave the neural tube at progressively more caudal levels. Cultures of neural crest cells from different axial levels can thus be prepared by explanting the last few segments of embryos at the appropriate developmental stage. Vagal neural crest is obtained from stage 10–11 (Hamburger and Hamilton, 1951) embryos; thoracic/upper lumbar crest, the

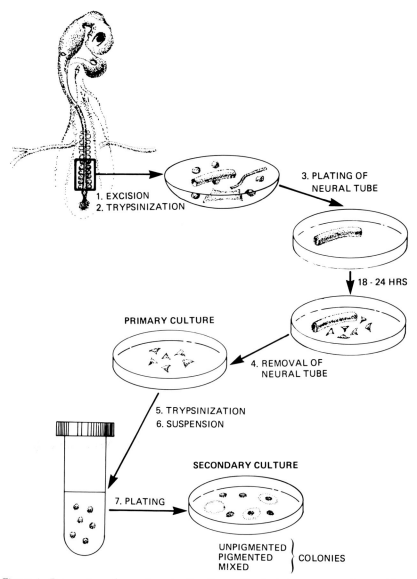

Figure 1. Preparation of neural crest cell cultures. The last six segments of stage 14 quail embryos are excised and trypsinized. Neural tubes are then placed into collagen-coated dishes. The neural crest cells migrate onto the dish. Eighteen to twenty-four hours after explantation, the neural tubes are removed. The emigrated neural crest cells stay in the dish, proliferate, and differentiate. For the preparation of secondary cultures, cells in 18-hr primary cultures are resuspended by trypsinization. About 50–100 cells are seeded into 35-mm collagen-coated dishes. Early in the second week of secondary culture, the unpigmented, pigmented, and mixed colonies are enumerated. At day 12, the plates are processed for histofluorescence and scored for adrenergic colonies by fluorescence microscopy.

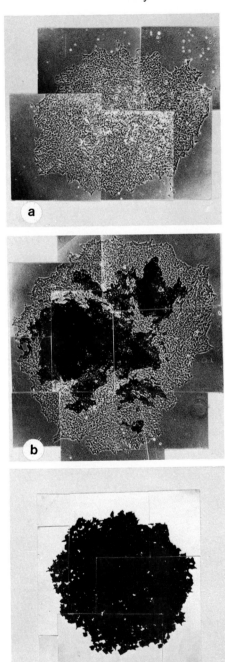

material used for our studies, from stage 14 embryos; and lumbosacral crest from stage 17 embryos. Neural tubes are separated from the surrounding tissues by trypsinization and transferred to collagen-coated culture dishes (Cohen and Konigsberg, 1975). After about 1 hr, when the explanted neural tubes are firmly attached to the collagen substratum, culture medium [a mixture of 75% α-modified minimal essential medium, 10% chick embryo extract, and 15% of a selected lot of horse serum (Sieber-Blum and Cohen, 1980)] is added. Two to three hours later, the mesenchymal neural crest cells begin to leave the neural tube and migrate onto the culture substratum. Eighteen hours after explantation, the neural tubes are removed. The crest cells that are left behind proliferate rapidly and differentiate into melanocytes and neurons (Fig. 1). Pigmented cells and catecholamine-containing neurons become typically recognizable after 4 days in culture.

4.2. Secondary Cultures

Primary neural crest cell cultures often contain a small number of cells that are not of neural crest origin, regardless of whether the neural tubes have been isolated by dissection or by trypsinization. Most of them are probably somitic, neural tube, or fibroblastic cells. Their initial concentration is low. However, during the course of a primary culture, they proliferate and eventually reach densities that could interfere with the development of neural crest cells. It is therefore desirable to remove contaminating noncrest cells as early as possible. This is most readily achieved by subculturing neural crest cells at low density. Two versions of this approach have been developed in this laboratory (Sieber-Blum and Cohen, 1980) and are described below.

4.2.1. Clones.
Clonal cultures are prepared by growing single, isolated neural crest cells in small cell culture wells. To this end, 18-hr primary cultures are trypsinized and the resulting single-cell suspension is diluted to a concentration of 16–20 cells/ml. Single drops of the suspension are then placed into the center of collagen-coated culture wells. Viable cells attach to the substratum and spread within 30 min. Small cell aggregates segregate into well-recognizable single cells within 1–2 hr. Every well is inspected with an inverted microscope at 30 min and again 2 hr after cloning. Wells containing more than one cell are excluded

←

Figure 2. Three types of colonies were observed after 9 days in clonal cultures on a collagen substratum: (a) unpigmented, (b) mixed, and (c) fully pigmented clones. Unpigmented cells tend to aggregate somewhat in the middle of the colony. Pigmented cells form a monolayer and stay flattened. In mixed clones, pigmented cells are always located on top of the unpigmented cells. Bar = 1 mm. (From Sieber-Blum and Cohen, 1980).

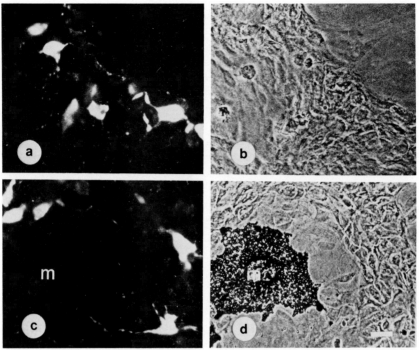

Figure 3. Adrenergic cells in neural crest cell clones. Some unpigmented and mixed clones contained catecholamine-producing cells, as characterized by formaldehyde-induced histofluorescence (FIF). (a) Adrenergic (FIF-positive) cells in an unpigmented clone; (b) same area under phase-contrast optics; (c) part of a mixed clone grown on collagen and fibronectin; fluorescent cells with processes and one melanocyte (m) are shown; (d) same area under phase-contrast optics. Note the difference in size of melanocytic and adrenergic cells. Phase-contrast micrographs were taken after processing for histofluorescence. Bar = 10 μm. (From Sieber-Blum and Cohen, 1980.)

from further evaluation. Each well is examined for a third time 18 hr after cloning and only those cells that have undergone at least one division are included in the final analysis.

Cloned neural crest cells proliferate with a generation time of about 12 hr and generate three types of clones—pigmented clones, unpigmented clones, and mixed clones (Fig. 2). Pigmented clones consist of melanocytes only, unpigmented clones of unpigmented cells only, and mixed clones of both melanocytes and unpigmented cells. Twenty to thirty percent of the unpigmented and mixed clones contain adrenergic neurons that can be identified (Fig. 3) with the formaldehyde/glyoxylic acid-induced histofluorescence (FIF) method of Lorén et al. (1976). Supplementation of the culture medium with cellular fibronectin can increase the frequency of catecholamine-positive unpigmented and mixed clones to as much as 85%.

Experiments with cloned quail neural crest cells have led to two major conclusions: (1) Contrary to widely accepted views, neural crest cells can differentiate into melanocytes and adrenergic neurons in the absence of continued interactions with noncrest cells. (2) The early embryo contains neural crest cells that are pluripotent. The term *pluripotent* is used without mechanistic connotations; it merely indicates that these cells can generate more than one type of differentiated progeny.

4.2.2. Colony Assay. The repeated microscopic inspections make "true" clonal cultures a rather laborious technique that is not very practical for routine investigations. For many applications, it is not crucial to prove the clonal nature of each individual colony. in such cases, sparse secondary cultures or so-called "colony assays" (Fig. 1) offer an acceptable substitute for true clonal cultures (Sieber-Blum and Cohen, 1980).

Single-cell suspensions that are essentially free of cell aggregates are prepared from 18-hr primary cultures as previously described. The density is adjusted to 50–100 cells/ml and 1-ml aliquots are placed into collagen-coated 35-mm culture dishes. The cells have to be resuspended frequently in order to maintain a homogeneous distribution. About 50 plates can be filled before the repeated pipetting begins to interfere with cell viability. Unpigmented, pigmented, and mixed colonies are scored by phase-contrast microscopy early in the second week of secondary culture. Occasionally, cultures contain colonies of noncrest origin such as somite cells or fibroblastlike cells. These noncrest cells are readily recognized by their typical flattened morphological appearance, and cultures containing such cells can be eliminated from further evaluation. On day 12 or 13 of secondary culture, the cultures are processed for FIF (Lorén *et al.*, 1976), and colonies containing one or more catecholaminergic cells are enumerated with the fluorescence microscope. Statistical evaluations of the colony assay are typically based on mean colony counts of 10 replicate dishes for each experimental group.

5. REGULATION OF *IN VITRO* NEURAL CREST CELL DEVELOPMENT BY HUMORAL FACTORS

5.1. Heart Cell-Conditioned Medium

Heart cell-conditioned medium contains an activity that promotes cholinergic differentiation and suppresses adrenergic and melanogenic

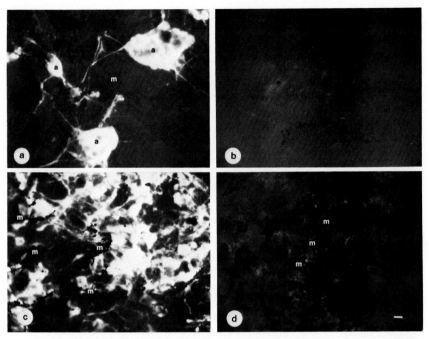

Figure 4. Effect of heart cell-conditioned medium (HCM) on neural crest cell differentiation. (a) Culture grown for 7 days in regular culture medium contains aggregates of adrenergic (FIF-positive) cells (a) with axons and numerous melanocytes (m); (b) culture at day 7 grown from day 1 to day 7 in the presence of HCM contains no adrenergic (FIF-positive) cells and few melanocytes; (c) culture exposed to HCM from day 1 to day 3, grown in regular culture medium for 7 additional days, contains numerous flattened adrenergic (FIF-positive) cells and melanocytes; (d) culture exposed to HCM from day 1 to day 4, grown for 7 additional days in regular culture medium, contains no adrenergic (FIF-positive) cells, but numerous melanocytes. Bar = 10 μm. (From Sieber-Blum and Kahn, 1982.)

differentiation (Sieber-Blum and Kahn, 1982). The stimulation of cholinergic differentiation is indicated by a more than fourfold increase in the specific activity of the enzyme choline acetyltransferase. The inhibition of terminal adrenergic differentiation is manifested by a complete absence of FIF-positive cells. The specific activity of the enzyme, dopamine-β-hydroxylase, however, remains unchanged. Inhibition of adrenergic differentiation becomes irreversible when the neural crest cell cultures are exposed to heart cell-conditioned medium for more than 48 hr (Fig. 4). By contrast, blockage of melanogenesis remains reversible throughout the entire 12-day culture period. Melanin granules appear about 12 hr after removal of the conditioned medium.

It remains to be established whether, under our culture conditions, heart cell-conditioned medium promotes the development of a distinct subpopulation of cholinergic precursor cells or whether it diverts adrenergic cells to the cholinergic pathway. Experiments with individual sympathetic neurons in microcultures have unequivocally shown that adrenergic neurons can become cholinergic under the influence of culture medium conditioned by nonneural cells (Potter *et al.*, 1980; see Chapter 5). These data emphasize the importance of environmental signals in the regulation of neurotransmitter synthesis during the last phases of neural crest differentiation.

5.2. Tumor-Promoting Phorbol Esters

Tumor-promoting phorbol esters have been shown to affect the proliferation and differentiation of many types of cultured cells (Diamond *et al.*, 1980), and it has been suggested that they achieve this by interacting with physiologic regulatory mechanisms (Weinstein *et al.*, 1977). Phorbol esters are, therefore, considered useful tools for the analysis of growth control at the cellular and molecular levels. Supplementation of the culture medium with tumor-promoting phorbol esters has profound effects on the *in vitro* development of quail neural crest cells (Sieber-Blum and Sieber, 1981). It accelerates cell growth in pigmented, unpigmented, and mixed colonies and all three types of colonies grow markedly larger (Fig. 5). Phorbol esters also cause transient and permanent changes in the morphological appearance of individual cells and colonies, many of which may be attributable to alterations in the adhesion of neural crest cells to the substratum and to other crest cells. The onset of pigmentation is delayed by 1 or 2 days, but the number of pigmented colonies is markedly increased. The increase in pigmented colonies is accompanied by an equivalent decrease in the number of unpigmented and mixed colonies, suggesting that tumor-promoting phorbol esters cause some neural crest cells to preferentially differentiate along the melanogenic pathway (Table I). The susceptibility of neural crest cells to the multiple effects of phorbol esters appears to be developmentally regulated. A temporary exposure to phorbol esters during the early phases of the culture period has no noticeable effects on the concentration of pigmented, unpigmented, mixed, and FIF-positive colonies. However, considerably shorter exposures of more mature cultures to the same concentration of phorbol esters completely eliminate FIF-positive cells. A close correlation exists between the ability of a phorbol ester to interfere with the *in vitro* development of quail neural crest cells and its ability to promote the formation of skin tumors in mice (Fig. 5,

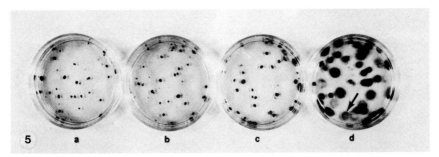

Figure 5. Effect of phorbol esters on the macroscopic appearance of neural crest cell colonies after 10 days in secondary culture. Only melanocyte-containing colonies are discernible since the cultures were not stained. (a) Control culture (no additions to the culture medium); (b) 10^{-7} M 4α-phorbol-12,13-didecanoate (inactive analog of the potent promoter 12-O-tetradecanoyl phorbol 13-acetate); (c) 10^{-7} M phorbol 12,13-diacetate (weak promoter); (d) 10^{-7} M 12-(O)-tetradecanoyl phorbol 13-acetate (potent promoter). The arrow points at a colony which had initially assumed the morphology of an unpigmented colony but gradually became pigmented. The grayish appearance indicates that this colony was still in the early phase of pigmentation. (From Sieber-Blum and Sieber, 1981.)

Table I). This may suggest that the interactions of phorbol esters with initiated cells and with normal cells may share some mechanisms in common.

6. *IN VITRO* DEVELOPMENT OF NEURAL CREST CELLS ON ARTIFICIAL SUBSTRATA AND EXTRACELLULAR MATRIX COMPONENTS

6.1. Basic Polyamino Acids

Basic polyamino acid substrata enhance the clonal growth of a number of different cell types (McKeehan and Ham, 1976) and promote neuronal expression (Letourneau, 1975a,b; Helfand et al., 1976; Kozak et al., 1978). Quail neural crest cells in sparse secondary cultures initially adhere well to culture dishes that have been coated with an aqueous solution of poly-D-ornithine or poly-DL-lysine (molecular weight 40,000) and they proliferate normally. However, after 6–7 days in culture, unpigmented cells frequently aggregate (Fig. 6) and eventually detach from the substratum. Aggregation and detachment of unpigmented cells are not caused by cell death, but rather due to relatively strong cell–cell adhesive forces competing with progressively weaker adhesive forces between cells and substratum. Unlike unpigmented cells, melanocytes

Table I. Effects of Tumor-Promoting and Nonpromoting Phorbol Esters on Neural Crest Cell Differentiation[a]

	U	M	P	C_A	U + M + P
TPA (10^{-7} M)	2.5 ± 0.27*	3.5 ± 0.43*	36.1 ± 1.10*	0*	42.1 ± 1.12
NA	7.3 ± 0.56	10.1 ± 0.67	24.0 ± 1.38	4.5 ± 0.45	41.4 ± 0.88
PDD (10^{-7} M)	1.8 ± 0.49*	1.8 ± 0.33*	52.8 ± 2.59*	0*	56.4 ± 0.88
NA	8.0 ± 0.95	8.5 ± 0.95	39.0 ± 2.26	3.2 ± 0.42	55.5 ± 2.75
PDA (10^{-7} M)	5.6 ± 0.58	9.1 ± 0.85	27.4 ± 1.89	2.8 ± 0.42	42.1 ± 1.73
NA	7.3 ± 0.56	10.1 ± 0.67	24.0 ± 1.38	4.5 ± 0.45	41.4 ± 0.88
4-O-Me-TPA (10^{-7} M)	3.5 ± 0.65	3.9 ± 0.62	18.2 ± 1.59	3.7 ± 0.79	25.6 ± 1.78
NA	2.8 ± 0.74	3.4 ± 0.72	19.6 ± 1.59	2.6 ± 0.52	25.8 ± 1.96
4α-PDD (10^{-7} M)	7.0 ± 0.61	9.1 ± 0.60	25.1 ± 2.00	5.3 ± 0.67	41.2 ± 1.70
NA	7.3 ± 0.56	10.1 ± 0.67	24.0 ± 1.38	4.5 ± 0.45	41.4 ± 0.88
PHR (10^{-7} M)	8.3 ± 0.82	8.1 ± 0.64	37.7 ± 1.89	3.6 ± 0.54	54.1 ± 2.41
NA	8.0 ± 0.95	8.5 ± 0.95	39.0 ± 2.26	3.2 ± 0.42	55.5 ± 2.75
DMSO (1.4×10^{-4} M)	7.6 ± 0.76	8.2 ± 0.63	40.0 ± 2.74	3.2 ± 0.42	55.8 ± 2.15
NA	8.0 ± 0.95	8.5 ± 0.95	39.0 ± 2.26	3.2 ± 0.42	55.5 ± 2.75

[a] Between 30 and 60 cells were seeded into each dish and the medium was supplemented as indicated. Unpigmented (U), mixed (M), and pigmented (P) colonies were scored after 10 days in secondary culture. On the 12th day, they were fixed and processed for catecholamine-specific histofluorescence, and U and M colonies containing adrenergic cells were enumerated. It was technically not possible to test all phorbol esters in the same experiment. Each experimental series, therefore, is listed separately together with the corresponding control (NA: no additions) series using the same preparation of cells. Data are expressed as means of 10 replicate plates ± S.E.M. Experimental values significantly different from the control series as judged by a two-sided Student's t test are marked with an asterisk ($p < 0.001$). C_A: colonies containing adrenergic cells. U + M + P: total number of colonies per plate. (Reproduced from Sieber-Blum and Sieber, 1981.)

remain flattened and firmly attached to the substratum and continue to proliferate (Sieber-Blum and Cohen, 1980). Covalent coupling of poly-DL-ornithine to gelatin-coated culture dishes reduces leakage of the polyamino acid during the culture period (Hawrot and Patterson, 1979). When sparse secondary cultures are established on dishes that have been treated by this method, pigmented, unpigmented, and mixed colonies are formed and all cells remain flattened throughout the culture period. However, adrenergic differentiation as indicated by the presence of FIF-positive cells is minimal (Table II).

6.2. Extracellular Matrix Components

Basic polyamino acids are thought to promote clonal growth by stimulating cells to increase the production of extracellular matrices

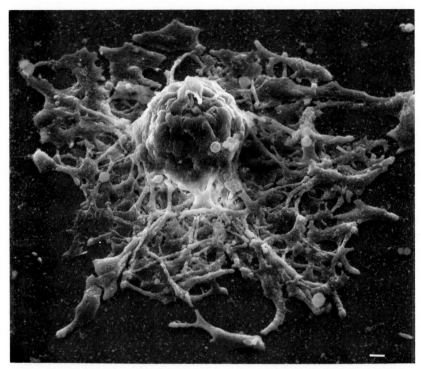

Figure 6. Scanning electron micrograph of a 7-day-old unpigmented colony grown on a poly-DL-ornithine-coated plate. Poly-DL-ornithine coating was performed at high pH in the absence of gelatin and glutaraldehyde. Unpigmented cells initially attach to the substratum but aggregate later and eventually detach from the plates. Bar = 10 μm.

(McKeehan and Ham, 1976). It is conceivable that poly-DL-ornithine and poly-D-lysine fail to promote clonal growth of quail neural crest cells because the latter are unable to synthesize the relevant extracellular matrix components. A number of observations support this view:

Extracellular matrices produced by noncrest cells promote clonal growth of neural crest cells (Sieber-Blum and Cohen, 1980). This can be demonstrated by growing secondary cultures on matrix-coated dishes. To this end, somitic cells or skin fibroblasts are grown on polyamino acid-coated culture dishes until the culture is about 50–70% confluent (extracellular matrices produced by 100% confluenct cultures contain an activity that inhibits clonal growth). The cells, but not the deposited matrix material, are then removed with EDTA and the matrix-covered dishes are used for sparse secondary cultures of neural crest cells. The coating with extracellular matrix increases the frequency of mixed col-

Table II. Growth and Differentiation of Neural Crest Cells on Different Substrata[a]

Substratum	Number of colonies (mean ± S.E.M.)				
	U	M	P	FIF-positive	Total
Poly-DL-ornithine	4.5 ± 0.50	6.1 ± 0.43	33.7 ± 1.21	0.1 ± 0.10	44.3 ± 1.48
Poly-DL-ornithine + matrix	3.6 ± 0.65	12.2 ± 0.89	37.9 ± 1.88	1.1 ± 0.38	53.7 ± 6.96
Collagen	4.3 ± 0.37	12.0 ± 0.77	38.7 ± 0.94	3.4 ± 0.22	55.0 ± 1.16
Collagen + CFN	4.8 ± 0.57	16.5 ± 1.14	39.7 ± 1.67	7.1 ± 0.48	61.0 ± 1.96

[a] Poly-DL-ornithine-coated plates were prepared according to the method of Hawrot and Patterson (1979). Extracellular matrix from chick embryo skin fibroblasts and collagen-coated plates were prepared as described by Sieber-Blum and Cohen (1980). Cellular fibronectin (CFN; 50 µg/plate) was added to the culture dishes before plating of the cells. Unpigmented (U), mixed (M), and pigmented (P) colonies were enumerated on day 7. FIF-positive cells were scored on day 12. Data represented as mean counts of 10 replicate dishes ± S.E.M.

onies about 2-fold and the frequency of FIF-positive colonies about 10-fold while the frequencies of unpigmented and pigmented colonies remain unchanged (Table II).

Extracellular matrices consist primarily of proteoglycans, collagen, and fibronectin (Yaoi and Kanaseki, 1972; Terry and Culp, 1974; Culp et al., 1978; Hay, 1981; Yamada, 1981). Both collagen and fibronectin appear to be capable of supporting adrenergic differentiation. Neural crest cells that are grown on a three-dimensional gel of collagen produce about as many FIF-positive colonies as cells cultured on fibroblast or somite cell-derived matrices. Addition of cellular fibronectin to collagen-coated dishes further increases the frequency of mixed colonies. FIF-positive colonies are about 70 times more numerous than in cultures grown on polyamino acid-coated dishes (Table II). By contrast, a coating of the dish with hyaluronate increases neither the plating efficiency of any of the three types of colony-forming crest cells nor the frequency of FIF-positive colonies.

In clonal cultures and sparse secondary cultures, adrenergic differentiation is poor in the absence of exogenous fibronectin. In primary cultures, however, extensive adrenergic differentiation occurs even in the absence of fibronectin. These strikingly different requirements for fibronectin are most likely due to the presence of fibronectin-producing cells in primary cultures and their absence in secondary cultures (Sieber-Blum et al., 1981). The presence of fibronectin in primary cultures can be demonstrated by immunologic techniques at both the light and the elecron microscopic level. Indirect immunofluorescence techniques detect fibronectin on large flattened cells at the periphery of the culture as early as 1 day after explantation. After 3 to 5 days in primary culture, fibronectin-specific fluorescence is also found on adrenergic cell aggregates and cell processes. On the other hand, no fibronectin is detectable on melanocytes (Fig. 7). Scanning electron microscopy shows a three-dimensional network of extracellular material on cell bodies and processes of adrenergic cell aggregates in primary cultures (Fig. 8). This extracellular material has been identified as fibronectin based on its reaction with an antifibronectin primary antibody and colloidal gold particles that had been coated with a suitable secondary antibody. Simultaneous observation of the carbon-coated specimen in the secondary and the backscattered electron detector mode allowed an unequivocal identification of the gold granules because of the large difference in atomic number between gold and carbon (Figs. 8c, d).

Neural crest cells in clonal cultures have little, if any, extracellular material adsorbed to their surfaces and no fibronectin is detected by immunofluorescence (Fig. 9) or by immunogold staining. This strongly

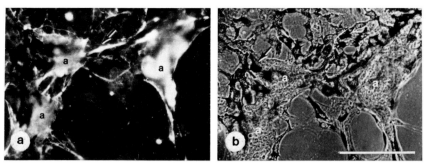

Figure 7. Effect of fibronectin on neural outgrowth from neural tube explants (primary cultures) on the 6th day of culture as detected by indirect immunofluorescence. (a) Intense fluorescence on aggregates of unpigmented cells (a) and interconnecting axons (arrow). (b) The same field under phase-contrast optics. Pigmented (arrow) and unpigmented cells are recognizable. The latter often form aggregates (a) that resemble ganglia. Bar = 100 μm. (From Sieber-Blum *et al.*, 1981.)

suggests that neural crest cells that form pigmented, unpigmented, and mixed colonies are not capable of synthesizing fibronectin.

In primary explants, strands of fibronectin seem to originate from large, flattened, unpigmented, FIF-negative cells at the periphery of the culture and to gradually advance toward processes and aggregates of adrenergic cells. Primary cultures that happen to contain few or none of these large flattened cells also show little or no reaction with antifibronectin antibodies, if one discounts the faint uniform background fluorenscence that is probably attributable to small amounts of fibronectin introduced by the serum and embryo extract. The identity of the large flattened cells that appear to be the main source of fibronectin in primary cultures has not been conclusively established. They could be as yet unidentified neural crest progeny or cells of noncrest origin that are closely associated with the neural crest *in vivo* and thus likely contaminants of primary explants. Cultures of skin fibroblasts, neural tubes, notochords, and somites from the same embryonic stage and the same axial level as the neural crest explants do form characteristic fibrillar patterns of fibronectin (Fig. 9). Identical patterns are produced when the cells are grown in a medium that has been depleted of fibronectin by affinity chromatography on insolubilized gelatin. This indicates that fibronectin is actually synthesized by these cells and not just sequestered from the culture medium. With respect to morphological appearance, location in primary neural crest explants, and amount of fibronectin synthesized, cultures of somitic cells closely resemble the large flattened fibronectin-producing cells in dense primary cultures. Occasionally, one

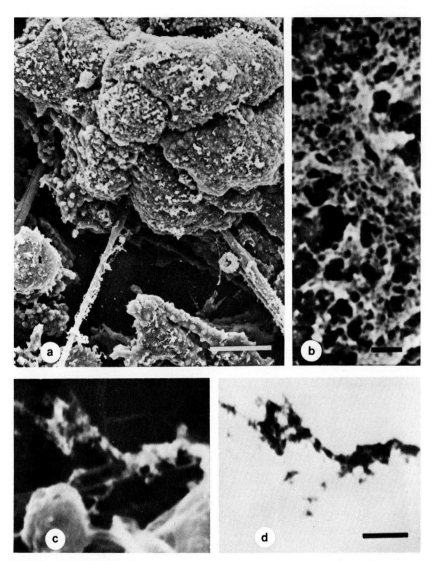

Figure 8. (a, b) Scanning electron micrographs of extracellular material on cell aggregates and axons. (b) A three-dimensional meshwork becomes apparent at higher magnification [field (b) different from (a)]. (c, d) Positive identification of extracellular material as cellular fibronectin by the immunogold staining technique. Colloidal gold granules coated with rabbit anti-goat IgG selectively cover fibers of extracellular material pretreated with anti-fibronectin serum. The backscatter electron detector was adjusted to selectively detect signals emitted by elements with high atomic numbers. (c) Secondary electron image of the carbon-coated specimen; (d) backscatter image; same field as (c). Bars: 10 µg (a), 1 µm (b–d). (From Sieber-Blum et al., 1981.)

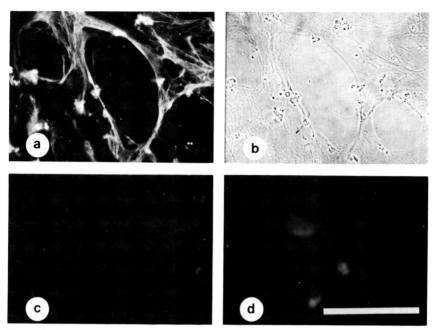

Figure 9. Somitic cells derived from the trunk region of stage 14–15 quail embryos synthesizing fibronectin *in vitro*. (a) Large amounts of fibronectin (some of it organized into large bundles) are detected by indirect immunofluorescence on the 4th day of culture. (b) Same area under phase-contrast optics. Somitic cells are extremely flattened and transparent when grown on a collagen substratum (shown) or on polylysine (not shown). (c) Unpigmented clones; (d) mixed clones. In clonal culture, no fibronectin is detectable. Bar = 100 μm. (From Sieber-Blum *et al.*, 1981.)

can also observe contracting myotubes in old primary cultures, which is a further indication that primary cultures are sometimes contaminated with somitic cells.

Two earlier reports by Cohen (1972) and Norr (1973) have shown that differentiation of chick neural crest cells into adrenergic neurons depends on the presence of somites and the ventral part of that neural tube (including the notochord). Nerve growth factor, however, may be substituted for ventral neural tube (Norr, 1973). In transfilter experiments, somites cease to stimulate adrenergic differentiation of neural crest cells when the thickness of the filter is increased from 25 μm to 150 μm. This suggests that the "inductive" agent is not a freely diffusible molecule but rather an extracellular matrix material such as fibronectin.

Addition of exogenous fibronectin to neural crest cell cultures affects the adhesion of cells to the substratum, the plating efficiency of cells in

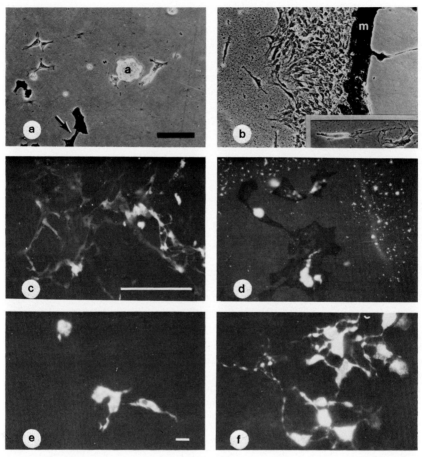

Figure 10. (a, b) Phenotypes of neural crest cell colonies grown on poly-D-lysine substrata in the absence (a) and in the presence (b) of exogenous cellular fibronectin (CFN). (a) After 14 days in culture in the absence of exogenous CFN, all large aggregates have detached from the substratum and only a few small aggregates ("a") and single unpigmented and pigmented (arrow) cells remain. (b) Part of a mixed colony consisting of melanocytes and unpigmented cells grown for 14 days in the presence of exogenous CFN. The cells are partially aggregated in a ringlike fashion (right-hand panel). Dark melanocytes (m) lay on top of the aggregated unpigmented cells. Some unpigmented cells continue to migrate and form a loose monolayer (left-hand panel). Exogenous CFN is recognizable as a granular precipitate on the polylysine substratum. It is sometimes arranged into fibers at the trailing end of unpigmented cells (inset). Bar = 100 μm; inset: 1.3× magnification of (a, b). (c, d) Interaction of unpigmented and pigmented cells in colonies with CFN at the 7th day in secondary culture. (c) Some colonies of unpigmented cells have fibers of CFN attached to their upper surfaces. (d) Pigmented colonies remove fibronectin from the culture dish and accumulate it in an aggregated form on their upper cell surfaces. Bar = 100 μm. (e, f) Adrenergic differentiation on collagen in the presence and absence of CFN (day 12 in secondary culture). (e) In the absence of exogenous CFN, only a few cells contain catecholamines after 12 days in secondary culture. Cell processes are rare and short. (f) When 60 μg CFN is added on days 0, 4, and 8 of secondary culture, adrenergic differentiation is enhanced. The number of catecholamine-positive colonies and the number of adrenergic cells in positive colonies increase. Cell processes are more numerous and longer, showing characteristic varicosities. Bar = 10 μm. (From Sieber-Blum *et al.*, 1981.)

Table III. Plating Efficiency and Differentiation in the Presence and Absence of Added Cellular Fibronectin[a]

Colonies	Mean number of colonies/plate ± S.E.M.		
	Without CFN	With CFN	p
Unpigmented	4.30 ± 0.30	4.80 ± 0.50	0.500 (NS)
Mixed	12.00 ± 0.70	16.50 ± 1.10	0.004
Pigmented	38.70 ± 0.90	39.70 ± 1.60	0.600 (NS)
Catecholamine-positive	3.40 ± 0.20	7.10 ± 0.50	≤0.001
Catecholamine-positive per unpigmented plus mixed	0.21 ± 0.02	0.34 ± 0.03	0.002

[a] One milliliter of the same cell suspension was pipetted into each of 10 plates coated with collagen and 10 plates coated with collagen plus cellular fibronectin. After 12 days of culture, the dishes were processed for histofluorescence, and the different types of colonies were counted. NS: not significant (two-sided Student's *t* test). (From Sieber-Blum *et al.*, 1981.)

secondary cultures, and the terminal differentiation of adrenergic cells. In cultures that contain no fibronectin or very low levels of fibronectin, unpigmented cells tend to aggregate and detach from the substratum. When the culture medium is supplemented with fibronectin, unpigmented cells remain attached to the culture dish and migrate on the fibronectin substratum (Figs. 10a, b). The added fibronectin is visible under phase-contrast optics as a fine granular precipitate that is sometimes arranged into characteristic fibrils at the trailing end of unpigmented cells (Figs. 10b, c). Melanocytes react differently to exogenous fibronectin. They clear their immediate surroundings of fibronectin granules and deposit them in large aggregates on their upper surfaces (Fig. 10d). Supplementation of the culture medium with exogenous fibronectin increases the plating efficiency of mixed colony-forming cells (Table III), stimulates the outgrowth of neuronal processes (Figs. 10e, f), and enhances the frequency of FIF-positive colonies (Table III). Simultaneous addition of antifibronectin antibodies neutralizes the stimulatory effect of fibronectin on adrenergic differentiation (Table IV).

Fibronectin has been shown to accelerate cell migration in several experimental systems. It is conceivable that fibronectin not only plays a role in the regulation of adrenergic differentiation but also in morphogenetic events where differential cell migration plays a crucial role. When neural crest cells leave the neural tube, prospective skin melanocytes migrate dorsolaterally in close proximity to the ectoderm. The other cells migrate dorsoventrally through an area that is rich in extracellular matrix. At the onset of neural crest cell migration, somites begin to disintegrate and sclerotome cells initiate their limited migration. It is

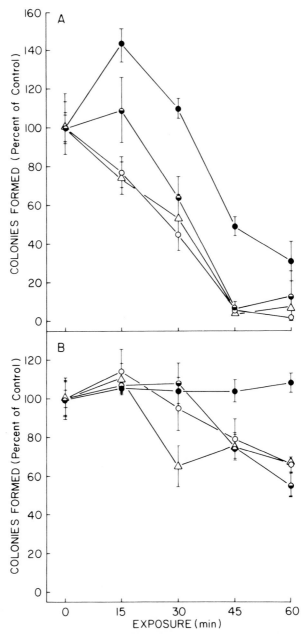

Figure 11. MC 540-mediated photosensitization of quail neural crest cells in sparse secondary culture. Photosensitization was performed 2 hr (A) or 24 hr (B) after plating of the cells. Progenitors of unpigmented (○) and mixed colonies (◑) were photosensitized at a

Table IV. Suppression of CFN-Promoted Adrenogenesis by Anti-CFN Antibodies[a]

	Mean number of colonies/plate ± S.E.M.		
Colonies	Without CFN	With CFN	With CFN + aCFN-ab
Catecholamine-positive per unpigmented plus mixed	0.55 ± 0.02[a]	0.79 ± 0.05[b]	0.53 ± 0.06[c]

[a] Procedures and abbreviations as in Table III. aCFN-ab: antibodies against cellular fibronectin. Equal amounts of CFN and anti-CFN antibodies were added simultaneously to the culture medium. The differences between (a) and (b) and between (b) and (c) are significant, $p = 0.0008$ and $p = 0.006$, respectively; the difference between (a) and (c) is not significant, $p = 0.79$. (From Sieber-Blum et al., 1981.)

conceivable that the neural crest cells that enter the somitic mesenchyme accelerate their migration, whereas migration of crest cells between somites becomes restricted. This may lead to the metamerization of the neural crest population that eventually leads to the formation of the segmented structures of neural crest origins such as the sensory and sympathetic ganglia (Weston, 1970; Erickson et al., 1980). Others (Thiery et al., 1982), however, did not find any neural crest cells within the sclerotome.

7. LINEAGE FORMATION BY NEURAL CREST CELLS

7.1. Membrane Heterogeneity among Early Neural Crest Cells

One of the most important objectives of current research on neural crest development is to determine when, where, and how neural crest cells choose between different lineages. Clonal analysis has shown that

faster rate than progenitors of pigmented (●) colonies. The decline of adrenergic FIF-positive colonies parallels the decline of unpigmented and mixed colonies. In 24 hr cultures (B) photosensitization typically had to kill 2 to 4 cells of the same clone (generation time approximately 12 hr) to prevent the formation of a colony. This, however, does not fully explain the markedly reduced sensitivity to MC 540-mediated photosensitization of older cultures. Recovery from trypsinization and differentiation-related plasma membrane changes may have played a role, also. In one-third of the experiments, brief (15 min) photosensitization caused a moderate (10–40%) increase in the number of colonies formed. Brief exposure to fluorescent light is known to have a mitogenic effect on some cells under certain experimental conditions (Parshad and Sanford, 1977). All data represent mean colony counts ± S.E.M. of 10 replicate dishes.

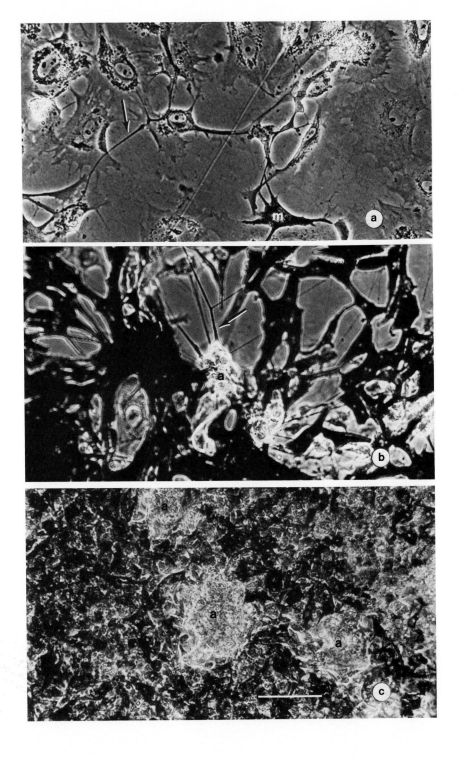

some early migratory crest cells form mixed colonies *in vitro* and are, therefore, at least bipotent (Sieber-Blum and Cohen, 1980). The majority of the clones, however, consist exclusively of pigmented or unpigmented cells. It is conceivable that these pure pigmented or pure unpigmented colonies are the progeny of committed precursor cells. However, one could also argue that all early migratory neural crest cells are equivalent (pluripotent) but that only a few of them are capable of expressing more than one differentiative option under *in vitro* culture conditions. We have recently addressed the question of equivalence or nonequivalence of early migratory neural crest cells with the lipophilic plasma membrane probe, merocyanine 540 (MC 540) (Sieber-Blum and Sieber, 1982, 1984). This probe is a potential-sensitive fluorescent dye that binds preferentially to fluidlike domains in the outer leaflet of the plasma membrane (Easton *et al.*, 1978; Waggoner, 1979; Lelkes and Miller, 1980; Lelkes *et al.*, 1980; Williamson *et al.*, 1981). Electrically excitable cells, leukemic cells, and immature blood cells appear to be particularly rich in high-affinity MC 540 binding sites (Easton *et al.*, 1978; Valinsky *et al.*, 1978; Schlegel *et al.*, 1980; Sieber *et al.*, 1981; Meagher *et al.*, 1983). Photoexcitation of membrane-bound dye leads to an increase in dye uptake, a breakdown of normal membrane functions, and eventually cell death. The exact mechanism of MC 540-mediated photosensitization is not understood. It probably involves the formation of reactive oxygen species that leads to the oxidation of vital plasma membrane components.

If all early migratory neural crest cells were equivalent, all three types of clonogenic cells should be photosensitized at the same rate. However, as Fig. 11 shows, progenitors of pigmented colonies are markedly less sensitive than the progenitors of unpigmented and mixed colonies. Even between the progenitors of mixed and pure unpigmented colonies, there is a slight difference in sensitivity. Figure 11A is based on an experiment where the MC 540-mediated photosensitization was performed 2 hr after plating in sparse secondary cultures. The same

←——————————————————————————————

Figure 12. Effect of blocked cell proliferation on *in vitro* neural crest cell differentiation. (a) Phase-contrast micrograph of a neural crest cell culture grown in the presence of cytosine 2 μg/ml arabinoside (ara-C) from day 0 to day 7. The selected area illustrates the typical morphological appearance of melanocytes ("m"), flattened unpigmented cells, and cells with neuronlike processes (arrow). The latter contain no catecholamines as judged by FIF. (b) Phase-contrast micrograph of neural crest cells grown in the presence of ara-C from day 3 to day 7. This culture contains numerous melanocytes and cell aggregates ("a") with processes (arrow) which are FIF-positive. (c) Section of a 7-day-old culture grown in the absence of ara-C. The culture is dense and contains neurons, cell aggregates ("a"), and scattered melanocytes. The average cell size is markedly smaller than in ara-C-treated cultures of the same age. Bar = 100 μm. (From Kahn and Sieber-Blum, 1983.)

rank order of sensitivity is obtained when the photosensitization is performed after 24 hr (Fig. 11B) in secondary culture. While these experiments do not prove that pigmented and unpigmented colonies are the progeny of unipotent precursor cells, they conclusively show that the cells giving rise to the three types of clones are not identical. They differ with regard to the number or affinity of MC 540 binding sites or their intrinsic sensitivity to reactive oxygen species produced by photoexcited membrane-bound dye molecules (Sieber-Blum and Sieber, 1984).

7.2. Competence for Terminal Differentiation

Progenitor cells have to undergo a certain number of divisions before they acquire competence for terminal differentiation. In the quail embryo, prospective melanocytes reach this stage before prospective adrenergic neurons. This has been shown with primary cultures of quail neural crest cells that were exposed to the cytostatic agent cytosine arabinoside (ara-C) for varying periods of time (Kahn and Sieber-Blum, 1983). At a concentration of 2 μg/ml, ara-C reduces thymidine incorporation by 97.3% and completely inhibits mitosis as judged by a microscopic examination of the culture dishes. When the drug is present during the entire 12-day culture period, adrenergic differentiation is completely suppressed. Pigmented cells, however, consistently appear in all drug-treated primary cultures. The addition of the drug can be delayed for up to 2 days without affecting the suppression of adrenergic differentiation. However, if the drug treatment is delayed for 3 days, a few FIF-positive adrenergic neurons with characteristic processes are formed (Fig. 12). Further delays in the addition of the drug gradually increase the frequency of FIF-positive cultures, until it reaches normal levels when the cultures are allowed to grow in drug-free medium for 6 or more days. Short-term (1–3 days) exposure of neural crest cell cultures to ara-C shows that the inhibition of differentiation is reversible. A delay in terminal differentiation occurs that is roughly equivalent to the length of the drug treatment (Kahn and Sieber-Blum, 1983).

ACKNOWLEDGMENTS

The authors have been supported by NIH Grants HD-15311 (M.S.-B.) and AM-27157 (F.S.). We thank Mrs. A. Fields for her help with the preparation of the manuscript.

REFERENCES

Ayer-LeLièvre, C., and Fontaine-Perus, J., 1982, The neural crest: Its relations with APUD and paraneuron concepts, Arch. Histol. Jpn. 45:409–427.

Bolender, D. L., Seliger, W., and Markwald, R., 1980, A histochemical analysis of polyanionic compounds found in the extracellular matrix encountered by migrating cephalic neural crest cells, *Anat. Rec.* **196:**401–412.

Bronner-Fraser, M., 1982, Distribution of latex beads and retinal pigment epithelial cells along the ventral neural crest pathway, *Develop. Biol.* **91:**50–63.

Cohen, A. M., 1972, Factors directing the expression of sympathetic nerve traits in cells of neural crest origin, *J. Exp. Zool.* **129:**167–182.

Cohen, A. M., and Hay, E. D., 1971, Secretion of collagen by embryonic neuroepithelium at the time of spinal cord–somite interaction, *Develop. Biol.* **26:**578–605.

Cohen, A. M., and Konigsberg, I. R., 1975, A clonal approach to the problem of neural crest determination, *Develop. Biol.* **46:**262–280.

Culp, L. A., Rollins, B. J., Buniel, J., and Hitri, S., 1978, Two functionally distinct pools of glycosaminoglycan in the substrate adhesion site of murine cells, *J. Cell Biol.* **79:**788–801.

Derby, M. A., 1978, Analysis of glycosaminoglycans within the extracellular environment encountered by migrating neural crest cells, *Develop. Biol.* **66:**321–336.

Diamond, L., O'Brien, T. A., and Baird, W. M., 1980, Tumor promoters and the mechanism of tumor promotion, *Adv. Cancer Res.* **32:**1–74.

Easton, T. G., Valinsky, J. E., and Reich, E., 1978, Merocyanine 540 as a fluorescent probe of membranes: Staining of electrically excitable cells, *Cell* **13:**475–486.

Erickson, C. A., Tosney, K. W., and Weston, J. A., 1980, Analysis of migratory behavior of neural crest and fibroblastic cells in embryonic tissues, *Develop. Biol.* **77:**142–156.

Fisher, M., and Solursh, M., 1977, Glycosaminoglycan localization and role in maintenance of tissue spaces in the early chick embryo, *J. Embryol. Exp. Morphol.* **42:**195–207.

Hamburger, V., and Hamilton, H., 1951, A series of normal stages in the development of the chick embryo, *J. Morphol.* **88:**49–92.

Hawrot, E., and Patterson, P. H., 1979, Long-term culture of dissociated sympathetic neurons, *Methods Enzymol.* **58:**574–584.

Hay, E. D., 1981, Collagen and embryonic development, in: *Cell Biology of Extracellular Matrix* (E. D. Hay, ed.), Plenum Press, New York, pp. 379–409.

Helfand, S. L., Smith, J. A., and Wessells, N. K., 1976, Survival and development in culture of dissociated parasympathetic neurons from ciliary ganglia, *Develop. Biol.* **50:**541–547.

Johnston, M. C., 1966, A radioautographic study of the migration and fate of cranial neural crest cells in the chick embryo, *Anat. Rec.* **156:**143–156.

Johnston, M. C., and Listgarten, M. A., 1972, Observations on the migration, interaction, early differentiation of orofacial tissues, in: *Developmental Aspects of Oral Biology* (H. C. Slavkin and L. A. Bavetta, eds.), Academic Press, New York, pp. 53–80.

Jonakait, G. M., Wolf, J., Cochard, P., Goldstein, M., and Black, I. B., 1979, Selective loss of noradrenergic phenotype characters in neuroblasts of the rat embryo, *Proc. Natl. Acad. Sci. USA* **76:**4683–4686.

Kahn, C. R., and Sieber-Blum, M., 1983, Cultured quail neural crest cells attain competence for terminal differentiation into melanocytes before competence to terminal differentiation into adrenergic neurons, *Develop. Biol.* **95:**232–238.

Kozak, L. P., Eppig, J. J., Dahl, D., and Bignami, A., 1978, Enhanced neuronal expression of reaggregating cells of mouse cerebellum cultured in the presence of poly-L-lysine, *Develop. Biol.* **64:**252–264.

Landis, S. C., and Keefe, D., 1983, Evidence for neurotransmitter plasticity *in vivo*: Developmental changes in properties of cholinergic sympathetic neurons, *Develop. Biol.* **98:**349–372.

Le Douarin, N., 1977, The differentiation of the ganglioblasts of the autonomic nervous system studied in chimeric avian embryos, in: *Cell Interactions in Differentiation* (M. Karkinen-Jääskelainen, L., Saxén, and L. Weiss, eds.), Academic Press, New York, pp. 171–190.

Le Douarin, N., 1980, Migration and differentiation of neural crest cells, *Curr. Top. Develop. Biol.* **16**:31–85.

Le Douarin, N., and Teillet, M.-A., 1973, The migration of neural crest cells to the wall of the digestive tract in avian embryos, *J. Embryol. Exp. Morphol.* **30**:31–48.

Le Douarin, N. M., and Teillet, M.-A., 1974, Experimental analysis of the migration and differentiation of neuroblasts of the autonomic nervous system and of neuroectodermal mesenchymal derivatives using a biological cell marking technique, *Develop. Biol.* **41**:162–184.

Le Douarin, N. M., Renaud, D., Teillet, M.-A., and Le Douarin, G. H., 1975, Cholinergic differentiation of presumptive adrenergic neuroblasts in interspecific chimeras after heterotopic transplantations, *Proc. Natl. Acad. Sci. USA* **72**:728–732.

Lelkes, P. I., and Miller, I. R., 1980, Perturbations of membrane structure by optical probes. I. Location and structural sensitivity of merocyanine 540 bound to phospholipid membranes, *J. Membr. Biol.* **52**:1–15.

Lelkes, P. I., Bach, D., and Miller, I. R., 1980, Perturbations of membrane structure by optical probes. II. Differential scanning colorimetry of dipalmitoyllecithin and its analogs interacting with merocyanine 540, *J. Membr. Biol.* **54**:141–148.

Letourneau, P. C., 1975a, Possible role for cell-to-substratum adhesion in neuronal morphogenesis, *Develop. Biol.* **44**:77–91.

Letourneau, P. C., 1975b, Cell-to-substratum adhesion and guidance of axonal elongation, *Develop. Biol.* **44**:92–101.

Linder, E., Vaheri, A., Ruoslahti, E., and Wartiovaara, J., 1975, Distribution of fibroblast surface antigen in the developing chick embryo, *J. Exp. Med.* **142**:41–49.

Lorén, I., Björklund, A., Falck, B., and Lindvall, O., 1976, An improved histofluorescence procedure for freeze-dried paraffin-embedded tissue based on combined formaldehyde–glyoxilic acid perfusion with high magnesium content and acid pH, *Histochemistry* **49**:177–192.

MeKeehan, W. L., and Ham, R. G., 1976, Stimulation of clonal growth of normal fibroblasts with substrata coated with basic polymers, *J. Cell Biol.* **71**:727–734.

Markwald, R. R., Fitzharris, T. P., Bank, H., and Bernanke, D. H., 1978, Structural analysis on the matrical organization of glycosaminoglycans in developing endocardial cushions, *Develop. Biol.* **62**:292–316.

Mayer, B. W., Hay, E. D., and Hynes, R. O., 1981, Immunocytochemical localization of fibronectin in embryonic chick trunk and area vasculosa, *Develop. Biol.* **82**:267–286.

Meagher, R. C., Sieber, F., and Spivak, J. L., 1983, Susceptibility to merocyanine 540-mediated photosensitization: A differentiation marker on murine hematopoietic progenitor cells, *J. Cell. Physiol.* **116**:118–124.

Newgreen, D., and Thiery, J.-P., 1980, Fibronectin in early avian embryos: Synthesis and distribution along the migration pathways of neural crest cells, *Cell Tissue Res.* **211**:269–291.

Noden, D. M., 1980, The migration and cytodifferentiation of cranial neural crest cells, in: *Current Research Trends in Prenatal Craniofacial Development* (R. M. Pratt and R. L. Christiansen, eds.), Elsevier/North-Holland, Amsterdam, pp. 3–25.

Noden, D. M., 1983, The role of the neural crest patterning of avian cranial skeletal, connective, and muscle tissues, *Develop. Biol.* **96**:144–165.

Norr, S. C., 1973, *In vitro* analysis of sympathetic neuron differentiation from chick neural crest cells, *Develop. Biol.* **34**:16–38.

Parshad, R., and Sanford, K. K., 1977, Proliferative response of human diploid fibroblasts to intermittent light exposure, *J. Cell. Physiol.* **92**:481–486.

Pintar, J. E., 1978, Distribution and synthesis of glycosaminoglycans during quail neural crest morphogenesis, *Develop. Biol.* **67**:444–464.

Potter, D. D., Landis, S. C., and Furshpan, E. J., 1980, Dual function during development of rat sympathetic neurons in culture, *J. Exp. Biol.* **89**:57–71.

Pratt, R. M., Larsen, M. A., and Johnston, M. C., 1975, Migration of cranial neural crest cells in a cell-free hyaluronate-rich matrix, *Develop. Biol.* **44**:298–305.

Schlegel, R. A., Phelps, B. M., Waggoner, A., Terada, L., and Williamson, P., 1980, Binding of merocyanine 540 to normal and leukemic erythroid cells, *Cell* **20**:321–328.

Sieber, F., Meagher, R. C., and Spivak, J. L., 1981, Differential sensitivity of mouse hematopoietic stem cells to merocyanine 540, *Differentiation* **19**:65–67.

Sieber-Blum, M., and Cohen, A. M., 1980, Clonal analysis of quail neural crest cells: They are pluripotent and differentiate *in vitro* in the absence of noncrest cells, *Develop. Biol.* **90**:96–106.

Sieber-Blum, M., and Kahn, C. R., 1982, Suppression of catecholamine and melanin synthesis and promotion of cholinergic differentiation of quail neural crest cells by heart cell conditioned medium, *Stem Cells* **2**:344–353.

Sieber-Blum, M., and Sieber, F., 1981, Tumor-promoting phorbol esters promote melanogenesis and prevent expression of the adrenergic phenotype in quail neural crest cells, *Differentiation* **20**:117–123.

Sieber-Blum, M., and Sieber, F., 1982, Plasma membrane heterogeneity in early avian neural crest cells, *J. Cell Biol.* **95**:43a.

Sieber-Blum, M., and Sieber, F., 1984, Membrane heterogeneity among early quail neural crest cells, *Develop. Brain Res.* **14**:241–246.

Sieber-Blum, M., Sieber, F., and Yamada, K. M., 1981, Cellular fibronectin promotes adrenergic differentiation of quail neural crest cells *in vitro*, *Exp. Cell Res.* **133**:285–295.

Solursh, M., and Morris, G. M., 1977, Glycosaminoglycan synthesis in rat embryos during the formation of the primary mesenchyme and neural folds, *Develop. Biol.* **57**:75–86.

Solursh, M., Fisher, M., Meier, S., and Singley, C. T., 1979, The role of extracellular matrix in the formation of sclerotome, *J. Embryol. Exp. Morphol.* **54**:75–98.

Terry, A. H., and Culp, L. A., 1974, Substrate attached glycoproteins from normal and virus-transformed cells, *Biochemistry* **13**:414–425.

Thiery, J.-P., Duband, J. L., and Delouvée, A., 1982, Pathways and mechanisms of avian trunk neural crest cell migration and localization, *Develop. Biol.* **93**:324–343.

Toole, B. P., 1972, Hyaluronate turnover during chondrogenesis in the developing chick limb and axial skeleton, *Develop. Biol.* **29**:321–329.

Toole, B. P., 1973, Hyaluronate and hyaluronidase in morphogenesis and differentiation, *Am. Zool.* **13**:1061–1065.

Toole, B. P., 1976, Morphogenetic role of glycosaminoglycans in brain and other tissues, in: *Neuronal Recognition* (S. H. Barondes, ed.), Plenum Press, New York, pp.275–329.

Toole, B. P., and Gross, J., 1971, The extracellular matrix of the regenerating newt limb: Synthesis and removal of hyaluronate prior to differentiation, *Develop. Biol.* **25**:57–77.

Toole, B. P., and Trelstad, R. L., 1971, Hyaluronate production and removal during corneal development in the chick, *Develop. Biol.* **26**:28–35.

Tosney, K. W., 1978, The early migration of neural crest cells in the trunk region of the avian embryo: An electron microscopic study, *Develop. Biol.* **62**:317–333.

Tosney, K. W., 1982, The segregation and early migration of cranial neural crest cells in the avian embryo, *Develop. Biol.* **89**:13–24.

Valinsky, J. E., Easton, T. G., and Reich, E., 1978, Merocyanine 540 as a fluorescent probe of membranes: Selective staining of leukemic and immature hemopoietic cells, *Cell* **13**:487–499.

Waggoner, A. S., 1979, Dye indicators of membrane potential, *Annu. Rev. Bioeng.* **8**:47–68.

Wartiovaara, J., Leivo, I., and Vaheri, A., 1979, Expression of the cell surface-associated glycoprotein, fibronectin, in the early mouse embryo, *Develop. Biol.* **69**:247–257.

Weinstein, I. B., Wigler, M., and Pietropaolo, C., 1977, The action of tumor-promoting agents in cell culture, in: *The Origins of Human Cancer*, Volume 4 (H. H. Hyatt, J. D. Watson, and J. A. Winsten, eds.), Cold Spring Harbor Laboratory, Cold Spring Harbor, New York, pp. 751–772.

Weston, J. A., 1970, The migration and differentiation of neural crest cells, *Adv. Morphog.* **8**:41–114.

Williamson, P. L., Massey, W. A., Phelps, B. M., and Schlegel, R. A., 1981, Membrane phase state and the re-arrangement of hematopoietic cell surface receptors, *Mol. Cell Biol.* **1**:123–125.

Yamada, K. M., 1981, Fibronectin and other structural proteins, in: *Cell Biology of Extracellular Matrix* (E. D. Hay, ed.), Plenum Press, New York, pp. 95–114.

Yaoi, Y., and Kanaseki, T., 1972, Role of microexudate carpet in cell division, *Nature* **237**:283–285.

7

Biochemical Differentiation in Serum-Free Aggregating Brain Cell Cultures

PAUL HONEGGER

1. INTRODUCTION

The basic methodology of rotation-mediated aggregating cell culture was introduced by Moscona (1961), who took advantage of the finding that dissociated immature cells *in vitro* reassemble spontaneously to form histotypic, three-dimensional structures (Moscona, 1960). Subsequent morphological investigations have revealed that such cell aggregates prepared from fetal brain form patterns of cell alignment similar to those *in vivo* (Moscona, 1965; DeLong, 1970; DeLong and Sidman, 1970; Garber and Moscona, 1972; Levitt *et al.*, 1976; Garber 1977), and undergo extensive morphological differentiation, including synaptogenesis and myelination (Seeds and Vatter, 1971; Kozak *et al.*, 1977; Matthieu *et al.*, 1978, 1981; Seeds and Haffke, 1978; Honegger *et al.*, 1979; Matthieu and Honegger, 1979; Trapp *et al.*, 1979, 1982; Lu *et al.*, 1980). The tissue-specific cellular organization and differentiation in aggregating brain cell cultures were further established by detailed biochemical studies which showed that the developmental expression of neuronal and glial characteristics closely resembles that *in vivo* (Seeds, 1971, 1973, 1975a,b;

PAUL HONEGGER • Institute of Physiology, University of Lausanne, Lausanne, Switzerland.

Seeds and Gilman, 1971; Schmidt, 1975; Honegger and Richelson, 1976, 1977a,b, 1979; Seeds *et al.*, 1977; Mathieu *et al.*, 1978, 1979; Honegger *et al.*, 1979; Wenger *et al.*, 1979; Honegger and Matthieu, 1980; Knodel and Richelson, 1980; Trapp *et al.*, 1981, 1982; Wehner *et al.*, 1982).

Originally, aggregating brain cell cultures were obtained from trypsin-dissociated cells. The replacement of the enzymatic dissociation technique by a purely mechanical procedure (Honegger and Richelson, 1976) greatly simplified the method and allowed one to grow numerous replicate cultures for highly reproducible biochemical work. A further significant improvement of the culture system was the recent introduction of a serum-free culture technique (Honegger *et al.*, 1979). This report describes the methodology of serum-free aggregating brain cell culture and reviews some recent findings which may serve to discern the potentialities and limitations of this culture system.

2. METHODOLOGY

2.1. Mechanical Dissociation of Brain Tissue

The preparation of mechanically dissociated aggregating brain cells requires relatively immature tissues, in order to minimize cell damage during dissociation and to obtain a high proportion of undifferentiated cells with maximal capacity for growth and differentiation *in vitro* (Honegger and Richelson, 1976; Lenoir and Honegger, 1983). For example, cultures of rat telencephalon are usually prepared from tissue of 15-day fetuses. The entire dissection and dissociation procedure is performed in ice-cold, sterile solution D [modified Puck's D solution (Wilson *et al.*, 1972)]: pH 7.4, 340 mOsm, containing 138 mM NaCl, 5.4 mM KCl, 0.17 mM Na_2HPO_4, 0.22 mM KH_2PO_4, 5.5 mM glucose, 58.4 mM sucrose, and 20 μg/ml gentamicin. The excised brains or brain parts are pooled in solution D and dissociated together. The tissue is then transferred to a nylon mesh bag (3.5 × 12 cm) with 200-μm pores (Nybolt 200/360, Swiss Silk Bolting Cloth Manufacturing, Zurich), submerged in solution D, and forced through the meshes by gently stroking the bag from the outside with a glass rod. The dispersed tissue is gently triturated with a 5-ml plastic pipette, and filtered by gravity flow through a second nylon mesh with 115-μm pores (Nybolt 11 P-115). The resulting cell suspension is sedimented by centrifugation ($180g_{av}$, 13 min, 4°C) and washed once or twice (depending on the quantity of tissue processed) in solution D by gentle trituration with subsequent centrifugation. After the last centrifugation the cells are resuspended in cold (4°C) culture

medium. The cell number is determined by use of either a hemocyto-
meter or an electronic cell counter. Cell viability (nigrosin exclusion)
usually averages 50%. The formation of uniform aggregates, showing a
narrow size distribution, requires a minimal cell density of $1.5–3 \times 10^7$
cells/ml, depending on the developmental stage of the tissue taken for
the preparation. For routine work the critical cell density, i.e., the lowest
cell number per flask that allows the formation of uniform aggregates,
should be determined at the outset by serial dilutions.

2.2. Culture Medium

Aggregating brain cell cultures are prepared and grown in strictly
serum-free conditions. The chemically defined culture medium consists
of Dulbecco's modified Eagle's medium (DMEM) (no pyruvate, 4.5 g/
liter glucose, GIBCO, catalog No. 320-1965) supplemented with nutritional factors, vitamins, hormones, and trace elements, as shown in
Table I.

2.3. Cell Aggregation

Aggregate formation is initiated by placing 3.5-ml aliquots of the
single-cell suspension into 25-ml DeLong flasks and incubating at 37°C
in an atmosphere of 10% CO_2 and 90% humidified air under constant
gyratory agitation. Gas-permeable closures are used to ensure an adequate gas supply. Optimal agitation is of utmost importance for obtaining uniform, reproducible cultures. The initial rotation speed is set
around 68 rpm. The exact setting depends on the dimensions of the
culture vessel and has to be determined empirically for each batch of
culture flasks. Since the dimensions of the culture flasks often vary considerably, it is important to use carefully matched flasks in each preparation. The vortex and shearing forces created in each flask by the
gyratory movement have to be such that on the one hand attachment
between single cells and small cell clusters is ensured and on the other
hand clumping of the final cell aggregates is prevented. Too forceful
agitation during the initial phase of cell aggregation leads to inhomo-
geneous cultures, due to substantial cell death and appearance of float-
ing fibrous material, e.g., DNA, in the medium.

2.4. Maintenance of Aggregating Brain Cell Cultures

Reaggregation of mechanically dissociated brain cells in serum-free
medium starts immediately after inoculation, and within 2 days small

*Table I. Constituents of the Chemically Defined Culture
Medium Used for Aggregating Brain Cell Cultures*

Nutritional factors and vitamins	
Choline chloride	1 mM
i-Inositol	51 μM
Nicotinamide	41 μM
Pyridoxal·HCl	25 μM
Thiamine·HCl	15 μM
L-Carnitine	12 μM
Folic acid	11 μM
Calcium pantothenate	11 μM
Linoleic acid	10 μM
Biotin	4 μM
Riboflavin	1.3 μM
Lipoic acid	1 μM
Vitamin B_{12}	1 μM
Retinol[a]	Trace
DL-α-Tocopherol[a]	Trace
Hormones	
Insulin (bovine)	0.8 μM
Triiodothyronine	30 nM
Hydrocortisone-21-phosphate	20 nM
Transferrin (human)	13 nM
Trace elements	
$Fe(NO_3)_3 \cdot 9H_2O$	250 nM
$Na_2SiO_3 \cdot 5H_2O$	250 nM
$ZnSO_4 \cdot 7H_2O$	50 nM
Na_2SeO_3	15 nM
$CuSO_4 \cdot 5H_2O$	10 nM
$CdSO_4 \cdot 8H_2O$	5 nM
$MnCl_2 \cdot 4H_2O$	5 nM
$(NH_4)_6 Mo_7O_{24}$	0.5 nM
$NiSO_4 \cdot 6H_2O$	0.25 nM
$SnCl_2 \cdot 2H_2O$	0.25 nM

[a] Retinol (5 μg/ml) and DL-α-tocopherol (10 μg/ml) are added to the basal medium by sonication followed by sterile filtration. Since a great proportion of these lipophilic vitamins are retained by the filter, only traces may be present in the medium. The final concentration in the medium has not been determined.

spherical aggregates of uniform size are formed. On day 2 the cultures are transferred to 50-ml DeLong flasks with the addition of 5 ml of fresh culture medium (thus giving a total of 8.5 ml of medium per flask). The rotation speed is gradually increased with increasing size of the aggregates (usually by 2 rpm/day up to the maximum speed of 75–80 rpm). As a rule, during agitation the aggregates should cover less than half of the bottom surface around the center of the flask. Media are replen-

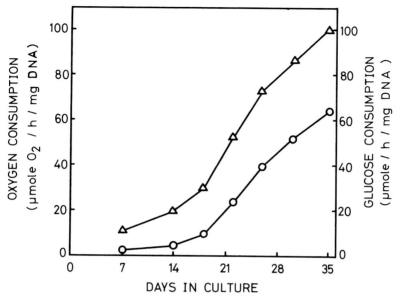

Figure 1. Consumption of oxygen and D-glucose in serum-free aggregating cell cultures of 15-day fetal rat telencephalon. Oxygen consumption (△) was measured in a Gilson Oxygraph using a Clark electrode and a 1.6-ml cell. Glucose consumption (○) was estimated by periodically measuring the glucose concentrations in the medium using the glucose dehydrogenase assay (Merckotest).

ished by replacing 5 ml of medium every 3 days until day 11, and every other day until day 19. On day 19, the cultures are split by dividing the aggregates of each flask into four equal parts, and distributing them to separate 50-ml DeLong flasks. Thereafter, media are replenished every other day, or daily if a considerable decrease in culture pH is observed. These changes in the culture scheme are required by the accelerating metabolic rate of the cultures. Typically, glucose and oxygen consumption (Fig. 1) as well as utilization of some amino acids (Table II) show a dramatic increase with time in culture, i.e., with progressing cellular differentiation. Both the more frequent replenishment and the reduction of the number of aggregates per flask on day 19 serve to meet the nutritional requirements of the cultures by replacing depleted nutrients and diminishing the accumulation of acidic and toxic metabolites. Thus, it is possible to maintain reaggregated brain cells for several months in culture. Electron microscopic examination of long-term cultures shows a tissuelike arrangement of highly differentiated neuronal and glial cells (Fig. 2). Many synaptic junctions and myelinated axons are found. Oc-

Table II. Amino Acid Concentrations in Fresh and Used Media of Aggregating Fetal Rat Brain Cells[a]

L-Amino acid	Concentration in fresh medium (μM)	Concentration in used medium (μM)		
		Day 5	Day 19	Day 29
Glutamine	2600	1870	3300	2920
Valine	800	654	370	330
Lysine	790	630	650	660
Isoleucine	730	520	250	230
Leucine	730	490	230	240
Threonine	620	620	590	380
Arginine	400	190	170	220
Tyrosine	380	320	330	320
Phenylalanine	370	300	310	310
Glycine	330	90	10	10
Serine	320	230	260	230
Cystine	310	260	5	5
Methionine	180	130	140	140
Histidine	160	120	130	140
Tryptophan	78		Not determined	
Alanine	0	330	100	150
Ornithine	0	80	30	30

[a] Cultures were prepared with mechanically dissociated cells of fetal (day 15 of gestation) rat (Wistar) whole brain. The used media collected at replenishment were analyzed. The amino acid concentration of the media were determined in a Biotronik BT 6700 amino acid analyzer, using a 0.6 × 36-cm column of DC6-A resin and a series of lithium citrate/lithium chloride buffers commonly used for the separation of biological fluids.

casionally, necrotic cells and loose myelin figures are observed, which may indicate inadequate culture conditions. A further optimization of long-term culture conditions is likely to be achieved, first by using a better balanced culture medium which contains an adequate supply of all required nutrients, vitamins, hormones, and growth factors, and second by avoiding wide fluctuations in nutrient levels, e.g., by a continuous flow of medium.

2.5. Culture Handling

Aggregating brain cell cultures are maintained in suspension culture and are therefore easy to handle. Aggregates cultured for more than 3 days settle quickly under the influence of gravity, thus allowing facile manipulations for medium replenishment and washing procedures. The transfer and sampling of cultures are done by simple pipetting. To ensure optimal conditions for both culture maintenance and handling it is

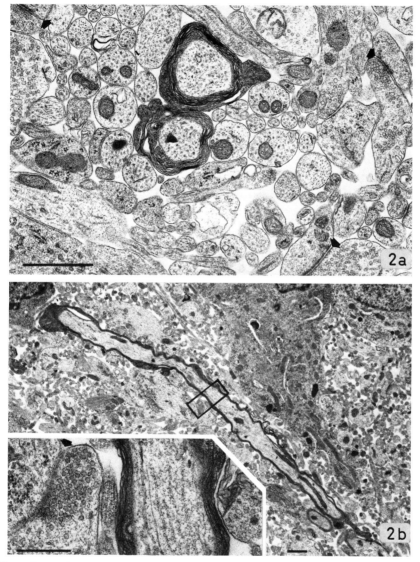

Figure 2. (a) Electron micrograph of two cross-sectioned myelinated fibers and three synaptic junctions (arrows) in an aggregate of fetal rat telencephalic cells after 40 days of culture in chemically defined medium. Bar = 1 μm. (b) Electron micrograph of a myelinated fiber in a 25-day telencephalic cell aggregate grown in chemically defined medium. Bar = 1 μm. Inset: magnification of the area indicated by the rectangle, showing a synapse (arrow) and part of the myelinated fiber. Bar = 0.5 μm.

important to grow aggregates of ideal size (300- to 400-μm diameter). The final size of the aggregates can be influenced to some extent through variation of inoculation cell density and shaking speed during the initial phase of aggregate formation. The aggregates tend to remain smaller with relatively high cell densities at inoculation, and slightly increased agitation after the first day of incubation.

3. CELLULAR GROWTH AND DIFFERENTIATION

3.1. Synthesis of DNA and Protein

Serum-free aggregating brain cell cultures show a restricted period of DNA synthesis and cell proliferation (Honegger et al., 1979; Lenoir and Honegger, 1983). Synthesis of DNA, determined by measuring the incorporation of [^{3}H]thymidine into a macromolecular fraction of the cultures, is significantly increased in the presence of insulin or insulin-like growth factors (IGF). This stimulatory effect appears to be mediated by a common binding site showing the highest affinity for the soma-tomedin IGF I (Lenoir and Honegger, 1983). At saturating levels of insulin (or IGF) the extent of mitotic activity in vitro depends on the developmental stage of the starting tissue. For example, the rate of DNA synthesis in cultures of 15-day fetal telencephalic cells (Fig. 3) is eightfold higher than in cultures prepared from the "hindbrain" (mesenceph-alon–diencephalon–rhombencephalon) of the same fetuses, and three- to fourfold higher than in cultures of 17-day fetal telencephalic cells (Lenoir and Honegger, 1983). The mitotic activity in aggregating brain cells is restricted to the first 2 weeks in culture (Fig. 3) and is followed by a prolonged period of cellular differentiation (see Section 3.2). Consequently, the total DNA content of the cultures increases steadily (Fig. 3) to reach a maximum after 2 weeks in vitro. During the third week a slight decrease in the DNA content is observed, indicating the occurrence of cell death during this culture period.

The increase in the total protein content of the cultures (Fig. 3) is a function of both the increase in cell number and the progression of cellular growth. Thus, in contrast to DNA synthesis, protein accumulation is found to continue during the third week in culture. Insulin appears to be more potent than IGF I in stimulating protein accumulation (Lenoir and Honegger, 1983). A further signficant increase in protein synthesis can be provoked by treating the cultures during the first week with epidermal growth factor (EGF) (5 ng/ml). EGF treatment causes on the one hand a partial inhibition of DNA synthesis and on the other

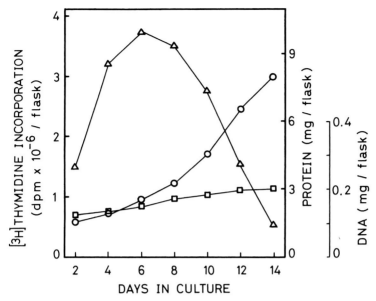

Figure 3. DNA synthesis (△), total DNA (□), and total protein (○) in serum-free aggregating cell cultures of 15-day fetal rat telencephalon. DNA synthesis was determined by measuring the incorporation of [³H]thymidine (36 nM, 49 Ci/mmole) into a macromolecular fraction after a 2-hr pulse. Total DNA and protein were determined as before (Lenoir and Honegger, 1983).

hand an increase in both the total protein content as well as the synthesis and release of extracellular soluble proteins (Guentert-Lauber and Honegger, 1984). These effects seem to be related to the enhanced glial differentiation induced by EGF (see Section 3.2.2).

3.2. Biochemical Differentiation

The maturation of brain cells is monitored most efficiently with the use of biochemical methods, by measuring the developmental expression of various cell type-specific characteristics. Biochemical parameters applied successfully to characterize cellular maturation in aggregating brain cell cultures grown either in the presence or absence of serum include: neurotransmitter-metabolizing enzymes (Seeds, 1973; Honegger and Richelson, 1976; Honegger et al., 1979); biosynthesis, storage, and release of neurotransmitters (Seeds et al., 1977; Honegger and Richelson, 1979); neurotransmitter receptors (Seeds et al., 1977; Knodel and Richelson, 1980; Wehner et al., 1982); neuron-specific enolase (Trapp

Table III. *Development of Neuronal and Glial Enzymatic Activities in Serum-Free Aggregating Cell Cultures of Fetal Rat Telencephalon*[a]

	Specific activity (nmole/min/mg protein)[b]						
	Days *in vitro*						
Enzyme[c]	Day 8	Day 11	Day 14	Day 19	Day 34	Day 54	Adult brain[d]
CAT	≤0.005	0.012	0.019	0.075	0.338	0.462	0.824
AChE	4.30	6.65	6.82	12.03	30.04	45.00	71.00
GAD	0.078	0.171	0.240	0.604	1.229	1.766	2.247
GLU-S	3.41	6.40	9.96	22.32	38.08	49.00	39.18
CNP	363	525	903	1771	2265	2055	5780

[a] Cultures were prepared with mechanically dissociated cells of 15-day fetal rat telencephalon. The specific activities of several enzymes were determined in homogenates of aggregates grown for different periods *in vitro*.
[b] Values show the mean of 3–4 culture flasks. Maximal variation from the mean of each value was < 10%.
[c] The activities of choline acetyltransferase (CAT), acetylcholinesterase (AChE), and glutamic acid decarboxylase (GAD) were measured as described elsewhere (Honegger and Lenoir, 1980). CAT activity was correlated for the portion of nonspecific activity, determined by omitting choline iodide in the reaction cocktail. AChE activity was corrected for the portion of pseudocholinesterase activity as before (Honegger and Richelson, 1976). The activity of 2′,3′-cyclic nucleotide 3′-phosphohydrolase (CNP) was determined according to Kurihara and Tsukada (1967); glutamine synthetase (GLU-S) activity was measured by a modification of the method of Pishak and Phillips (1979).
[d] Homogenates of adult rat forebrain were used for comparison.

et al., 1981); neuron-specific protein D_2 (Jørgensen *et al.*, 1984); myelin basic protein (Matthieu *et al.*, 1978; Almazan *et al.*, 1984, 1985); biosynthesis of cerebrosides and sulfatides (Seeds *et al.*, 1977; Matthieu *et al.*, 1979); myelin-associated enzymes (Matthieu *et al.*, 1980); glutamine synthetase (Honegger and Guentert-Lauber, 1983); and glial fibrillary acidic protein (L. Eng, J.-M. Matthieu and P. Honegger, unpublished results).

Periodic assays of different neuronal and glial marker enzymes in serum-free aggregating cell cultures of fetal rat telencephalon show great increases in their specific and total activities over several weeks in culture, up to levels comparable with those found in normal adult rat brain (Table III).

The final levels of enzymatic activities *in vitro* depend on both the cellular composition as well as the developmental stage of the starting tissue. Compared to their counterparts prepared from the mesencephalon–diencephalon–rhombencephalon part of the 15-day fetal rat brain, aggregating cell cultures of fetal telencephalon show specific enzymatic activities (Table III) which are about twice as high for glutamine synthetase (GLU-S), considerably higher for both choline acetyltransferase

(CAT) and 2′,3′-cyclic nucleotide 3′-phosphohydrolase (CNP), slightly lower for glutamic acid decarboxylase (GAD), and 60% lower for acetylcholinesterase (AChE). Furthermore, catecholaminergic characteristics (e.g., tyrosine hydroxylase activity; biosynthesis of catecholamines) are present in "hindbrain" cell cultures but absent in aggregates of fetal telencephalic cells. The proportions of the different cell types in culture, and thus the levels of marker enzyme activities, are also influenced by the mitotic activity occurring during the first 2 weeks in culture (Section 3.1). Aggregating cell cultures of fetal rat telencephalon grown in the absence of insulin show a significant reduction in both the DNA synthesis and the specific activities of GAD, GLU-S, and CNP, as well as a moderate decrease in CAT activity (Lenoir and Honegger, 1983; Honegger and Guentert-Lauber, 1984). These results, suggesting the presence of proliferating precursor cells of both neurons and glial cells, are supported by autoradiographic examinations on the electron microscopic level showing that both neurons and glial cells are capable of incorporating radiolabeled thymidine into their DNA (P. Honegger and P. Favrod, unpublished results).

After cessation of the mitotic activity *in vitro*, the expression of the differentiated characteristics progresses rapidly, as shown by the developmental increase in marker enzyme activities (Table III) similar to that observed *in vitro*. The changes in biochemical characteristics related to cellular differentiation are also in accord with the extensive morphological maturation *in vitro* (Fig. 2): the increase in the activities of neuronal marker enzymes is accompanied by both the growth of neuropil and the appearance of numerous morphologically mature synapses; the rapid rise in CNP activity observed after 2 weeks in culture is paralleled by both the accumulation of myelin basic protein (Almazan *et al.*, 1984, 1985) and the formation of myelin lamellae around axons.

Thus, for routine work using aggregating brain cell cultures, cellular differentiation can be monitored reliably by determining the specific activities of a set of marker enzymes. As shown below, this approach led to the detection of several environmental factors influencing specifically the maturation of brain cells *in vitro*.

3.2.1. Cholinergic Differentiation. The development of cholinergic neurons in serum-free aggregating brain cell cultures is greatly influenced by several environmental factors:

a. *Triiodothyronine* (T_3) enhances the developmental increase in CAT activity in a time- and concentration-dependent way (Honegger and Lenoir, 1980). Addition of optimal amounts of T_3 (3×10^{-8} M) is most effective at an early developmental stage of the cultures, resembling the response of hypothyroid rats to thyroid hormone treatments.

Table IV. Distribution of T_3- and NGF-Sensitive Cholinergic
Neurons in 15-Day Fetal Rat Brain[a]

Brain region used for culture preparation	CAT specific activity (pmoles/min/mg protein)		
	$-T_3$	$+T_3$	$+T_3 + NGF$
Upper telencephalon	3	7	27
Lower telencephalon	26	228	498
Hindbrain	55	49	50

[a] Three regions of 15-day fetal rat brain were dissected by two divisions of the brain, one separating the telencephalon from the hindbrain (mesencephalon–diencephalon–rhombencephalon) and a longitudinal one separating the telencephalon into an upper half, representing the cortical region, and a lower half containing the basal brain region. Each brain part was used to prepare serum-free aggregating cell cultures. Aggregates were grown in three different media: without T_3; with T_3 (30 nM); with both T_3 (30 nM) and NGF (10 ng/ml). CAT was measured in homogenates of 19-day cultures. Values show the mean of 4 culture flasks.

Since no effect was found on either cell survival or mitotic activity *in vitro*, it has been concluded that T_3 specifically stimulates the differentiation of cholinergic neurons (Honegger and Lenoir, 1980). This view is supported by observations *in vivo* (Legrand, 1967; Lauder, 1978) showing that T_3 influences the formation of neuropil in the developing cerebellum. Experiments *in vitro* have shown that thyroid hormone regulates the biosynthesis and assembly of microtubule-associated proteins essential for neurite formation (Fellous *et al.*, 1979; Mareck *et al.*, 1980). Furthermore, it has been shown that T_3 treatment increases the activity of Na^+,K^+-ATPase in aggregating cultures derived from fetal rat brain (Atterwill *et al.*, 1983). This may point to a modulatory role of T_3 in the biosynthesis of specific CNS proteins, similar to that described in hepatocytes (Seelig *et al.*, 1981).

   b. *Nerve growth factor* (NGF), a polypeptide essential for the development and maintenance of the peripheral sympathetic and sensory nervous system, also stimulates the developmental increase in CAT activity of cultured fetal rat telencephalic cells (Honegger and Lenoir, 1982). This effect is dose-dependent, showing half-maximal stimulation at medium concentrations of approximately 10^{-10} M 2.5S NGF. Further experiments have shown that this stimulatory effect of NGF is strictly dependent on the presence of T_3 in the culture medium (Honegger, 1983). Recently, it has been possible to localize the T_3- and NGF-sensitive cholinergic neurons in a relatively restricted region of the fetal rat telencephalon (Table IV). This finding suggests that only a distinct population of cholinergic CNS neurons is sensitive to T_3 and NGF, and allows the preparation of cultures enriched in such neurons for further investigations. Experiments *in vivo* (Gnahn *et al.*, 1983) have confirmed the stimulatory action of NGF on rat forebrain cholinergic neurons during their development.

c. *Elevated potassium ion concentrations* (30 mM KCl) in the culture medium significantly increase the levels of CAT activity in cultured telencephalic cells (Honegger, 1983). As has been shown for NGF, this stimulatory effect requires the presence of T_3 in the culture medium. The combined treatment with NGF and high potassium does not produce an additive effect, suggesting a common molecular mechanism of action, e.g., an alteration of ion fluxes across the plasma membrane. However, the voltage-dependent sodium channel appears not to be involved, since NGF stimulates CAT also in the presence of tetrodotoxin (Honegger, 1983). Another possible target that needs further examination is the Na^+,K^+-ATPase. It has been shown that the function of this enzyme is affected by NGF or by depolarizing levels of potassium ions in cultured cells of both rat pheochromocytoma (Boonstra *et al.*, 1981) and chick embryo dorsal root ganglion (Skaper and Varon, 1980). According to Boonstra *et al.* (1981) the activation of Na^+,K^+-ATPase may occur through a rapid increase in amiloride-sensitive Na^+ influx.

d. *A macromolecular extract*, prepared from conditioned media of either homologous cultures or astroglial monolayer cultures, added at a concentration of 2.8 μg protein/ml to aggregating cell cultures of fetal rat telencephalon, causes an increase in CAT activity both in the presence and absence of T_3 (Honegger and Guentert, 1983). This finding suggests that extracellular soluble proteins (presumably of astroglial origin) stimulate the development of cultured cholinergic forebrain neurons in a way distinct from the action of NGF or NGF-like proteins. This view is supported by a recent report (Crutcher and Collins, 1982) showing the existence of two different hippocampal factors which accelerate neurite growth in cultures of either sympathetic or parasympathetic neurons.

3.2.2. Astroglial Differentiation. Serum-free aggregating brain cell cultures treated with EGF (5 ng/ml show a slight decrease in DNA synthesis and a concomitant great increase in GLU-S activity (Fig. 4). This EGF-induced developmental rise in GLU-S activity is dose-dependent; maximal stimulation is obtained with daily additions of 3 ng/ml EGF. The sensitivity of the cells to EGF is restricted to the first 2 weeks in culture, coinciding with the period of active cellular proliferation (Honegger and Guentert, 1984). The EGF-dependent increase in GLU-S activity occurs also in the absence of hydrocortisone, which demonstrates

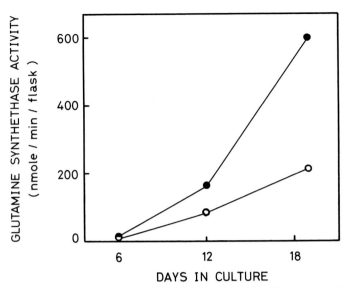

Figure 4. Development of glutamine synthetase in aggregating cell cultures of 15-day fetal rat telencephalon. ○, cultures grown in standard chemically defined medium; ●, cultures treated in addition with EGF (5 ng/ml) between day 2 and day 8 *in vitro.*

that it is unrelated to the glucocorticoid induction of GLU-S observed in aggregating cell cultures of chick neural retina (Morris and Moscona, 1970, 1971) and in astroglial monolayer cultures (Hallermayer *et al.*, 1981; Juurlink *et al.*, 1981). It has been shown in the CNS that GLU-S is localized exclusively in astrocytes (Norenberg, 1979; Norenberg and Martinez-Hernandez, 1979). Thus, since astrocytes constitute the preponderant cell type in aggregating brain cell cultures (Trapp *et al.*, 1979; Honegger *et al.*, 1979), it can be concluded that the EGF-triggered increase in GLU-S activity reflects an enhancement of astroglial differentiation. This finding is in agreement with recent reports showing that in certain cell types EGF stimulates the expression of differentiated characteristics (Johnson *et al.*, 1980; Murdoch *et al.*, 1982), but it is in contrast with the observation in astroglial monolayer cultures that EGF causes an increase in the mitotic activity (Leutz and Schachner, 1981; Simpson *et al.*, 1982). This disparity in astroglial responses to EGF suggests that EGF initiates a sequence of molecular events prerequisite to both mitotic activity and cellular differentiation, e.g., activation of protein synthesis, and that the ultimate cellular response is controlled by other environmental factors. In contrast to monolayer cultures, aggregating cell cultures show restricted mitotic activity and extensive cellular differentiation, similar to the situation *in vivo*. Therefore, it seems likely that the enhancement of astroglial differentiation we observe represents the histotypic response to EGF.

3.2.3. Oligodendroglial Differentiation. Thyroid hormone (30 nM T_3) treatment of serum-free aggregating cell cultures of rat telencephalon greatly enhances both the development of the myelin-related enzymes galactosylceramide sulfotransferase and CNP (Honegger and Matthieu, 1980) as well as the accumulation of myelin basic protein (Almazan *et al.* 1984, 1985). Maximal stimulation of CNP is obtained with T_3 treatments starting as late as 20 days after culture initiation. This contrasts with the T_3-dependent increase in CAT activity (Section 3.2.1) which depends on an early developmental stage of the cultures. Thus, the oligodendroglial response to T_3 is distinct from the T_3-induced enhancement of cholinergic differentiation (Honegger and Matthieu, 1980). Since T_3 has no apparent effect on either cell survival or mitotic activity, it can be concluded that thyroid hormones markedly influence the maturation of oligodendrocytes. This view is supported by earlier observations on cerebellar explant cultures (Hamburgh, 1966) as well as by a recent report of Bhat *et al.* (1979) showing a T_3-dependent stimulation of myelin-associated glycolipid synthesis in cultures of dissociated brain cells.

Treatment of aggregating brain cells with EGF enhances the development of CNP in a time- and concentration-dependent manner, comparable to the stimulation of GLU-S (Honegger and Guentert, 1984). However, due to the disproportionality in cell number between oligodendrocytes and astrocytes (Trapp *et al.*, 1979), the interpretation of the stimulatory effect on CNP is more difficult. The observation (Honegger and Guentert, 1984) that the EGF-induced increase in CNP activity is dependent on the presence of insulin would suggest a mitogenic effect of EGF on oligodendrocytes, whereas the finding Almazan *et al.* 1984, 1985 that EGF stimulates the accumulation of myelin basic protein in parallel to the increase in CNP activity would speak for an enhancement of oligodendroglial maturation. At any rate, several observations suggest that the response of oligodendrocytes to EGF occurs indirectly, through astroglial stimulation: in contrast to astrocytes, oligodendrocytes in monolayer culture display few (if any) specific EGF binding sites (Leutz and Schachner, 1982; Simpson *et al.*, 1982). Moreover, in monolayer culture astrocytes appear to support the growth and maintenance of oligodendrocytes (McCarthy and de Vellis, 1980; P. Honegger, unpublished observations). Finally, aggregating brain cell cultures treated with a macromolecular fraction prepared from conditioned media of homologous cultures show a significant increase in CNP activity and a slight decrease in the activity of GLU-S, the astroglial marker; this effect is even more pronounced after addition of an extract prepared from EGF-treated cultures (Guentert and Honegger, 1984). In view of these findings, it is tempting to speculate that the development of oligodendrocytes is controlled by the influence of differentiating astrocytes, either through direct cell–cell contact or via extracellular soluble macromolecules. Since it has been suggested (Raff *et al.*, 1983) that both "fibrous" (type 2) astrocytes and oligodendrocytes develop from a common progenitor cell, it is conceivable that a regulatory astroglial factor present in EGF-stimulated cultures induces these progenitor cells to become oligodendrocytes.

4. EVALUATION OF THE CULTURE SYSTEM

The present evidence indicates that serum-free aggregating cell cultures of mechanically dissociated fetal brain possess a number of unique features and, therefore, offer an attractive CNS model for studies *in vitro*. Most characteristically, and in contrast to dispersed monolayer cell cultures, aggregating cell cultures form regular three-dimensional cell arrangements. This particular configuration allows close cell–cell interactions through cell surface constituents and/or molecular transfers, and thus appears to be responsible for both the histotypic cellular organization and maturation as well as the long-term maintenance of highly differentiated cells. Moreover, it has been shown that the response of a given cell type to an exogenous stimulus, e.g., EGF, may be decisively influenced by the cell arrangement in culture and thus by the cellular microenvironment. Specific interactions during the phase of aggregate formation, which includes cell aggregation, migration, and sorting out, may explain the absence of fibroblasts in brain cell aggregates without using antimitotic drugs.

In comparison with explant cultures, i.e., cultured tissue fragments of about 1-mm^3 volume which retain a high degree of cellular organization and also undergo extensive cellular maturation, aggregating brain cell cultures have the advantages of both high yield and excellent reproducibility, allowing reliable and detailed biochemical studies. Furthermore, explants adhere to the culture surface and may become necrotic, whereas brain cell aggregates remain in suspension, thus being much easier to manipulate, and continue to be healthy for prolonged culture periods.

The disadvantage of an aggregate culture system with differentiating characteristics similar to the tissue *in vivo* is, obviously, the great structural complexity of the cultures which hinders direct observation and manipulation of individual cells and renders some biochemical data difficult to interpret. However, many of these obstacles can be circumvented by using correlative biochemical, immunohistochemical, and electron microscopic analysis. In addition, complementary approaches can be used such as modification of the cellular composition of the cultures, e.g., eliminating a class of cells either by selective adsorption or by a cytotoxic reaction, or intervention in specific molecular processes, e.g., blocking the synthesis of DNA or proteins or altering the influence of hormones. Also, it can be expected that further research will aid in developing new strategies and better tools to monitor the behavior of a specific cell type in aggregating brain cell cultures.

Thus, taking both the advantages and the disadvantages into account, it appears that the unique features of aggregating brain cell cultures are worth their price. As has been suggested earlier (Seeds, 1973; Honegger and Richelson, 1976, 1977a,b, 1979; Honegger and Haller, 1980; Matthieu et al., 1980), this system lends itself to developmental, pharmacological, toxicological, and virological investigations. The recent introduction of a serum-free culture method has further simplified and improved the technique as well as opened new interesting avenues in brain research.

ACKNOWLEDGMENTS

I would like to thank my colleagues, G. Almazan, P. du Pasquier, P. Favrod, B. Guentert, D. Lenoir, J.-M. Matthieu, and E. Raddatz, for participating in the studies described here and permitting me to present unpublished work. I am also indebted to Dr. E. Bachmann, Laboratoire Central, CHUV, for the amino acid analyses. Ms. J. Braissant and Ms. C. Albin provided expert assistance with the manuscript. Research in the author's laboratory was supported by Swiss National Science Foundation Grants 3.117.77 and 3.641.80.

REFERENCES

Almazan, G., Honegger, P., Guentert-Lauber, B., and Matthieu, J.-M., 1984, Brain cell aggregate culture: Effect of T3 and bGH on myelination, *Trans. Am. Soc. Neurochem.* **15**:258.

Almazan, G., Honegger, P, and Matthieu, J.-M., 1985, Triiodothyronine stimulation of oligodendroglial differentiation and myelination: A developmental study (submitted).

Atterwill, C. K., Kingsbury, A. E., and Balázs, R., 1983, Effects of thyroid hormone on neural development in vitro, in: *Drugs and Hormones in Brain Development* (M. Schlumpf and W. Lichtensteiger, eds.), Karger, Basel, pp. 50–61.

Bhat, N. R., Sarlève, L. L., Subba Rao, G., and Pieringer, R. A., 1979, Investigations on myelination in vitro: Regulation by thyroid hormone in cultures of dissociated brain cells from embryonic mice. *J. Biol. Chem.* **254**:9342–9344.

Boonstra, J., Van der Saag, P. T., Moolenaar, W. H., and De Laat, S. W., 1981, Rapid effects of nerve growth factor on the Na^+,K^+-pump in rat pheochromocytoma cells, *Exp. Cell Res.* **131**:452–455.

Crutcher, K. A., and Collins, F., 1982, In vitro evidence for two distinct hippocampal growth factors: Basis of neuronal plasticity?, *Science* **217**:67–68.

DeLong, G. R., 1970, Histogenesis of fetal mouse isocortex and hippocampus in reaggregating cell cultures, *Develop. Biol.* **22**:563–583.

DeLong, G. R., and Sidman, R. L., 1970, Alignment defect of reaggregating cells in cultures of developing brains of reeler mutant mice, *Develop. Biol.* **22**:584–600.

Fellous, A., Lennon, A. M., Francon, J., and Nunez, J., 1979, Thyroid hormone and neurotubule assembly in vitro during brain development, *Eur. J. Biochem.* **101**:365–376.

Garber, B. B., 1977, Cell aggregation and recognition in the self-assembly of brain tissues, in: *Cell, Tissue and Organ Cultures in Neurobiology* (S. Fedoroff and L. Hertz, eds.), Academic Press, New York, pp. 515–537.

Garber, B. B., and Moscona, A. A., 1972, Reconstruction of brain tissue from cell suspensions. I. Aggregation patterns of cells dissociated from different regions of the developing brain, *Develop. Biol.* **27**:217–234.

Gnahn, H., Hefti, F., Heumann, R., Schwab, M. E., and Thoenen, H., 1983, NGF-mediated increase of choline acetyltransferase (ChAT) in the neonatal rat forebrain: Evidence for a physiological role of NGF in the brain?, *Develop. Brain Res.* **9**:45–52.

Guentert-Lauber, B., and Honegger, P., 1984, Epidermal growth factor (EGF) stimulation of cultured brain cells. II. Increased production of extracellular soluble proteins, *Develop. Brain Res.* **11**:253–260.

Hallermayer, K., Harmening, C., and Hamprecht, B., 1981, Cellular localization and regulation of glutamine synthetase in primary cultures of brain cells from newborn mice, *J. Neurochem.* **37**:43–52.

Hamburgh, M., 1966, Evidence for a direct effect of temperature and thyroid hormone on myelogenesis in vitro, *Develop. Biol.* **13**:15–30.

Honegger, P., 1983, Nerve growth factor-sensitive brain neurons, in: *Drugs and Hormones in Brain Development* (M. Schlumpf and W. Lichtensteiger, eds.), Karger, Basel, pp. 36–42.

Honegger, P., and Guentert, B., 1983, Cholinergic differentiation in serum-free aggregating fetal brain cells, in: *Hormonally Defined Media, A Tool in Cell Biology* (G. Fischer and R. J. Wieser, eds.), Springer-Verlag, Berlin, pp. 203–214.

Honegger, P., and Guentert-Lauber, B., 1984, Epidermal growth factor (EGF) stimulation of cultured brain cells. I. Enhancement of the developmental increase in glial enzymatic activity, *Develop. Brain Res.* **11**:245–251.

Honegger, P., and Haller, O., 1980, Gene expression for myxovirus resistance in mouse brain aggregating cell cultures: A model system in developmental neurobiology, in: *Multidisciplinary Approach to Brain Development* (C. Di Benedetta et al., eds.), Elsevier/North-Holland, Amsterdam, pp. 407–408.

Honegger, P., and Lenoir, D., 1980, Triiodothyronine enhancement of neuronal differentiation in aggregating fetal rat brain cells cultured in a chemically defined medium, *Brain Res.* **199**:425–434.

Honegger, P., and Lenoir, D., 1982, Nerve growth factor (NGF) stimulation of cholinergic telencephalic neurons in aggregating cell cultures, *Develop. Brain Res.* **3**:229–238.

Honegger, P., and Matthieu, J.-M., 1980, Myelination of aggregating fetal rat brain cell cultures grown in a chemically defined medium, in: *Neurological Mutations Affecting Myelination* (N. Baumann, ed.), Elsevier/North-Holland, Amsterdam, pp. 481–488.

Honegger, P., and Richelson, E., 1976, Biochemical differentiation of mechanically dissociated mammalian brain in aggregating cell culture, *Brain Res.* **109**:335–354.

Honegger, P., and Richelson, E., 1977a, Biochemical differentiation of aggregating cell cultures of different fetal rat brain regions, *Brain Res.* **133**:329–339.

Honegger, P., and Richelson, E., 1977b, Kainic acid alters neurochemical development in fetal rat brain aggregating cell cultures, *Brain Res.* **138**:580–584.

Honegger, P., and Richelson, E., 1979, Neurotransmitter synthesis, storage and release by aggregating cell cultures of rat brain, *Brain Res.* **162**:89–101.

Honegger, P., Lenoir, D., and Favrod, P., 1979, Growth and differentiation of aggregating fetal brain cells in a serum-free defined medium, *Nature* **282**:305–308.

Johnson, L. K., Baxter, J. D., Vlodavsky, I., and Gospodarowicz, D., 1980, Epidermal growth factor and expression of specific genes: Effects on cultured rat pituitary cells are dissociable from the mitogenic response, *Proc. Natl. Acad. Sci. USA* **77**:394–398.

Jørgensen, O. S., Honegger, P., and Matthieu, J.-M., 1984, The neuronal adhesion protein D$_2$ in differentiating aggregates of brain cells, *Develop. Brain Res.* **14**:41–49.

Juurlink, B. H. J., Schousboe, A., Jørgensen, O. S., and Hertz, L., 1981, Induction by hydrocortisone of glutamine synthetase in mouse primary astrocyte cultures, *J. Neurochem.* **36**:136–142.

Knodel, E., and Richelson, E., 1980, Methionine-enkephalin immunoreactivity in fetal rat brain cells in aggregating culture and in mouse neuroblastoma cells, *Brain Res.* **197**:565–570.

Kozak, L., Eppig, J., Dahl, D., and Bignami, A., 1977, Ultrastructural and immunohistological characterization of a cell culture model for the study of neuronal–glial interactions, *Develop. Biol.* **59**:206–227.

Kurihara, T., and Tsukada, Y., 1967, The regional and subcellular distribution of 2′,3′-cyclic nucleotide 3′-phosphohydrolase in the central nervous system, *J. Neurochem.* **14**:1167–1174.

Lauder, J. M., 1978, Effects of early hypo- and hyperthyroidism on development of rat cerebellar cortex. IV. The parallel fibers, *Brain Res.* **142**:25–39.

Legrand, J., 1967, Variations, en fonction de l'âge, de la réponse du cervelet à l'action morphogénétique de la thyroïde chez le Rat, *Arch. Anat. Microsc. Morphol. Exp.* **56**:291–307.

Lenoir, D., and Honegger, P., 1983, Insulin-like growth factor I (IGF I) stimulates DNA synthesis in fetal rat brain cell cultures, *Develop. Brain Res.* **7**:205–213.

Leutz, A., and Schachner, M., 1981, Epidermal growth factor stimulates DNA-synthesis of astrocytes in primary cerebellar cultures, *Cell Tissue Res.* **220**:393–404.

Leutz, A., and Schachner, M., 1982, Cell type-specificity of epidermal growth factor (EGF) binding in primary cultures of early postnatal mouse cerebellum, *Neurosci. Lett.* **30**:179–182.

Levitt, P., Moore, R. Y., and Garber, B. B., 1976, Selective cell association of catecholamine neurons in brain aggregates in vitro, *Brain Res.* **111**:311–320.

Lu, E. J., Brown, W. J., Cole, R., and de Vellis, J., 1980, Ultrastructural differentiation and synaptogenesis in aggregating rotation cultures of rat cerebral cells, *J. Neurosci. Res.* **5**:447–463.

McCarthy, K. D., and de Vellis, J., 1980, Preparation of separate astroglial and oligodendroglial cell cultures from rat cerebral tissue, *J. Cell Biol.* **85**:890–902.

Mareck, A., Fellous, A., Francon, J., and Nunez, J., 1980, Changes in composition and activity of microtubule-associated proteins during brain development, *Nature* **284**:353–355.

Matthieu, J.-M., and Honegger, P., 1979, An in vitro model to study brain development: Brain aggregating cell cultures, in: *Models for the Study of Inborn Errors of Metabolism* (F. A. Hommes, ed.), Elsevier/North-Holland, Amsterdam, pp. 259–278.

Matthieu, J.-M., Honegger, P., Trapp, B. D., Cohen, S. R., and Webster, H., 1978, Myelination in rat brain aggregating cell cultures, *Neuroscience* **3**:565–572.

Matthieu, J.-M., Honegger, P., Favrod, P., Gautier, E., and Dolivo, M., 1979, Biochemical characterization of a myelin fraction isolated from rat brain aggregating cell cultures, *J. Neurochem.* **32**:869–881.

Matthieu, J.-M., Honegger, P., Favrod, P., Poduslo, J. F., Constantino-Ceccarini, E., and Kristic, R., 1980, Myelination and demyelination in aggregating cultures of rat brain cells, in: *Tissue Culture in Neurobiology* (E. Giacobini, A. Vernadakis, and A. Shahar, eds.), Raven Press, New York, pp. 441–459.

Matthieu, J.-M., Honegger, P., Favrod, P., Poduslo, J. F., and Kristic, R., 1981, Aggregating brain cell cultures: A model to study brain development, in: *Physiological and Biochemical Basis for Perinatal Medicine* (M. Monset-Couchard and A. Minkowski, eds.), Karger, Basel, pp. 359–366.

Morris, J. E., and Moscona, A. A., 1970, Induction of glutamine synthetase in embryonic retina: Its dependence on cell interactions, *Science* **167**:1736–1738.

Morris, J. E., and Moscona, A. A., 1971, The induction of glutamine synthetase in cell aggregates of embryonic neural retina: Correlations with differentiation and multicellular organization, *Develop. Biol.* **25**:420–444.

Moscona, A. A., 1960, Patterns and mechanisms of tissue reconstruction from dissociated cells, in: *Developing Cell Systems and Their Control* (D. Rudnick, ed.), Ronald Press, New York, pp. 45–70.

Moscona, A. A., 1961, Rotation-mediated histogenetic aggregation of dissociated cells: A quantifiable approach to cell interactions in vitro, *Exp. Cell Res.* **22**:455–475.

Moscona, A. A., 1965, Recombination of dissociated cells and the development of cell aggregates, in: *Cells and Tissues in Culture*, Volume 1 (E. N. Willmer, ed.), Academic Press, New York, pp. 489–529.

Murdoch, G. H., Potter, E., Nicolaisen, A. K., Evans, R. M., and Rosenfeld, M. G., 1982, Epidermal growth factor rapidly stimulates prolactin gene transcription, *Nature* **300**:192–194.

Norenberg, M. D., 1979, The distribution of glutamine synthetase in the rat central nervous system, *J. Histochem. Cytochem.* **27**:756–762.

Norenberg, M. D., and Martinez-Hernandez, A., 1979, Fine structural localization of glutamine synthetase in astrocytes of rat brain, *Brain Res.* **161**:303–310.

Pishak, M. R., and Phillips, A. T., 1979, A modified radioisotopic assay for measuring glutamine synthetase activity in tissue extracts, *Anal. Biochem.* **94**:82–88.

Raff, M. C., Miller, R. H., and Noble, M., 1983, A glial progenitor cell that develops in vitro into an astrocyte or an oligodendrocyte depending on culture medium, *Nature* **303**:390–396.

Schmidt, G. L., 1975, Development of biochemical activities associated with myelination in chick brain aggregate cultures, *Brain Res.* **87**:110–113.

Seeds, N. W., 1971, Biochemical differentiation in reaggregating brain cell cultures, *Proc. Natl. Acad. Sci. USA* **68**:1858–1861.

Seeds, N. W., 1973, Differentiation of aggregating brain cell cultures, in: *Tissue Culture of the Nervous System* (G. Sato, ed.), Plenum Press, New York, pp. 35–53.

Seeds, N. W., 1975a, Expression of differentiated activities in reaggregating brain cell cultures, *J. Biol. Chem.* **250**:5455–5458.

Seeds, N. W., 1975b, Cerebellar cell surface antigens of mouse brain, *Proc. Natl. Acad. Sci. USA* **72**:4110–4114.

Seeds, N. W., and Gilman, A. G., 1971, Norepinephrine stimulated increase of cyclic AMP levels in developing mouse brain cell cultures, *Science* **174**:292–293.

Seeds, N. W., and Haffke, S. C., 1978, Cell junction and ultrastructural development of reaggregated mouse brain cell cultures, *Develop. Neurosci.* **1**:69–79.

Seeds, N. W., and Vatter, A. E., 1971, Synaptogenesis in reaggregating brain cell culture, *Proc. Natl. Acad. Sci. USA* **68**:3219–3222.

Seeds, N. W., Marks, M. J., and Ramirez, G., 1977, Aggregate cultures: A model for studies of brain development, in: *Cell Culture and Its Application* (R. Acton and D. Lynn, eds.), Academic Press, New York, pp. 23–37.

Seelig, S., Liaw, C., Towle, H. C., and Oppenheimer, J. H., 1981, Thyroid hormone attenuates and augments hepatic gene expression at a pretranslational level, *Proc. Natl. Acad. Sci. USA* **78**:4733–4737.

Simpson, D. L., Morrison, R., de Vellis, J., and Herschman, H. R., 1982, Epidermal growth factor binding and mitogenic activity on purified populations of cells from the central nervous system, *J. Neurosci. Res.* **8**:453–462.

Skaper, S. D., and Varon, S., 1980, Properties of the sodium extrusion mechanism controlled by nerve growth factor in chick embryo dorsal root ganglionic cells, *J. Neurochem.* **34**:1654–1660.

Trapp, B. D., Honegger, P., Richelson, E., and Webster, H. D., 1979, Morphological differentiation of mechanically dissociated fetal rat brain in aggregating cell cultures, *Brain Res.* **160**:117–130.

Trapp, B. D., Marangos, P. J., and Webster, H. D., 1981, Immunocytochemical localization and development profile of neuron specific enolase (NSE) and non-neuronal enolase (NNE) in aggregating cell cultures of fetal rat brain, *Brain Res.* **220**:121–130.

Trapp, B. D., Webster, H., Johnson, D., Quarles, R. H., Cohen, S. R., and Murray, M. R., 1982, Myelin formation in rotation-mediated aggregating cell cultures: Immunocytochemical, electron microscopic, and biochemical observations, *J. Neurosci.* **2**:986–993.

Wehner, J. M., Feinmann, R. D., and Sheppard, J. R., 1982, β-Adrenergic response in mouse CNS reaggregate cultures, *Brain Res.* **255**:207–217.

Wenger, D., Wharton, C., and Seeds, N. W., 1979, Sphingomyelinase activities in neuronal cell cultures, *Life Sci.* **24**:679–684.

Wilson, S. H., Schrier, B. K., Farber, J. L., Thompson, E. J., Rosenberg, R. N., Blume, A. J., and Nirenberg, M. W., 1972, Markers for gene expression in cultured cells from the nervous system, *J. Biol. Chem.* **247**:3159–3169.

8

PC12 Cells as a Model of Neuronal Differentiation

GORDON GUROFF

1. DEVELOPMENT OF PC12 CELLS

In 1975 Tischler and Greene reported the culture of a norepinephrine-producing pheochromocytoma previously observed and carried in New England Deaconess rats by Warren and his co-workers (Warren and Chute, 1972; DeLellis *et al.*, 1973). The tumor cells grew readily under standard culture conditions and exhibited a formaldehyde-induced fluorescence characteristic of the presence of catecholamines. Many of the cells produced short processes which were evident within 24 hr of plating. In the presence of nanogram quantities of nerve growth factor (NGF), more processes were evident and within 1 to 2 weeks of plating there were up to 20 times more processes in the presence of NGF.

This initial report was followed closely by a series of studies in which Greene and his co-workers examined the properties of a particular clone from this tumor, the PC12. This clone has, for reasons specified later, become not only the premiere tool for the study of NGF action but also an increasingly acceptable model for the study of catecholamine biosynthesis and secretion, as well as for neuronal differentiation itself.

GORDON GUROFF • Section on Growth Factors, National Institute of Child Health and Human Development, National Institutes of Health, Bethesda, Maryland 20205.

The first studies of this clone established the characteristics of the cells and the outlines of their NGF responsiveness (Greene and Tischler, 1976; Greene and Rein, 1977a; Dichter *et al.*, 1977). It was shown, for example, that the cells had 40 chromosomes, 38 autosomes and an XY pair. The doubling time was determined to be about 92 hr in RPMI 1640 medium containing 10% heat-inactivated horse serum and 5% fetal calf serum. The cells appeared rounded or polygonal and tended to clump; they attached rather poorly to the plastic tissue culture dishes, but more firmly if they were grown on collagen. They contained dense-core granules, 40 to 350 nm in diameter, which were similar to those seen in both adrenal chromaffin cells and sympathetic neurons. The cells contained catecholamines, as visualized by the formaldehyde-induced fluorescence technique, and accordingly had levels of some of the catecholamine-synthesizing enzymes comparable to or greater than those found in the adrenal medulla. In contrast to adrenal cells, and, indeed, to the tumor from which they were cloned, they had much more dopamine than they did norepinephrine. The cells also synthesized and released acetylcholine and contained choline acetyltransferase (CAT), the enzyme catalyzing the synthesis of acetylcholine, as well as a number of small agranular vesicles thought to contain acetylcholine. The levels of CAT in these cells appeared to be dependent on the density of the culture, higher levels of enzyme being associated with higher density cultures. Overall, thus, these cells displayed many of the properties of adrenal medullary cells and some of the properties, as well, of sympathetic neurons.

Upon treatment with NGF the cells hypertrophied and began to form processes. These processes were quite evident in the cultures after several days and continued to elongate for several weeks (Fig. 1). They were similar in appearance to the processes produced by sympathetic neurons in culture and reached lengths of 500–1000 μm; they were fine, profusely branched, and had growth cones and numerous varicosities. In addition to these morphological changes, the cells exhibited a markedly decreased growth rate and some increase in CAT and the content of acetylcholine. Most interestingly, virtually all the cells in culture became electrically excitable and were much more sensitive to depolarization with acetylcholine than were untreated cells. Thus, generally speaking, NGF-treated PC12 cells exhibited many of the properties of mature, terminally differentiated sympathetic neurons.

One of the most striking observations, however, was that the effects of NGF, apparently producing a differentiation from an adrenal medullary cell to a mature sympathetic neuron, were completely and rapidly reversible. Within 24 hr of the removal of NGF, most of the cells lost

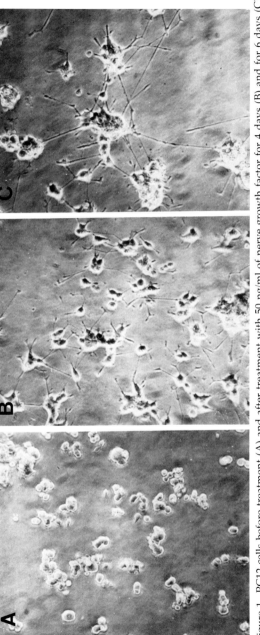

Figure 1. PC12 cells before treatment (A) and after treatment with 50 ng/ml of nerve growth factor for 4 days (B) and for 6 days (C).

their processes. This degeneration of processes was accompanied by a somewhat slower return to a normal rate of cell division and, in general, a resumption of the properties of the original adrenal medullary chromaffinlike cells.

2. GENERAL CHARACTERISTICS

Since these original studies were published, the PC12 clone has been widely and generously distributed. Consequently, there have been a large number of papers published concerning various aspects of the biology of these cells. By far the largest proportion of these investigations concerned the actions of NGF, and these will be covered in a later section. A substantial number, however, have dealt with the properties of PC12 in the absence of NGF.

2.1. Transmitter Content

It was shown early on (Greene and Rein, 1977b) that untreated PC12 cells will take up catecholamines from the medium by a system that has a K_m of about 2 μM and resembles the uptake$_1$ system of sympathetic neurons. They store these catecholamines (norepinephrine and dopamine) in chromaffin-type granules and will release them in a Ca^{2+}-dependent fashion in response to the addition of high concentrations of K^+. They can also be released by treatment of the cells with veratridine or with nicotinic cholinergic agonists such as carbachol (Greene and Rein, 1977c).

The cells also store and release acetylcholine. They take up choline by a Na^+-dependent system with a K_m of 12 μM that is fairly insensitive to inhibition by hemicholinium (Melega and Howard, 1981). The acetylcholine produced is stored in granules which are, on the basis of sucrose density gradient separation, different from those which contain catecholamines (Schubert and Klier, 1977) but are nevertheless classified as dense-core. Since virtually all the cells contain catecholamines, as evidenced by their fluorescence, it has been concluded that at least some of them contain both transmitters, dopamine and acetylcholine, in different granules. Acetylcholine is secreted from the cells, along with dopamine, upon depolarization with high levels of K^+ or with nicotinic cholinergic agonists.

2.2. Transmitter-Synthesizing Enzymes

The enzymes for the metabolism of the catecholamines are present in PC12 cells. Tyrosine hydroxylase was observed in the early studies and has now been inspected from a number of vantage points. It can be induced by glucocorticoids (Edgar and Thoenen, 1978) and its specific activity increases with the density of the culture (Lucas *et al.*, 1979). Indeed, the mRNA for the enzyme has been isolated from PC12 cells and translated in a reticulocyte system (Baetge *et al.*, 1981); the formal demonstration that the synthesis of the mRNA for tyrosine hydroxylase is increased by treatment of the cells with glucocorticoids has come from these experiments. The dopamine-β-hydroxylase from PC12 cells has been found to be a glycoprotein containing two subunits of molecular weights 73,000 and 77,000 which occur near-equal amounts in the molecule (Sabban *et al.*, 1983). The enzyme secreted from the cells appears to be a single subunit of slightly different molecular weight than either of the subunits of the cellular form (McHugh *et al.*, submitted). Detailed studies on the other enzymes of catecholamine biosynthesis or catabolism have not been done, but whole cells have been studied as a tool by which to understand the overall regulation of catecholamine metabolism (Greene and Rein, 1978). In these studies it has been shown that one reason these cells produce such a large excess of dopamine is that they may have a relative insufficiency of ascorbic acid, a cofactor for the enzyme dopamine-β-hydroxylase which converts dopamine to norepinephrine.

CAT is present in these cells and its level is regulated by cell density, by conditioned media of various cell types, and by cAMP derivatives, as well as by NGF (Schubert *et al.*, 1977). Acetylcholinesterase (AChE) is also present; in untreated cells there are three forms of the enzyme— 4, 6.5, and 10S (Rieger *et al.*, 1980). The specific activity of these forms is unaffected by the density of the culture, but, as discussed below, NGF treatment increases the specific activity and also leads to the appearance of another molecular form. The induction of AChE activity in these cells can also be produced by medium conditioned by C6 glioma cells or by extracts of chick embryo or rat or human brain (Lucas *et al.*, 1981). It is not known whether these other agents induce the same new molecular form that NGF induces, but it is known that the conditioned medium and the tissue extracts act by a different mechanism than does NGF.

2.3. Receptors

The cells contain, of course, receptors for NGF. These will be discussed in detail in a later section. They also have a number of other receptors on their cell membranes. Primary among these are the acetylcholine receptors. PC12 cells have nicotinic acetylcholine receptors and the binding of acetylcholine or nicotinic cholinergic agonists leads to the release of catecholamines (Greene and Rein, 1977c). These receptors are similar to those seen on sympathetic neurons (Patrick and Stallcup, 1977a,b). The cells also have muscarinic cholinergic receptors as revealed by the saturable, high-affinity binding of the receptor agonist quinuclidinyl benzilate (Jumblatt and Tischler, 1982), and these receptors are comparable to those found on adrenal medullary cells.

There are receptors for the mitogen epidermal growth factor (EGF) on these cells (Huff and Guroff, 1979; Huff *et al.*, 1981), and EGF has some interesting actions on the cells, to be discussed later. The receptors are specific for EGF and bind with an affinity of 1.9×10^{-9} M. There are the order of 80,000 such receptors per cell. The EGF receptors are distinct from the NGF receptors, and it has been shown (Pevzner *et al.*, 1982) that both receptors can be found on the same individual cells.

Receptors for adenosine are also present on the cells (Guroff *et al.*, 1981). These receptors are of the R_a class and are linked to adenylate cyclase. There are also receptors of some kind for the tumor promoter 12-O-tetradecanoylphorbol-13-acetate (End *et al.*, 1982b). More recently, it has been reported that receptors for enkephalin can be found in low numbers on a subclone of PC12 (PC12h) (Inoue and Hatanaka, 1982) and that the number of such receptors is dramatically increased by treatment of the cultures with NGF.

2.4. Electrophysiology

Ion flux measurements (Arner and Stallcup, 1981) have defined a number of ion channels in PC12 membranes. Among the channels found are (1) voltage-dependent Na^+ channels, (2) voltage-dependent Ca^{2+} channels, (3) acetylcholine receptor channels, (4) voltage-dependent K^+ channels, and (5) Ca^{2+}-dependent K^+ channels. Standard electrophysiological measurements on PC12 cells are difficult because the cells are quite small, but cells fused by treatment with polyethylene glycol give rise to large multinuclear cells which can be used for such measurements (O'Lague and Huttner, 1980). These fused cells exhibit resting membrane potentials of -50 to -65 mV. Electrophysiological measurements give evidence for the presence of (1) voltage-sensitive K^+ conductance, (2) Ca^{2+}-dependent K^+ conductance, and (3) voltage-dependent Ca^{2+} conductance. Cells treated with NGF show all of the above-mentioned phenomena and display a Na^+-dependent action potential mechanism not seen in untreated cells.

3. ACTIONS OF NGF

It would be difficult to overemphasize the significance of the PC12 model for studies on the actions of NGF. Suffice it to say that before this model became available there were no completely acceptable *in vitro* studies on this peptide. Indeed, for 25 years after the discovery of the factor, every *in vitro* experiment was subject to a crucial criticism. That is, since NGF is required for the very survival of target cells in culture, any effects seen in treated cells had to be compared against a control not given NGF which was, in fact, dying. Even short-term experiments in which the deleterious effects of NGF deprivation were still reversible were not completely without taint. The advent of PC12 provided a cell which, while showing a profound response to NGF, did not die in its absence. It is not surprising, then, that most of the recent mechanistic studies have been done with this model.

3.1. NGF Receptors

The NGF receptors on the plasma membrane of these cells are of two types (Landreth and Shooter, 1980; Schechter and Bothwell, 1980). Of the approximately 60,000 receptors on the surface of each cell, some 75% are characterized by a fast dissociation rate ($t_{1/2}$ 30 sec) and a sensitivity to digestion by brief exposure to trypsin. The remainder have a much slower association time and a very much slower dissociation time ($t_{1/2}$ 1800 sec) and are resistant to digestion by trypsin. Both kinds of receptors are specific for NGF. Some data indicate that both types of receptors have equilibrium constants of about 2×10^{-10} M (Schechter and Bothwell, 1980), while other experiments (Landreth and Shooter, 1980) show that the trypsin-sensitive receptor has a lower affinity (K_{eq} 1×10^{-9} M), and there are some conflicting data about the relationship of these receptor classes to one another; one group (Landreth and Shooter, 1980) has found evidence that the rapidly dissociating, trypsin-sensitive receptor is converted in the presence of NGF to the slow-dissociating, trypsin-resistant form, while no evidence for this ligand-induced conversion could be obtained by another group (Schechter and Bothwell, 1980).

The binding of NGF to its receptors is followed by the clustering of these originally diffusely distributed receptors into patches (Levi *et al.*, 1980). Using rhodamine-labeled NGF, clustering of about 70–80% of the total receptors on PC12 cells occurs. These clusters are then subjected to an energy-dependent endocytosis, similar to that previously shown to occur for insulin and for EGF among others, and this endocytosis seems to account for the loss of surface receptors known as down-regulation. The internalization of NGF leads to its localization primarily or even exclusively to the lysosomes where it is degraded (Rohrer et al., 1982; Hogue-Angeletti et al., 1982). Indeed, although there are clearly receptors for NGF associated with the nucleus of PC12 cells (Yankner and Shooter, 1979), the weight of evidence suggests that they are not physiologically significant (Heumann et al., 1981).

3.2. Rapid, Membrane-Associated Actions

The binding of NGF to its receptors leads to a large number of alterations in the cell. These can be divided roughly into two classes. First, there are a number of rapid changes occurring at or near the membrane. These are measured in minutes or even seconds and do not seem to require intracellular mediation and certainly not transcription. Then, there are a number of longer-term changes in the overall biology of the cells, most of which appear to require changes in the transcriptional events in the cells.

Perhaps the most rapid of the former class, the membrane-associated effects, are changes in the structure of the membrane itself (Connolly et al., 1979). Within a very few seconds after the addition of NGF to the culture medium, the surface morphology, initially quite complex, becomes simplified and within hours, even in the continued presence of NGF, becomes complex again. The changes involve the appearance of ruffles within 30 sec. These ruffles become quite prominent by about 3 min and almost disappear by about 7 min. As the ruffles become prominent, the microvilli originally seen on the cells disappear. Also within 3 min there is a threefold increase in the density of pits on the cell surface. As indicated above, these alterations are transient and disappear completely within a few hours.

In view of the changes in morphology it is not surprising that the properties of the membrane change. One of the changes involves the adhesiveness of the cells (Schubert and Whitlock, 1977). Within 10 min after the addition of NGF, and perhaps substantially earlier than that, there is an increase in the affinity of the cells for the plastic tissue culture surface and an increase in the adhesion of the cells to each other as well.

NGF has been reported to produce increases in the cAMP levels in the cells (Schubert and Whitlock, 1977). These increases were moderate (< twofold) and transient (baseline again within 22 min). Such increases in PC12 cells due to NGF have not been observed by others (Hatanaka et al., 1978).

Another somewhat controversial observation has been that the early effects of NGF include an increase in the transmembrane movements of calcium ions. Schubert *et al.* (1978) reported that NGF stimulates the efflux of $^{45}Ca^{2+}$ from PC12 cells preloaded with the isotope. The effects seen were small and the concentration of NGF used was quite high. Under similar conditions, others could not replicate these findings (Landreth *et al.*, 1980), nor did they see any effect of NGF on the influx of calcium.

It has also been reported (Boonstra *et al.*, 1981) that NGF causes a rapid increase in the activity of the Na^+,K^+ pump of the cells. This increase can be blocked by amiloride, an inhibitor of Na^+ flux, and mimicked by monensin, a Na^+ ionophore. These latter observations suggest that the stimulation of the pump is triggered by an NGF-induced increase in Na^+ influx. Such an influx of Na^+ has also been reported to be a consequence of EGF and insulin actions on their respective target cells.

The actions of NGF on uptake are not limited to the transport of ions. The model amino acids α-aminoisobutyric acid and aminocyclo-pentane-1-carboxylic acid were both taken up about 50% faster into PC12 cells 24 hr after treatment of the cells with NGF (McGuire and Greene, 1979). Some increase was seen as little as 15 min after treatment with the factor and this increase was not blocked by inhibitors of RNA synthesis. In the same experiments it was shown that NGF has no effect on the uptake of nucleosides or of norepinephrine.

An effect of NGF on the metabolism of phospholipids in PC12 cells has been seen (Traynor *et al.*, 1982). The incorporation of inorganic phosphate into phosphatidylinositol and phosphatidic acid was increased some two- to threefold after NGF treatment. The stimulation of the incorporation of phosphate into the other phospholipids was smaller, and the overall phospholipid composition of the cells did not change even after long treatment with the factor. The stimulation, appearing initially after about 10 min, is one of the longer of the "short-term effects" and the authors consider that these changes cannot be responsible for the rather faster alterations in such things as cellular adhesion.

3.3. Changes in Phosphorylation

Also following the binding of NGF to its receptor are a number of alterations in the phosphorylation of various cellular proteins. A number of cytoplasmic and nuclear proteins exhibit increased labeling in NGF-treated cells following the addition of labeled inorganic phosphate to the medium (Yu *et al.*, 1980; Halegoua and Patrick, 1980). Among these are tyrosine hydroxylase, the ribosomal protein S6, and certain chromosomal proteins. Increases in the soluble proteins were evident within 15 to 30 min after the addition of NGF; the nuclear proteins showed the effect somewhat more slowly. Recently, it has been shown that a specific soluble protein exhibits decreased phosphorylation and that this decrease is reflected in a cell-free system prepared from NGF-treated cells and phosphorylated with [^{32}P]-ATP (End *et al.*, 1982a, 1983b). This cell-free system may provide a tool by which the molecular actions of NGF on phosphorylation can be understood.

3.4. Long-Term, Transcription-Dependent Alterations

Perhaps the most rapid, transcription-dependent response to NGF treatment reported in PC12 cells is the increase in ornithine decarboxylase (Greene and McGuire, 1978; Hatanaka *et al.*, 1978; Huff and Guroff, 1979). This enzyme, generally thought to be rate-limiting for the synthesis of polyamines, seems to be involved in the regulation of macromolecular synthesis. The exact role of ornithine decarboxylase in such processes is as yet uncertain, but the induction of this enzyme is nevertheless an excellent indicator of impending transcriptional change and a facile probe for the action of various effectors on their target cells. NGF causes an exuberant induction of ornithine decarboxylase in PC12 cells. Clearly this increase is dependent on RNA synthesis (Greene and McGuire, 1978) and on protein synthesis as well (Hatanaka *et al.*, 1978). The role of the induction in the NGF response is not so clear. It has been shown (Greene and McGuire, 1978) that inhibition of the induction or of the action of ornithine decarboxylase does not prevent the subsequent neurite formation which is characteristic of the action of NGF on these cells.

Although the parent PC12 clone shows no increase in tyrosine hydroxylase activity upon the addition of NGF, the subclone PC12h demonstrates an approximately twofold increase in specific activity in cells cultured in the presence of 50 ng/ml (or lower) of NGF (Hatanaka, 1981). Although this increase has not been formally shown to require transcription, the author considers it likely that it is due to the induction of new enzyme synthesis, because the assays for enzyme activity are done in the presence of saturating levels of all cofactors and substrates, and so it is considered unlikely that some posttranslational change altering the properties of existing enzyme molecules is responsible for the increases seen in activity. Nevertheless, it could be that this increase is indeed due to the phosphorylation of the existing tyrosine hydroxylase molecules, rather than to an increase in tyrosine hydroxylase synthesis.

No definitive experiments on this point have appeared. It is interesting that in the preparation of the several subclones used in this study (Hatanaka, 1981), none were found which lacked either tyrosine hydroxylase or CAT, thus providing another argument favoring the dual-transmitter potential of single PC12 cells.

The increases seen in the specific activity of CAT due to NGF have been well documented (Greene and Rein, 1977a; Schubert et al., 1977; Edgar and Thoenen, 1978). The specific activity of the enzyme rises on the order of twofold when cells in a rapidly growing culture are treated with NGF. Since, as mentioned before, the activity of this enzyme in PC12 cells varies with cell density, in older, more crowded cultures the uninduced levels of enzyme are greater and the effect of NGF is smaller.

The increases seen in the specific activity of AChE have also been extensively studied (Rieger et al., 1980; Lucas et al., 1980; Greene and Rukenstein, 1981; Inestrosa et al., 1981). The overall activity of this enzyme rises about threefold upon treatment of the cells with NGF. In addition, NGF induces a form of the enzyme not seen in untreated cultures. In untreated cultures there are three forms of the enzyme— 4, 6.5, and 10S. The specific activities of all these forms increase after NGF treatment, and a minor form (16S), comprising about 2–3% of the total, appears. This latter form seems to be associated with neurite formation in some way since, in spinner cultures in which the cells cannot attach and therefore cannot form neurites, the overall increase in activity due to NGF is still seen, but the 16S form does not appear. There is some evidence (Inestrosa et al., 1981) that the 16S form is analogous to the asymmetric tailed form of the enzyme that is associated with muscle end-plates. Clearly, the increases in the activity of AChE are dependent on transcription, since they are blocked by low concentrations of actinomycin D (Greene and Rukenstein, 1981). It is of interest that unlike the enzymes tyrosine hydroxylase and CAT, whose activities increase as the density of the cultures increases, the specific activity of AChE does not fluctuate with cell density.

There are a number of other proteins in PC12 cells which have been seen to increase when the cells are treated with NGF. Among these are the neuronal marker, neuron-specific enolase (Vinores et al., 1981). This increase occurs after about 2 days of NGF treatment and, under some conditions, can be as much as six- or eightfold. The level of the protein increases with cell density and, as in the cases mentioned above, the NGF effect on its concentration decreases as the basal level rises. Small increases in the concentration of the pharmacologically active peptide neurotensin have also been reported (Tischler et al., 1982a) upon treatment with NGF. This action is augmented markedly by the presence of dexamethasone; up to 100-fold increases in an immunoreactive material identified as neurotensin have been seen in monolayer cultures, somewhat less in spinner cultures. There has also been a report (Levi et al., 1978) that the enzyme tyrosyl-tubulin ligase increases some twofold upon treatment with NGF. This enzyme, which catalyzes the posttranslational modification of tubulin, may participate in the events involved in neurite outgrowth.

One protein whose synthesis is clearly stimulated by treatment with NGF is the NGF-inducible large external (NILE) glycoprotein (McGuire et al., 1978; Salton et al., 1983). This 230,000-dalton surface marker was initially seen as a spot with increased radioactivity because of an increase in the incorporation of radioactive fucose or glucosamine after treatment of the cells with NGF. It was found that this increase was blocked by inhibitors of transcription and more recently it has been shown by immunological means that there is indeed an approximately threefold increase in the incorporation of radioactive amino acids into the protein, indicating that the effect of NGF is, in fact, a transcriptional one. A survey of the distribution of this glycoprotein reveals its presence on the surface of a variety of neuronal cell types in the CNS and PNS. Since it is detectable in several species using an antibody prepared against rat NILE, it is thought that the molecule has been structurally conserved. Antibodies prepared against the protein apparently do not prevent neurite outgrowth (Salton et al., 1983), nor do they alter action potentials in the cells. The function of this protein is obviously of great interest.

Clearly then, the synthesis of a number of proteins is increased when the cells are differentiated with NGF. There are, however, many fewer than one might expect from the global changes in structure and function that take place. Studies with one-dimensional (McGuire and Greene, 1980) or two-dimensional (McGuire et al., 1978; Garrels and Schubert, 1979) gels, the latter looking at 700 or 800 individual proteins, indicate that none appear or disappear when the cells are treated. Indeed, very few spots change at all; some quantitative change was apparent in about 5% of the proteins spots and, with computer assistance, it could be seen that there were minor alterations in the amounts of another 20 to 25% of the proteins (Garrels and Schubert, 1979). But, again, in spite of profound changes in the properties of the cells, the synthesis of specific cellular proteins was not altered qualitatively and very few of the proteins even changed quantitatively.

The limited number of alterations in the protein composition of the cells upon treatment with NGF would seem to predict an equally limited alteration in the RNA metabolism of the cell. The hybridization experiments which may be needed to specify the number of new mRNAs found have not been reported so it is not known whether the limited number of changes seen in the protein economy are matched by an equally limited number of changes in the mRNA economy. But, overall, NGF leads to an increase in the amount of RNA present in PC12 cells within 1 day of treatment (Gunning *et al.*, 1981). This increase is largely (95% at least) accounted for by increases in rRNA and tRNA. There is a corresponding increase in the total amounts of protein per cell, although, as mentioned above, little change in the protein population. These overall increases in protein and RNA content contribute to or perhaps underlie the hypertrophy of the cell body reported in several studies (Dichter *et al.*, 1977; Greene and McGuire, 1978).

The DNA synthesis in the cells appears to continue unaltered for about 4 days. Then, in concert with the decreases seen in cell division, the synthesis of DNA shows a progressive decrease (Gunning *et al.*, 1981). It is of interest here that the decreased synthesis of DNA, and by implication the decreased capacity for cell division, is not coincident with the appearance of the capability for neurite outgrowth (Gunning *et al.*, 1981). Autoradiography shows that cells in the process of differentiation still incorporated thymidine into their DNA. It can be concluded, then, that cells which have differentiated morphologically can continue to synthesize DNA.

3.5. Neurite Outgrowth

The characteristic morphological change seen due to NGF treatment, neurite outgrowth, has been the subject of substantial investigation since it is the hallmark of neuronal differentiation and, of course, one of the most prominent and distinguishing features of neuronal growth. The characteristics of these neurites have been mentioned before. They are long, thin, branched, and vesiculated. They are also very slender (1 μm in diameter), with varicosities, some fascicles, microspikes (about 0.14 μm in diameter), and growth cones. They contain arrays of microtubules that are oriented parallel to their long axes (Luckenbill-Edds *et al.*, 1979). Neurite growth under standard conditions can proceed at 30–50 μm/day and continues as long as NGF is present in the medium. Even after 1 or 2 days, the neurites may be more than 100 μm in length (Fujii *et al.*, 1982). This neurite response has been adapted to serve as a quantitative assay for NGF (Greene, 1977).

The mechanism by which NGF causes the cells to elaborate neurites is quite unknown. It was not even clear for a while after the initial observations whether the process required the synthesis of new RNA. Now it seems likely that NGF-induced neurite outgrowth in PC12 cells involves at least two stages; the first of these is transcription-dependent, the second is transcription-independent. The experiments supporting this concept, the so-called "priming model" (Burstein and Greene, 1978; Greene et al., 1982), involve the treatment of naive cells with NGF so as to produce outgrowth. This generation of neurites proceeds with a lag time of some 24 hr and can be blocked by the presence of low concentrations of actinomycin D or other inhibitors of RNA synthesis. When cells bearing neurites, as a consequence of having been treated with NGF, are removed from the tissue culture surface, the neurites are broken off and the cells round up. When these cells are put down again and exposed to NGF, they regenerate their neurites and this regeneration is much faster than the original generation and is not affected by inhibitors of RNA synthesis. These latter cells are "primed" and the interpretation which has been given for these data is as follows. Neurite generation requires the NGF-dependent synthesis of proteins and hence the synthesis of RNA. It also requires some, perhaps unrelated, NGF actions at the membrane which do not require the synthesis of RNA. Once the cells have been treated with NGF, they build up these transcription-dependent products and can regenerate neurites in a faster and RNA synthesis-independent fashion, requiring only the second locus of NGF action, that at the membrane. Thus, the current concept of NGF action on neurite outgrowth indicates that there are two sites at which NGF action is required. One is at the nucleus and is transcription-dependent; the other is at the membrane and there the action of NGF is transcription-independent.

3.6. Synapse Formation

By whatever mechanism these neurites are produced there is no question that they are functional. Coculture of the PC12 cells with a clonal line of rat skeletal muscle cells (L6) provided morphological evidence of synapse formation (Schubert et al., 1977). Furthermore, intracellular recordings made from the muscle cells indicated the occurrence of miniature end-plate potentials which could be abolished by the addition of 0.1 μM α-bungarotoxin or by 4.4 μM d-tubocurarine. These data show that the PC12 cells make functional synapses on the clonal muscle cells and that these synapses are cholinergic.

3.7. Antigenic Alterations

Antisera prepared against PC12 cells recognize some antigens which are unique to brain and PC12 cells, some which are unique to adrenal medulla and PC12 cells, and some which are unique only to PC12 cells (Lee *et al.*, 1977). Using a cytotoxicity assay, some differences were found in the antisera prepared against untreated PC12 cells and antisera prepared against NGF-treated PC12 cells (Lee *et al.*, 1980a). When antisera were prepared against cultures of sympathetic neurons from newborn rats, they recognized antigens unique to these neurons and PC12 cells (Lee *et al.*, 1980b). Interestingly, these antisera also revealed antigenic differences between untreated PC12 cells and those treated with NGF.

3.8 Effect of Dexamethasone

It has been reported (Chiba *et al.*, 1981) that treatment of PC12 cells with dexamethasone, while eliciting no gross changes at the light microscopic level, does cause the appearance of a population of intensely fluorescing cells containing dense-core vesicles, an increased number of glycogen particles, and bearing a small number of short processes. These cells resemble the small intensely fluorescent (SIF) cells seen in sympathetic ganglia. Combined treatment with dexamethasone and NGF inhibited but did not completely prevent the neurite formation normally seen with NGF alone.

4. SUBCLONES

The PC12 cell line is characteristically very plastic. After multiple passages in culture the cells become quite heterogeneous and a number of apparently different cell types can be seen. This plasticity has been a source of some concern among individuals working with the line since if the lines diverge in different laboratories under the different culture conditions, then it is difficult to expect the data from different laboratories to be exactly congruent.

The spontaneous plasticity of the line has been used to advantage to isolate subclones of PC12 (Greene and Rein, 1977a; Greene and Rukenstein, 1981) for the inspection of the linkage of specific properties of the parent. Ethyl methanesulfonate mutagenesis has also been employed (Bothwell *et al.*, 1980) for the isolation of some 40 NGF-unresponsive mutants, some of which have been shown to lack NGF receptors. Also, some of these clones were shown to form neurites while continuing to proliferate. Another series of subclones (Hatanaka, 1981), isolated by subcloning from standard cultures, provided evidence for the multiple neurotransmitter nature of single PC12 cells and yielded a subclone which demonstrated an NGF-dependent induction of tyrosine hydroxylase, a property not demonstrated by the parent PC12 clone. There are, in fact, clones for which NGF, instead of inhibiting cell proliferation, actually appears to be a mitogen (Burstein and Greene, 1983).

5. COMPARISON WITH ADRENAL CHROMAFFIN CELLS IN CULTURE

The adrenal chromaffin cell in culture is becoming an increasingly useful model for studies of catecholamine secretion and metabolism. There are some differences, discussed below, between the rat adrenal medullary cells and those of bovine origin. For technical reasons the bovine system is the one in most abundant use at the present time (Trifaro, 1982).

The cells are derived from enzyme-dissociated adrenal medullary tissue and are sometimes purified through Percoll gradients before being plated on collagen-coated tissue culture dishes in the presence of 10% fetal calf serum (Fenwick et al., 1978; Mizobe et al., 1979; Trifaro and Lee, 1980; Kilpatrick et al., 1980). They can be kept in culture for a relatively long period (2–4 weeks) and will maintain their metabolic and secretory properties.

The bovine cells will spontaneously grow a small number of processes which have varicosities and growth cones (Unsicker et al., 1980). The surface of the cell is smooth with a few filipodia at the edges of the growth cones. There are a number of spherical structures in the cells, on the order of 200 nm in diameter, which correspond to the secretory granules, since they appear to possess catecholamine fluorescence (Trifaro, 1982).

The cells contain all three catecholamines—dopamine, norepinephrine, and epinephrine. The total content of catecholamines decreases by about 50% immediately after plating, but remains stable then for about 3 weeks. The cells will take up catecholamines by a system which has many of the characteristics of neuronal catecholamine uptake (Trifaro, 1982). The affinity of the uptake system is high and it has an absolute requirement for Na^+. The generation of neurites does not seem to influence either the qualitative or the quantitative aspects of the uptake of the catecholamines.

The cells have acetylcholine receptors and will release catecholamine in a Ca^{2+}-dependent fashion in response to the addition of nicotinic cholinergic agonists (Mizobe et al., 1979). Depolarization of the cells with 56 mM K^+ will also lead to the release of catecholamines. The presence of concanavalin A blocks the release of catecholamines induced by acetylcholine, but does not inhibit the depolarization-induced release (Trifaro, 1982). It has been reported that substance P and somatostatin (Mizobe *et al.*, 1979), and the opiate agonists (Kumakura *et al.*, 1980) also inhibit the release of catecholamines induced by the nicotinic cholinergic agonists, but the meaning of these observations is not completely clear. Bovine adrenal medullary cells also bind muscarinic cholinergic agonists, but do not release catecholamines. In fact, there is some evidence that the action of the muscarinic agonists is to inhibit the release produced by the nicotinic agonists (Derome *et al.*, 1981).

The cells contain a number of enkephalins (Trifaro, 1982). Leu- and met-enkephalins are known to be present as well as a number of others, including their biosynthetic precursors (Rossier *et al.*, 1980); and the cells have been used to study the biosynthesis of many of these opiate peptides. These peptides are also released from the cells by depolarization or by the action of nicotinic cholinergic agonists.

It has been shown that the cells possess tyrosine hydroxylase, dopamine-β-hydroxylase, and phenylethanolamine-N-methyltransferase. The levels of these enzymes are stable for a week or more in culture and then decline (Kilpatrick *et al.*, 1980). The regulation of tyrosine hydroxylase in these cells is controlled by many different factors. It has been shown, for example, that treatment of the cells with reserpine causes, as one of its effects, a more than twofold increase in tyrosine hydroxylase activity, which is prevented by inhibitors of RNA synthesis or of protein synthesis (Wilson *et al.*, 1981). The cells also contain AChE, which can be secreted from the cells in a Ca^{2+}-dependent fashion in response to nicotinic cholinergic agonists (Mizobe and Livett, 1983).

The effect of NGF on these bovine cells has until recently been thought to be minimal. Indeed, the classic NGF-induced response, that of neurite outgrowth, has been seen in the absence of exogenous NGF in many of these cultures (Unsicker *et al.*, 1980; Trifaro and Lee, 1980), and NGF has been without much effect. More recently, perhaps due to differing culture conditions or differing strains of animals, other workers (Naujoks *et al.*, 1982) have prepared cultures of bovine adrenal medullary cells which exhibit very minimal outgrowth in the absence of NGF. Cells from early fetal animals show a substantial neurite outgrowth in the presence of 1 μg/ml of either mouse or bovine NGF. Cells from fetal animals or from calves showed a three- to fourfold increase in the specific activity of tyrosine hydroxylase and that increase was prevented by cycloheximide, indicating that NGF causes an increase in the synthesis of the protein itself. As expected, the cells have receptors for NGF, receptors which have a dissociation constant in the nanomolar range; and they decrease in number, but not in affinity for the ligand, as the animal develops. Cells from adult animals have much lower numbers of receptors per cell and exhibit no discernible response to NGF in culture.

Cultures made from the adrenals of other species have not been so heavily used, although a substantial amount of work has been done with cultures from rats. Adrenal medullary cells from postnatal rats can be cultured by much the same methodology used to prepare bovine cultures (Unsicker and Chamley, 1977). The cultures contain large numbers of chromaffin cells, Schwann cells, and a small number of cells identified as neurons. The chromaffin cells were round after plating but became polygonal after 2 or 3 days in culture. They contained dense-core structures indicative of the presence of amine-containing vesicles.

The response of these cultures from postnatal animals to NGF has been studied (Unsicker et al., 1978). NGF in amounts ranging from 4 to 12 ng/ml causes the outgrowth of processes within 2 to 3 days. These processes are long, thin, and terminate in what appear to be growth cones. The presence of dexamethasone inhibits this fiber outgrowth. In cells treated with NGF, the tyrosine hydroxylase levels increase about 50% and dexamethasone does not prevent this increase; levels of tyrosine hydroxylase in the presence of both NGF and dexamethasone are higher than with NGF alone.

Some studies have also been done with adrenal medullary cells from young adult rats (Tischler et al., 1982b). These cultures appear to have somewhat different characteristics than the cultures prepared from the adrenals of postnatal animals. First, very little process outgrowth is noted from the chromaffin cells in these cultures even upon the addition of NGF. This little bit of spontaneous outgrowth is not affected by dexamethasone. Second, in the presence of NGF, a population of neurons is present and these cells exhibit the outgrowth of processes; thus, NGF is required either for the survival of these cells or for their outgrowth. The presence of dexamethasone has no effect on this process outgrowth. Finally, although these cells, when freshly prepared, contain relatively large amounts of epinephrine, smaller amounts of norepinephrine, and very little dopamine, over a culture period of 30 days they lose their ability to store epinephrine almost completely. Losses in the content of the other catecholamines are substantial but not as precipitous as the loss of epinephrine. In spite of this, these adult cells appear to retain some capacity to store and synthesize epinephrine, while cultures from younger rats appear to lose this ability entirely.

In summary, then, aside from the obvious intellectual serenity conveyed by the fact that these chromaffin cells are "normal" cells, fetal or postnatal adrenal medulla cells in dispersed cultures differ from PC12 in at least the following major ways:

1. They have a finite lifetime in culture.
2. Their catecholamine content is different; they contain phenyle-thanolamine-N-methyltransferase and retain the capacity, for some period of time at least, to synthesize and store epinephrine. In addition, their dopamine content is low in comparison to their norepinephrine level.
3. They contain large amounts of opiatelike peptides and the bio-chemical machinery for their synthesis; PC12 cells do not (L. Eiden, personal communication).
4. Some induction of tyrosine hydroxylase can be seen in the pres-ence of NGF; this is not evident in parent PC12 cells.

Other differences certainly exist but the responses of these two systems have not been explored in enough detail to be able to state them as general rules at this time.

6. COMPARISON WITH SYMPATHETIC NEURONS IN CULTURES

Methods for the preparation of long-term cultures of dissociated sympathetic neurons from neonatal rats have been available for some time (Mains and Patterson, 1973a,b,c). Basically, the method involves mechanical dissociation of superior cervical ganglia followed by plating of the cell clumps on a collagen-coated surface. In the early work, the medium used for plating was kept on the cells for a few days and then changed to a medium containing serum from adult rats and designed to promote the long-term growth of the cells. The conditions can be adjusted, primarily by the omission of bicarbonate and growth in air, to discourage the survival of nonneuronal cells in the culture.

Under these conditions, the cultures contain few nonneuronal cells and also few of the SIF cells seen in the ganglia *in vivo*. The cells will synthesize dopamine, norepinephrine, and acetylcholine. During the first few hours of culture some of the cells will begin to elaborate pro-cesses and eventually these neurites will develop into an intricate mesh-work of processes terminating in growth cones. In some older cultures the processes can be as much as 30 μm thick and probably exist as bundles rather than as single processes. In spite of the extended life of these cultures, neuronal cell division is not seen. NGF is absolutely and continually required for the survival of these cells. In the presence of NGF, these neurons will survive in such cultures for many weeks.

Sympathetic neurons have nicotinic acetylcholine receptors and where side-by-side comparisons have been made with a number of ligands (Patrick and Stallcup, 1977a), these receptors are indistinguishable from those found on PC12 cells. The cells also have receptors for NGF. While the gross outlines of NGF binding to sympathetic neurons seem the same as those of NGF binding to PC12 cells, e.g., specificity, saturability, and high affinity, there appear to be some differences in detail (Herrup and Thoenen, 1979). It should be noted, however, that the literature on sympathetic neurons contains some discrepancies in the characteristics of NGF binding when measured in different laboratories (Vinores and Guroff, 1980).

The electrophysiological responses of sympathetic neurons in culture (O'Lague *et al.*, 1978) seem to be quite similar to those seen in fused PC12 cells (O'Lague and Huttner, 1980), even to the development of a Na^+-dependent spike mechanism in many of the cells treated with NGF (Dichter *et al.*, 1977; O'Lague and Huttner, 1980).

Sympathetic neurons in culture will make cholinergic synapses with skeletal muscle (Nurse and O'Lague, 1975). During such a coculture there is a marked increase in the specific activity of CAT (Patterson and Chun, 1974; Johnson *et al.*, 1976), an effect which can be mimicked by the presence of conditioned medium (Patterson and Chun, 1977). Similar changes are seen in PC12 cells under similar circumstances (Schubert *et al.*, 1977). One difference is that PC12 cells seems to possess a much higher basal level of CAT than do sympathetic neurons (Schubert *et al.*, 1977).

Upon exposure to NGF in culture, sympathetic neurons exhibit marked and immediate changes in the structure of the surface membrane (Connolly *et al.*, 1981). When these neurons have been deprived of NGF for a few hours, and then NGF is added back, microvilli and small ruffles appear within 30 sec on a cellular surface which was previously smooth. After about 7 min the surface is smooth again. During this time also, there is an increase, and then a decrease, in the number of coated pits observable. Rapid changes, some of them similar to these, have been seen on PC12 cell membranes after the addition of NGF (Connolly *et al.*, 1979).

Sympathetic neurons from fetal animals in dispersed cell culture differ from PC12 cells in at least the following major ways:

1. They have a finite lifetime in culture.
2. They do not appear to respond to EGF or adenosine, as do PC12 cells.
3. They require NGF for survival.

4. They cannot be prepared in a form that has never been exposed to NGF; this means that unlike PC12 cells, they cannot be used as a fully credible model for the immediate actions of NGF. This changes the characteristics and the interpretation of some of their responses to NGF (Burstein and Greene, 1978; Greene *et al.*, 1982).

7. PC12 CELLS AS A MODEL FOR THE EARLY EVENTS IN NEURONAL DIFFERENTIATION

It may be that the PC12 cells offer a window on a period in the natural history of sympathetic neurons that has been unavailable until this time. This is obviously the most difficult area to judge because of the unavailability of appropriate normal cells with which to compare the findings.

For example, one question which might be explored using PC12 cells is the possible function of NGF in the terminal differentiation of sympathetic neurons. In the PC12 cells, as mentioned above, NGF causes the cells to stop dividing and to differentiate. Inquiries into the mechanism of this effect in PC12 cells may have been facilitated by the observation that the cells also respond to EGF, a potent mitogen for most of its target cells. The observation, then, that the same cells respond to a mitogen and to a terminal differentiating agent led to studies on what would happen if both agents were present simultaneously. The answer is that cells treated with NGF become increasingly unresponsive to EGF (Huff and Guroff, 1979; Huff *et al.*, 1981). The mechanism by which they become unresponsive appears to be that the cells lose their capacity to bind the mitogen. That is, over a period of 72 hr the number of EGF receptors decreases by at least 80%, and in some experiments it is difficult to detect any EGF receptors at all.

The data suggest that a mechanism by which NGF instructs PC12 cells to stop dividing is to stop the synthesis of the receptor for the mitogen or mitogens to which they normally respond. It can be speculated that a mechanism by which NGF acts on normal neurons is to differentiate them by blinding them to the mitogens to which they normally respond.

This postulate about the action of NGF has been tested in cultures of neural crest cells from embryonic chicks (End *et al.*, 1983a), cells which might be, like PC12 cells about to be treated with NGF, at the point of decision about becoming neurons. Under the conditions used these cells did not have any EGF receptors, so the test gave a negative, but rather unsatisfactory answer. Of course, it may be that the system is inappropriate or the mitogen is the wrong one. Thus, the postulate is still unproven. The data do indicate, however, the possibility that the changes in PC12 cells could be used to predict actions which might occur in neurons just at the point of decision.

8. CONCLUSION

Clearly, the PC12 cells are a unique and very interesting model applicable to a number of different questions. First and foremost, they lend themselves admirably to studies on the mechanisms of action of NGF. Second, they are a reasonable tool by which to study the biosynthesis and secretion of catecholamines. Finally, they may be a useful system with which to investigate or even predict the changes which occur during the differentiation of normal sympathetic neurons.

There are, of course, some cautions to be observed. The obvious and often-mentioned conceptual difficulties of dealing with a tumor cell rather than a normal one need no elaboration here. It should be pointed out that these cells respond to a number of effectors to which normal adrenal cells or sympathetic neurons may not be sensitive, e.g., EGF, adenosine, and some less well-characterized factors (Edgar *et al.*, 1979; Lucas *et al.*, 1981; Rieske *et al.*, 1981). It should also be mentioned that these cells grow neurites in response to changes in the environment which are independent of the presence of NGF (Fujii *et al.*, 1982; see Chapter 1).

Thus, while the PC12 cells remain a powerful tool for the study of a number of interesting aspects of neural crest, chromaffin cell, and sympathetic neuron development and function, they are a tool which must be used with a certain amount of care and caution.

REFERENCES

Arner, L. S., and Stallcup, W. B., 1981, Two types of potassium channels in the PC12 cell line, *Brain Res.* **215**:419–425.

Baetge, E. E., Kaplan, B. B., Reis, D. J., and Joh, T. H., 1981, Translation of tyrosine hydroxylase from poly(A)-mRNA in pheochromocytoma cells is enhanced by dexamethasone, *Proc. Natl. Acad. Sci. USA* **78**:1269–1273.

Boonstra, J., VanderSaag, P. T., Moolenaar, W. H., and DeLaat, S. W., 1981, Rapid effects of nerve growth factor on the Na^+, K^+-pump in rat pheochromocytoma cells, *Exp. Cell Res.* **131**:452–455.

Bothwell, M. A., Schechter, A. L., and Vaughn, K. M., 1980, Clonal variants of PC12 pheochromocytoma cells with altered response to nerve growth factor, *Cell* **21:**857–866.

Burstein, D. E., and Greene, L. A., 1978, Evidence for RNA synthesis-dependent and -independent pathways in stimulation of neurite outgrowth by nerve growth factor, *Proc. Natl. Acad. Sci. USA* **75:**6059–6063.

Burstein, D. E., and Greene, L. A., 1983, Nerve growth factor has both mitogenic and anti-mitogenic action, *Develop. Biol.* **94:**477–482.

Chiba, T., Murata, Y., and Koike, T., 1981, Plasticity of pheochromocytoma (PC12) cells demonstrated by nerve growth factor or glucocorticoid treatment: A catecholamine fluorescence and electron microscopic investigation, *Biomed. Res.* **2:**618–628.

Connolly, J. L., Greene, L. A., Viscarello, R. R., and Riley, W. D., 1979, Rapid sequential changes in surface morphology of PC12 pheochromocytoma cells in response to nerve growth factor, *J. Cell Biol.* **82:**820–827.

Connolly, J. L., Green, S. A., and Greene, L. A., 1981, Pit formation and rapid changes in surface morphology of sympathetic neurons in response to nerve growth factor, *J. Cell Biol.* **90:**176–180.

DeLellis, R. A., Merk, F. B., Deckers, P., Warren, S., and Balogh, K., 1973, Ultrastructure and *in vitro* growth characteristics of a transplantable rat pheochromocytoma, *Cancer* **32:**227–235.

Derome, G., Tseng, R., Mercier, P., Lemaire, L., and Lemaire, S., 1981, Possible muscarinic regulation of catecholamine secretion mediated by cyclic GMP in isolated bovine adrenal chromaffin cells, *Biochem. Pharmacol.* **30:**855–860.

Dichter, M. A., Tischler, A. S., and Greene, L. A., 1977, Nerve growth factor-induced increase in electrical excitability and acetylcholine sensitivity of a rat pheochromocytoma cell line, *Nature* **268:**501–504.

Edgar, D. H., and Thoenen, H., 1978, Selective enzyme induction in a nerve growth factor-responsive pheochromocytoma cell line (PC12), *Brain Res.* **154:**186–190.

Edgar, D., Barde, Y.-A., and Thoenen, H., 1979, Induction of fibre outgrowth and choline acetyltransferase in PC12 pheochromocytoma cells by conditioned media from glial cells and organ extracts, *Exp. Cell Res.* **121:**353–361.

End, D., Hanson, M., Hashimoto, S., and Guroff, G., 1982a, Inhibition of the phosphorylation of a 100,000-dalton soluble protein in whole cells and cell-free extracts of PC12 pheochromocytoma cells following treatment with nerve growth factor, *J. Biol. Chem.* **257:**9223–9225.

End, D., Tolson, N., Yu, M., and Guroff, G., 1982b, Effects of 12-O-tetradecanoyl-13-acetate (TPA) on rat pheochromocytoma (PC12) cells: Interactions with epidermal growth factor and nerve growth factor, *J. Cell. Physiol.* **111:**140–148.

End, D., Pevzner, L., Lloyd, A., and Guroff, G., 1983a, Identification of nerve growth factor receptors in primary cultures of neural crest cells, *Develop. Brain Res.* **7:**131–136.

End, D., Tolson, N., Hashimoto, S., and Guroff, G., 1983b, Nerve growth factor-induced decrease in the cell-free phosphorylation of a soluble protein in PC12 cells, *J. Biol. Chem.* **258:**6549–6555.

Fenwick, E. M., Fajdiga, P. B., Howe, N. B. S., and Livett, B. G., 1978, Functional and morphological characterization of isolated bovine adrenal medullary cells, *J. Cell Biol.* **76:**12–30.

Fujii, D. K., Massoglia, G. L., Savin, N., and Gospodarowicz, D., 1982, Neurite outgrowth and protein synthesis by PC12 cells as a function of a substratum and nerve growth factor, *J. Neurosci.* **8:**1157–1175.

Garrels, J. C., and Schubert, D., 1979, Modulation of protein synthesis by nerve growth factor, *J. Biol. Chem.* **254:**7978–7985.

Greene, L. A., 1977, A quantitative bioassay for nerve growth factor (NGF) activity employing a clonal pheochromocytoma cell line, *Brain Res.* **133**:350–353.

Greene, L. A., and McGuire, J. C., 1978, Induction of ornithine decarboxylase by nerve growth factor dissociated from affects on survival and neurite outgrowth, *Nature* **276**:191–194.

Greene, L. A., and Rein, G., 1977a, Synthesis, storage and release of acetylcholine by a noradrenergic pheochromocytoma cell line, *Nature* **268**:349–351.

Greene, L. A., and Rein, G., 1977b, Release, storage and uptake of catecholamines by a clonal cell line of nerve growth factor (NGF) responsive pheochromocytoma cells, *Brain Res.* **129**:247–263.

Greene, L. A., and Rein, G., 1977c, Release of [^{3}H]-norepinephrine from a clonal line of pheochromocytoma cells (PC12) by nicotinic cholinergic stimulation, *Brain Res.* **138**:521–528.

Greene, L. A., and Rein, G., 1978, Short-term regulation of catecholamine biosynthesis in a nerve growth factor responsive clonal line of rat pheochromocytoma cells, *J. Neurochem.* **30**:549–555.

Greene, L. A., and Rukenstein, A., 1981, Regulation of acetylcholinesterase activity by nerve growth factor, *J. Biol. Chem.* **256**:6363–6367.

Greene, L. A., and Tischler, A. S., 1976, Establishment of a noradrenergic clonal line of rat adrenal pheochromocytoma cells which respond to nerve growth factor, *Proc. Natl. Acad. Sci. USA* **73**:2424–2428.

Greene, L. A., Burstein, D. E., and Black, M. M., 1982, The role of transcription-dependent priming in nerve growth factor promoted neurite outgrowth, *Develop. Biol.* **91**:305–316.

Gunning, P. W., Landreth, G. E., Layer, P., Ignatius, M., and Shooter, E. M., 1981, Nerve growth factor induced differentiation of PC12 cells: Evaluation of changes in RNA and DNA metabolism, *J. Neurosci.* **1**:368–379.

Guroff, G., Dickens, G., End, D., and Londos, C., 1981, The action of adenosine analogs on PC12 cells, *J. Neurochem.* **37**:1431–1439.

Halegoua, S., and Patrick, J., 1980, Nerve growth factor mediates phosphorylation of specific proteins, *Cell* **22**:571–581.

Hatanaka, H., 1981, Nerve growth factor mediated stimulation of tyrosine hydroxylase activity in a clonal rat pheochromocytoma cell line, *Brain Res.* **222**:225–233.

Hatanaka, H., Otten, U., and Thoenen, H., 1978, Nerve growth factor-mediated selective induction of ornithine decarboxylase in rat pheochromocytoma: A cyclic AMP-independent process, *FEBS Lett.* **92**:313–316.

Herrup, K., and Thoenen, H., 1979, Properties of the nerve growth factor receptor of a clonal line of rat pheochromocytoma (PC12) cells, *Exp. Cell Res.* **121**:71–78.

Heumann, R., Schwab, M., and Thoenen, H., 1981, A second messenger required for nerve growth factor biological activity?, *Nature* **292**:838–840.

Hogue-Angeletti, R., Stieber, A., and Gonatas, N. K., 1982, Endocytosis of nerve growth factor by PC12 cells studied by quantitative ultrastructural autoradiography, *Brain Res.* **241**:145–156.

Huff, K. R., and Guroff, G., 1979, Nerve growth factor-induced reduction in epidermal growth factor responsiveness and epidermal growth factor receptors in PC12 cells: An aspect of cell differentiation, *Biochem. Biophys. Res. Commun.* **89**:175–180.

Huff, K., End, D., and Guroff, G., 1981, Nerve growth factor-induced alteration in the response of PC12 pheochromocytoma cells to epidermal growth factor, *J. Cell Biol.* **88**:189–198.

Inestrosa, N. C., Reiness, C. G., Reichardt, L. F., and Hall, Z. W., 1981, Cellular localization of the molecular forms of acetylcholinesterase in rat pheochromocytoma PC12 cells treated with nerve growth factor, *J. Neurosci.* **1**:1260–1267.

Inoue, N., and Hatanaka, H., 1982, Nerve growth factor induces specific enkephalin binding sites in a nerve cell line, *J. Biol. Chem.* **257**:9238–9241.

Johnson, M., Ross, D., Meyers, M., Rees, R., Bunge, R., Wakshull, E., and Burton, H., 1976, Synaptic vesicle cytochemistry changes when cultured sympathetic neurons develop cholinergic interactions, *Nature* **262**:308–310.

Jumblatt, J. E., and Tischler, A. S., 1982, Regulation of muscarinic ligand binding sites by nerve growth factor in PC12 phaeochromocytoma cells, *Nature* **297**:152–154.

Kilpatrick, D. L., Ledbetter, F. H., Larson, K. A., Kirshner, A. G., Slepetes, R., and Kirshner, N., 1980, Stability of bovine adrenal medulla cells in culture, *J. Neurochem.* **35**:679–692.

Kumakura, K., Karoum, F., Guidotti, A., and Costa, E., 1980, Modulation of nicotinic receptors by opiate receptor agonists in cultured adrenal chromaffin cells, *Nature* **283**:489–492.

Landreth, G. E., and Shooter, E. M., 1980, Nerve growth factor receptors on PC12 cells: Ligand-induced conversion from low- to high-affinity states, *Proc. Natl. Acad. Sci. USA* **77**:4751–4755.

Landreth, G., Cohen, P., and Shooter, E. M., 1980, Ca^{2+} transmembrane fluxes and nerve growth factor action on a clonal cell line of rat phaeochromocytoma, *Nature* **283**:202–204.

Lee, V., Shelanski, M. L., and Greene, L. A., 1977, Specific neural and adrenal medullary antigens detected by antisera to clonal PC12 and pheochromocytoma cells, *Proc. Natl. Acad. Sci. USA* **74**:5021–5025.

Lee, V. H., Greene, L. A., and Shelanski, M. L., 1980a, Differential cytotoxic activities of antisera against nerve growth factor-treated and untreated clonal pheochromocytoma cells, *Neuroscience* **5**:1979–1987.

Lee, V. M., Shelanski, M. L., and Greene, L. A., 1980b, Characterization of antisera raised against cultured rat sympathetic neurons, *Neuroscience* **5**:2239–2245.

Levi, A., Castellani, L., Calissano, P., Deanin, G. G., and Gordon, M. W., 1978, Studies on NGF-induced differentiation in PC12 pheochromocytoma cells: Specific rise in tyrosyl tubulin ligase activity induced by nerve growth factor, *Bull. Mol. Biol. Med.* **3**:425–505.

Levi, A., Schechter, Y., Neufeld, E. J., and Schlessinger, J., 1980, Mobility, clustering, and transport of nerve growth factor in embryonal sensory cells and in a sympathetic neuronal cell line, *Proc. Natl. Acad. Sci. USA* **77**:3469–3473.

Lucas, C. A., Edgar, D., and Thoenen, H., 1979, Regulation of tyrosine hydroxylase and choline acetyltransferase activities by cell density in the PC12 rat pheochromocytoma clonal cell line, *Exp. Cell Res.* **121**:79–86.

Lucas, C. A., Czlonkowska, A., and Kreutzberg, G. W., 1980, Regulation of acetylcholinesterase by nerve growth factor in the pheochromocytoma PC12 cell line, *Neurosci. Lett.* **18**:333–337.

Lucas, C. A., Czlonkowska, A., and Kreutzberg, G. W., 1981, Regulation of acetylcholinesterase activity in pheochromocytoma PC12 clonal cell line by C6 glioma conditioned medium and brain homogenates, *Biol. Cell.* **41**:91–96.

Luckenbill-Edds, L., VanHorn, C., and Greene, L. A., 1979, Fine structure of initial outgrowth of processes induced in a pheochromocytoma cell line (PC12) by nerve growth factor, *J. Neurocytol.* **8**:493–511.

McGuire, J. C., and Greene, L. A., 1979, Rapid stimulation by nerve growth factor of amino acid uptake by clonal PC12 pheochromocytoma cells, *J. Biol. Chem.* **254:**3362–3367.

McGuire, J. C., and Greene, L. A., 1980, Stimulation by nerve growth factor of specific protein synthesis in rat PC12 pheochromocytoma cells, *Neuroscience* **5:**179–189.

McGuire, J. C., Greene, L. A., and Furano, A. V., 1978, NGF stimulates incorporation of fucose or glucosamine into an external glycoprotein in cultured rat PC12 pheochromocytoma cells, *Cell* **15:**357–365.

McHugh, E. M., McGee, R., Jr., and Fleming, P. J., 1985, Multiple forms of dopamine β-hydroxylase in rat pheochromocytoma cells, submitted.

Mains, R. E., and Patterson, P. H., 1973a, Primary cultures of dissociated sympathetic neurons. I. Establishment of long-term growth in culture and studies of differentiated properties, *J. Cell Biol.* **59:**329–345.

Mains, R. E., and Patterson, P. H., 1973b, Primary cultures of dissociated sympathetic neurons. II. Initial studies on catecholamine metabolism, *J. Cell Biol.* **59:**346–360.

Mains, R. E., and Patterson, P. H., 1973c, Primary cultures of dissociated sympathetic neurons. III. Changes in metabolism with age in culture, *J. Cell Biol.* **59:**361–366.

Melega, W. P., and Howard, B. D., 1981, Choline and acetylcholine metabolism in PC12 secretory cells, *Biochemistry* **20:**4477–4483.

Mizobe, F., and Livett, B. G., 1983, Nicotine stimulates secretion of both catecholamines and acetylcholinesterase from cultured adrenal chromaffin cells, *J. Neurosci.* **3:**871–876.

Mizobe, F., Kozouk, V., Dean, D. M., and Livett, B. G., 1979, Pharmacological characterization of adrenal paraneurons: Substance P and somatostatin as inhibitory modulators of the nicotinic response, *Brain Res.* **178:**555–556.

Naujoks, K. W., Korsching, P., Rohrer, H., and Thoenen, H., 1982, Nerve growth factor-mediated induction of tyrosine hydroxylase and of neurite outgrowth in cultures of bovine adrenal chromaffin cells: Dependence on developmental stage, *Develop. Biol.* **92:**365–379.

Nurse, C. A., and O'Lague, P. H., 1975, Formation of cholinergic synapses between dissociated sympathetic neurons and skeletal myotubes of the rat in cell culture, *Proc. Natl. Acad. Sci. USA* **72:**1955–1959.

O'Lague, P. H., and Huttner, S. L., 1980, Physiological and morphological studies of rat pheochromocytoma cells (PC12) chemically fused and grown in culture, *Proc. Natl. Acad. Sci. USA* **77:**1701–1705.

O'Lague, P. H., Potter, D. D., and Furshpan, E. J., 1978, Studies on rat sympathetic neurons developing in culture. I. Growth characteristics and electrophysiological properties, *Develop. Biol.* **67:**384–403.

Patrick, J., and Stallcup, B., 1977a, α-Bungarotoxin binding and cholinergic receptor function in a rat sympathetic nerve line, *J. Biol. Chem.* **252:**8629–8633.

Patrick, J., and Stallcup, B., 1977b, Immunological distinction between acetylcholine receptor and the α-bungarotoxin-binding component on sympathetic neurons, *Proc. Natl. Acad. Sci. USA* **74:**4689–4692.

Patterson, P. H., and Chun, L. L. Y., 1974, The influence of nonneuronal cells in catecholamine and acetylcholine synthesis and accumulation in cultures of dissociated sympathetic neurons, *Proc. Natl. Acad. Sci. USA* **71:**3607–3610.

Patterson, P. H., and Chun, L. L. Y., 1977, The induction of acetylcholine synthesis in primary cultures of dissociated rat sympathetic neurons. I. Effects of conditioned medium, *Develop. Biol.* **56:**263–280.

Pevzner, L., End, D., and Guroff, G., 1982, Simultaneous visualization of the binding of nerve growth factor and epidermal growth factor to single rat pheochromocytoma (PC12) cells through indirect immunohistofluorescence, *Acta Histochem.* **71**:183–190.

Rieger, F., Shelanski, M. L., and Greene, L. A., 1980, The effects of nerve growth factor on acetylcholinesterase and its multiple forms in cultures of rat PC12 pheochromocytoma cells: Increased total specific activity and appearance of the 16S molecular form, *Develop. Biol.* **76**:238–243.

Rieske, E., Kreutzberg, G. W., Czlonkowska, A., and Lucas, C. A., 1981, Induction of fiber outgrowth in PC12 pheochromocytoma cells by a neuronotrophic factor occurring in human tumors, *Acta Neuropathol.* **53**:221–225.

Rohrer, H., Schafer, T., Korsching, S., and Thoenen, H., 1982, Internalization of nerve growth factor by pheochromocytoma PC12 cells: Absence of transfer to the nucleus, *J. Neurosci.* **2**:687–697.

Rossier, J., Trifaro, J. M., Lewis, R. V., Lee, R. W. H., Stern, A., Kimura, S., Stein, S., and Udenfriend, S., 1980, Studies with [^{35}S]methionine indicate that the 22,000-dalton [Met]enkephalin-containing protein in chromaffin cells is a precursor of [Met]enkephalin, *Proc. Natl. Acad. Sci. USA* **77**:6889–6891.

Sabban, E. L., Goldstein, M., and Greene, L. A., 1983, Regulation of the multiple forms of dopamine-β-hydroxylase by nerve growth factor, dexamethasone, and dibutyryl cyclic AMP in the PC12 pheochromocytoma cell line, *J. Biol. Chem.* **258**:7819–7823.

Salton, S. R. J., Richter-Landsberg, C., Greene, L. A., and Shelanski, M. L., 1983, Nerve growth factor inducible large external (NILE) glycoprotein: Studies of a central and peripheral neuronal marker, *J. Neurosci.* **3**:441–454.

Schechter, A. L., and Bothwell, M. A., 1980, Nerve growth factor receptors in PC12 cells: Evidence for two receptor classes with differing cytoskeletal association, *Cell* **24**:867–874.

Schubert, D., and Klier, F. G., 1977, Storage and release of acetylcholine by a clonal cell line, *Proc. Natl. Acad. Sci. USA* **74**:5184–5188.

Schubert, D., and Whitlock, C., 1977, Alteration of cellular adhesion by nerve growth factor, *Proc. Natl. Acad. Sci. USA* **74**:4055–4058.

Schubert, D., Heinemann, S., and Kidokoro, Y., 1977, Cholinergic metabolism and synapse formation by a rat nerve cell, *Proc. Natl. Acad. Sci. USA* **74**:2579–2583.

Schubert, D., LeCorbiere, M., Whitlock, C., and Stallcup, W., 1978, Alterations in the surface properties of cells responsive to nerve growth factor, *Nature* **273**:718–723.

Tischler, A. S., and Greene, L. A., 1975, Nerve growth factor-induced process formation by cultured rat pheochromocytoma cells, *Nature* **258**:341–342.

Tischler, A. S., Lee, Y. C., Slayton, V. W., and Bloom, S. R., 1982a, Content and release of neurotensin in PC12 pheochromocytoma cell cultures: Modulation by dexamethasone and nerve growth factor, *Regul. Peptides* **3**:415–421.

Tischler, A. S., Perlman, R. L., Nunnemacher, G., Morse, G. M., DeLellis, R. A., Wolfe, H. J., and Sheard, B. E., 1982b, Long-term effects of dexamethasone and nerve growth factor on adrenal medullary cells cultured from young adult rats, *Cell Tissue Res.* **225**:525–542.

Traynor, A. E., Schubert, D., and Allen, W. R., 1982, Alterations of lipid metabolism in response to nerve growth factor, *J. Neurochem.* **39**:1677–1683.

Trifaro, J. M., 1982, The cultured chromaffin cell: A model for the study of biology and pharmacology of paraneurones, *Trends Pharm. Sci.* **3**:389–392.

Trifaro, J. M., and Lee, R. W. H., 1980, Morphological characteristics and stimulus–secretion coupling in bovine adrenal chromaffin cell cultures, *Neuroscience* **5**:1533–1546.

Unsicker, K., and Chamley, J. H., 1977, Growth characteristics of postnatal rat adrenal medulla in culture, *Cell Tissue Res.* **177**:247–268.

Unsicker, K., Krisch, B., Otten, U., and Thoenen, H., 1978, Nerve growth factor-induced fiber outgrowth from isolated rat adrenal chromaffin cells: Impairment by glucocorticoids, *Proc. Natl. Acad. Sci. USA* **75**:3498–3502.

Unsicker, K., Griesser, G.-H., Lindmar, R., Loffelholz, K., and Wolf, U., 1980, Establishment, characterization, and fiber outgrowth of isolated bovine adrenal medullary cells in long-term cultures, *Neuroscience* **5**:1445–1460.

Vinores, S., and Guroff, G., 1980, Nerve growth factor: Mechanism of action, *Annu. Rev. Biophys. Bioeng.* **9**:223–257.

Vinores, S. A., Marangos, P. J., Parma, A. M., and Guroff, G., 1981, Increased levels of neuron-specific enolase in PC12 pheochromocytoma cells as result of nerve growth factor treatment, *J. Neurochem.* **37**:597–600.

Warren, S., and Chute, R. N., 1972, Pheochromocytoma, *Cancer* **29**:327–331.

Wilson, S. P., Abou-Donea, M. M., Chang, K., and Viveros, O. H., 1981, Reserpine increases opiate-like peptide content and tyrosine hydroxylase activity in adrenal medullary chromaffin cells in culture, *Neuroscience* **6**:71–79.

Yu, M. W., Tolson, N. W., and Guroff, G., 1980, Increased phosphorylation of specific nuclear proteins in superior cervical ganglia and PC12 cells in response to nerve growth factor, *J. Biol. Chem.* **255**:10481–10492.

Yankner, B. A., and Shooter, E. M., 1979, Nerve growth factor in the nucleus: Interaction with receptors on the nuclear membrane, *Proc. Natl. Acad. Sci. U.S.A.* **76**:1269–1273.

9

Neural Differentiation of Pluripotent Embryonal Carcinoma Cells

BERNARD EDDÉ and MICHEL DARMON

The use of the teratocarcinoma of the mouse (Pierce, 1967; Stevens, 1967) for the study of neural differentiation offers two major advantages. First, it allows one to obtain large amounts of cells corresponding to the very early stages of neural differentiation, and second, since teratocarcinoma stem cells [embryonal carcinoma (EC) cells] can differentiate into other cell types, it offers the opportunity to study the segregation of the neuronal lineage and to evaluate which changes are specific for the neural pathway.

Various EC cell lines and various culture conditions have been used in order to obtain neuronal differentiation. For certain cell lines, such as PCC3 (Nicolas *et al.*, 1975), differentiation was obtained simply by either allowing the cells to grow at high densities or to form three-dimensional aggregates. Other cell lines require the addition of "inducers" such as retinoic acid (Kuff and Fewell, 1980; Jones-Villeneuve *et al.*, 1982; Paulin *et al.*, 1982) or culture in hormonally defined media (Darmon *et*

BERNARD EDDÉ • Unité de Génétique Cellulaire, Institut Pasteur, 75724 Paris Cedex 15; and Laboratoire de Biochimie Cellulaire, Collège de France, 75231 Paris Cedex 05, France.   MICHEL DARMON • Unité de Génétique Cellulaire, Institut Pasteur, 75724 Paris Cedex 15; and Département de Biologie Cellulaire, Centre International de Recherches Dermatologiques Sophia Antipolis, 06565 Valbonne, France.

al., 1981a). In this chapter we will review the results obtained with the cell lines presently used for studying the neuronal differentiation of teratocarcinomas.

1. DESCRIPTION OF THE CELLULAR SYSTEMS

1.1. PCC7-S AzaR1, Clone 1009

The 1009 cell line is a subclone derived from the PCC7-S cell line which was established from a spontaneous mouse teratocarcinoma (Fellous *et al.*, 1978). 1009 cells are multipotential since multidifferentiated tumors can be obtained after injection of these cells into syngeneic mice (Fellous *et al.*, 1978). Pfeiffer *et al.* (1981) described a way to reproducibly obtain neural derivatives with this cell line. When 1009 cells were grown at relatively low densities (5×10^4 cells/cm^2) they remained undifferentiated. If they were allowed to reach high densities, multilayered areas developed which then differentiated into neurite-bearing cells. Since abundant cell death was observed under these conditions, other methods have been attempted to obtain neural derivatives. Pfeiffer and co-workers found that the formation of aggregates was an efficient way to obtain high cell densities with limited cell death. 1009 cells were cultured in bacteriological petri dishes to prevent attachment. Under these conditions they formed aggregates 400–500 μm in diameter. Such aggregates, when cultured in this way for up to 7 days, did not show any apparent sign of differentiation. However, when they were allowed to attach on tissue culture dishes and provided they were older than 4 days, aggregates were found to send out numerous processes whose number and length increased with time. Bundles of processes forming bridges between individual aggregates appeared later. More recently, Paulin *et al.* (1982) showed that the aggregation step was not necessary if 1009 cells were cultured in the presence of retinoic acid (10^{-7} M) and dibutyryl cAMP (10^{-3} M). This treatment not only reduced the cell death usually observed when the cells grew to confluency as monolayers but provoked extensive neural differentiation.

Several criteria were used to identify the cell types derived from the 1009 cell line. Cell processes and networks could be strongly stained by the Bodian silver impregnation technique. Electron microscopy analysis showed that the processes had the morphology of rather mature neuronal axons. Particularly, they were characterized by the presence of abundant microtubules and the absence of endoplasmic reticulum. However, myelination and synapse formation were not observed. At the biochemical level, differentiation was accompanied by large increases in acetylcholinesterase (AChE) and choline acetyltransferase (CAT) activities (Pfeiffer *et al.*, 1981). Immunofluorescence techniques showed the presence of neurofilament proteins in neuronal derivatives but not in the original EC cell population. Some glial cells expressing the glial fibrillary acidic protein (GFA) and some fibroblastic cells containing vimentin were also found in these cultures (Paulin *et al.*, 1982).

1.2. P19 Cell Line

The P19 cell line, derived from a teratocarcinoma obtained after grafting a $7\frac{1}{2}$-day mouse embryo, is a multipotential EC line of normal male karyotype (Rossant and McBurney, 1982). Jones-Villeneuve *et al.* (1982) showed that aggregation and treatment with retinoic acid were both required for the differentiation of this cell line into neural derivatives. When aggregates of P19 cells were plated on tissue culture dishes, the great majority of the cells remained undifferentiated although surrounded by a small amount of endodermlike cells. Unlike 1009 cells, P19 cells cannot differentiate spontaneously into neural derivatives. However, treatment of P19 aggregates with retinoic acid (5×10^{-7} M) provoked neuronal differentiation. Within 24 hr after plating retinoic acid-treated aggregates on tissue culture dishes, a flat layer resulting from the migration of fibroblastlike cells formed at the periphery of the aggregates. Neuronal derivatives appeared later and their processes grew rapidly over the fibroblastic cell layer. Processes were frequently arranged in bundles. Interestingly, the appearance of neuronlike cells was found to be dependent on retinoic acid concentration (Edwards and McBurney, 1982). Neurons were characterized by AChE activity, the presence of microtubule networks, and the 160K neurofilament protein. In contrast, fibroblastlike cells were only stained with antisera directed against vimentin. A population of glial cells detected by the presence of GFA was found to appear at the junction of the fibroblastic layer and the aggregates 4–5 days after plating (Jones-Villeneuve *et al.*, 1982).

1.3. C17S1, Clone 1003

The 1003 cell line is a pseudotetraploid clone derived from the C17S1 mouse cell line (McBurney, 1976) and selected for its ability to grow in the absence of feeder-layers (Muramatsu *et al.*, 1978). 1003 cells form multidifferentiated tumors after injection into syngeneic mice (H. Jakob and J. Gaillard, unpublished results). They can be maintained in an undifferentiated state in conventional serum-containing medium at low densities. However, confluent cultures show sparse differentiation limited to the formation of keratin-containing epithelial cells, probably endodermal (2–5% of the total cell population). As an attempt to understand the discrepancy existing between the extensive differentiation of 1003 cells *in vivo* and the very limited differentiation found *in vitro*, Darmon *et al.* (1981a) tried to define a serum-free medium which would allow both growth and differentiation of 1003 cells. When F12/DME (1:1) medium was supplemented with insulin, transferrin, selenium, and fibronectin, the growth of 1003 cells was as fast as with a 10% fetal calf serum supplement. However, extensive differentiation was observed by day 4–5. The cells formed rosettes of neuroepithelium and just before confluency (days 6–9) neuronlike cells bearing processes appeared (Fig. 1b). Processes extended as a function of time and days 10–12 were marked by the formation of aggregates from which very long thick fibers extended.

Identification of neurons was ascertained using morphological, biochemical, and immunocytochemical criteria: AChE and CAT activities, veratridine-stimulatable sodium channels, 70K and 200K neurofilament proteins, and the N6 cell-surface neuron-specific antigen (Darmon *et al.*, 1981a, 1982a,c,d). Since AChE and CAT activities could be detected but not tyrosine hydroxylase activity, neurons derived from 1003 seem to be mainly of cholinergic phenotype. However, a few neurons (approximately 1/1000) were stained with anti-tyrosine hydroxylase antiserum. See Chapter 1 for additional details about the neuronal properties of 1003 cells in serum-free defined medium.

1.4. F9 Cell Line

F9 is a clonal cell line derived from the OTT 6050 mouse teratocarcinoma (Artz *et al.*, 1973). It was recently reported that retinoic acid and dibutyryl cAMP induced differentiation of F9 cells into neuronlike cells and provoked an increase in AChE activity (Kuff and Fewell, 1980). More evidence for neuronal differentiation was provided by Liesi *et al.* (1984) who showed that in long-term cultures other markers such as neurofilament proteins appeared.

F9 cells were maintained as undifferentiated stem cells in serum-containing medium. To induce differentiation, the cells were plated at low densities onto gelatin-coated dishes and cultured in 3% fetal calf serum. Retinoic acid (10^{-7} M) was added at day 2 and dibutyryl cAMP (10^{-3} M) at day 3. Neuronlike cells appeared within 7 days of culture. These cells were found AChE-positive but tyrosine hydroxylase-negative and did not express neurofilament proteins until 14 days of culture.

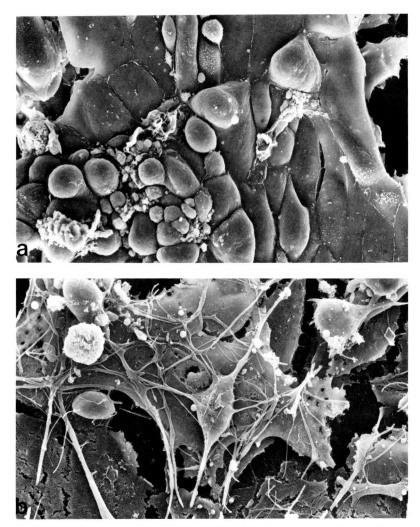

Figure 1. Scanning electron micrographs of 1003 cells in (a) serum-containing or (b) serum-free defined medium. (From Darmon *et al.*, 1981a.)

When nerve growth factor (NGF) (1 IU/ml) was added to the retinoic acid- and dibutyryl cAMP-containing medium, neuronal differentiation occurred earlier and was more extensive: neurofilament proteins were expressed within 10 days and, moreover, tyrosine hydroxylase was found in all neuronlike cells. Some cells showed Leu-enkephalin-like immunofluorescence, but double-labeling was not performed. The addition of NGF alone or in combination with only retinoic acid or dibutyryl cAMP was inefficient. Liesi *et al.* (1984) suggest that a "treatment with retinoic acid and dibutyryl cyclic AMP is a prerequisite for the ability of NGF to induce the differentiation of F9 cells in an adrenergic direction."

2. BIOCHEMICAL STUDIES

The cellular systems described in Section 1 have been used to study the molecular changes accompanying cell specialization and differentiation. Two different approaches have been attempted. In the first one, changes relative to the expression of specific intermediate filament proteins were detected with specific antibodies at the single-cell level by immunofluorescence techniques. In the other, two-dimensional electrophoresis was used to compare the total protein patterns.

2.1. Changes in Intermediate Filament Proteins during 1003 Differentiation

Contrary to their *in vivo* normal equivalents (inner cells of blastocysts), EC cells (including 1003 cells) were found to be stained by antivimentin antibodies (Paulin *et al.*, 1982; Darmon *et al.*, 1982a). After 4–5 days in serum-free defined medium, 1003 cells had formed typical rosettes of neuroepithelium. At that stage, neuronal antigens were not yet expressed but the cells displayed veratridine-stimulatable sodium channels (Darmon *et al.*, 1981a). Neuroepithelial cells contained vimentin but in higher amounts than undifferentiated 1003 cells (Darmon *et al.*, 1982a). A few days later (6–7 days after plating) neuroepithelial cells had differentiated into preneurons, cells with a rounder shape and a small neuritic process. Most of these cells still contained vimentin but, in addition, some of them were double-labeled with anti-70K neurofilament antibodies. A transient stage of differentiation defined by cells containing both vimentin and neurofilament proteins has also been described in the chick embryo (Tapscott *et al.*, 1981) and in the rat embryo (Bignami *et al.*, 1982). During 1003 differentiation a progressive transformation into morphologically identifiable neurons occurred during the following days. Most neurons were then heavily labeled with anti-70K neurofilament antibodies and did not contain vimentin. Elements decorated by anti-200K neurofilament antibodies appeared also as patches in the neurites; this labeling was still discontinuous after 14 days of culture in serum-free medium. It is noteworthy that electron microscopic studies (Sharp *et al.*, 1982) have shown that the 200K protein is periodically arranged along neurofilaments, contrary to other components which seem to be continuous. Unlike neurons derived from the 1009 cell line (Paulin *et al.*, 1982), neurons derived from the 1003 cell line were not decorated with anti-160K neurofilament antibodies.

2.2. Specific Changes in Protein Patterns of 1003 and 1009 Cells during Neural Differentiation

Modulation of protein expression has been investigated during neural differentiation of 1003 and 1009 cell lines (Eddé *et al.*, 1983) by two-dimensional electrophoresis (O'Farrell, 1975). Protein patterns of EC cells and their neural derivatives were found to differ both quantitatively and qualitatively. The changes observed were very similar during neural differentiation of either 1003 or 1009. Since neural differentiation of EC cell lines was always accompanied by the appearance of a minority of other cell types, it was impossible to exclude a priori that some of the changes in protein patterns were due to the contribution of nonneural cells. In the case of 1003, clones of nonneural cells could be derived: 10035 C1 of mesenchymal phenotype (Darmon *et al.*, 1982b) and 10031 D4 of fibroblastic phenotype (Darmon and Serrero, 1983). These cell lines were used as controls to determine which changes were specific for neural differentiation. This comparative analysis included other nonneural differentiated cells derived from teratocarcinomas such as PYS-2 (parietal yolk sac; Jakob *et al.*, 1973), 3 TDM-1 (trophoblastoma; Nicolas *et al.*, 1976), and 1168 (myoblastic; Darmon *et al.*, 1981b). The results of these studies showed that two obvious changes occurred specifically during neural differentiation: (1) the appearance of an additional β-tubulin isoform (β'-tubulin) and (2) a severalfold accumulation of the brain isozyme of creatine kinase (BCK). EC cell lines express the two α-tubulin isoforms (α1 and α2) and the β-tubulin isoform, which are present in all types and tissues studied. β'-tubulin was found to appear after neural differentiation in the form of an additional minor spot at the side of the β-tubulin spot. β'-tubulin was not found in any of the nonneural derivatives tested but was found in several neural cell lines and tissues (see below). BCK was synthesized at low levels in EC cell lines. It increased severalfold during neural differentiation of 1003 and 1009 cells but was not detectable in the nonneural derivatives analyzed. These changes were found to occur as early as the appearance of neuroepithelial cells, a moment at which the 70K neurofilaments and the N6 surface antigen were not yet detectable. β'-tubulin and BCK thus provide interesting markers for the early steps of neural differentiation.

Studies of adult mouse tissues showed that β'-tubulin is actually present in the nervous system. Moreover, this isoform is expressed by cell lines derived from the neural crest, such as neuroblastomas (Eddé *et al.*, 1982), and by primary cultures of neurons but not glial cells prepared from mouse brain (Moura-Neto *et al.*, 1983). BCK, very abundant in the mouse brain, was not found in the liver, kidneys, or spleen. However, BCK was found in the intestine and uterus (Adamson, 1976). Surprisingly, in this latter tissue, BCK and the neuron-specific enolase are the major components of the set of estrogen-induced proteins (Reiss and Kaye, 1981). Since BCK is accumulated during brain development (Soreq *et al.*, 1982; Vayssière, 1982), and taking into account the presence of estrogen receptors of high affinity in the brain, it remains to be determined whether the synthesis of BCK is also regulated in the nervous system by estrogen signals.

3. CONCLUSION

Although a quantification of the various neural cell types eventually obtained is difficult, a gross estimate indicates that neurons account for the majority in differentiated cultures of the EC cell line described by Darmon *et al.* (1981a). More than 60% of 1003 cells cultured in serum-free defined medium contained neurofilament proteins. Jones-Villeneuve *et al.* (1982) have reported that almost 100% of retinoic acid-treated aggregates of P19 cells exhibit extensive neuronal differentiation. Unfortunately, this measurement does not indicate the proportion of neurons in each differentiating aggregate. Attempts have been made to identify the cells accompanying neurons using immunofluorescent detection of specific antigens. Not only is this useful to draw conclusions about the specificity of biochemical results, but it may give some insight about the segregation of the various lineages. Differentiation of 1009 and P19 cells led to the formation of some astrocytes (GFA-positive cells). Moreover, neuronal differentiation is accompanied in the three cell lines described above by the appearance of fibroblastlike cells containing vimentin. During P19 differentiation, these cells seem to form a continuous layer on which neuronal processes extend, suggesting that a direct interaction may be necessary for neurite formation. In contrast, in the case of 1003 cultures, neurite extension was as extensive in areas of the dishes devoid of fibroblastlike cells as in areas where neurons were attached to them.

Because of their multipotentiality, EC cell lines should allow the study of the segregation of the neuronal lineage during the first steps of differentiation. As a prerequisite to such studies, it is important to determine whether neural derivatives appearing *in vitro* are generated by a direct induction of pluripotential EC cells or whether they differentiate from preexisting cells secondarily selected by the culture conditions. Such a selection process would imply that the nondifferentiated population contains not only EC cells but also some cells engaged in differentiation, which would survive and grow while the EC cells would die. However, the following observations indicate that a selection process is unlikely to be responsible for the formation of neural cells. (1) The differentiation of P19 cells occurs without detectable cell death. When P19 cells are plated in serum-containing medium at low densities, the number of colonies counted after 10 days is little if any affected by the addition of retinoic acid until 10^{-6} M. Moreover, aggregates grown in the presence of 5×10^{-7} M retinoic acid for 9 days contained 80% of the number of cells found in the untreated aggregates over the same period. (2) Although cell death occurs during differentiation of 1003 cells and thus some selection might occur, it cannot explain by itself the formation of neurons in serum-free medium. Using immunofluorescence techniques allowing the screening of more than 10^5 cells, no cells were found in the initial population to bear neural markers such as the neuron–glial antigen NG2 (Stallcup, 1982), the neuronal antigen N6 (Stallcup et al., 1981), or the 70K and 200K neurofilaments. The appearance of these markers during neuronal differentiation cannot therefore be explained by a process of selection and thus must result from an induction of differentiation by serum deprivation.

The observations reported above clearly exclude the possibility that differentiated cells are present in EC cultures and are selected either by retinoic acid or by serum deprivation. However, they do not exclude the hypothesis that EC cell cultures contain some cells which are apparently identical to stem cells (i.e., no markers are yet available to discriminate them) but are already committed to certain pathways of differentiation. This hypothesis seems nevertheless unlikely since cloning experiments performed with P19 and 1003 cells yield only cell lines of EC phenotype having potentialities similar to those of the parental cell lines. Moreover, in the case of the 1003 cell line the absence in the population growing in serum-containing medium of the NG2 antigen, which appears to characterize precursors of the neuronal and glial lineages (Stallcup, 1981), allows us to hypothesize that not even neuron–glial precursors are present in the initial cell population.

Interestingly, both 1003 and P19 cell lines have been found to further respond to variations in the culture conditions by developing various pathways of differentiation. If laminin, instead of fibronectin, is used as an attachment factor, neuronal differentiation of 1003 cells occurs, but at low cell densities (1–3 $\times$ 10^3 cells/cm^2) it is accompanied by the formation of large patches of multinucleated myotubes (up to 40% of the area of the dish). The muscular nature of these structures was ascertained by staining with antibodies directed against embryonic muscular myosin (Darmon, 1982). Moreover, if 1003 cells were first cultured in serum-free medium and serum was readded between days 2 and 4, neuroepithelial and neuronal differentiation were completely prevented while the majority of the cells differentiated into fibroblastic cells. Tumorigenic properties of 1003 cells and their various derivatives were analyzed. When injected into syngeneic mice, 1003 EC cells produced teratocarcinomas containing undifferentiated cells, neuroepithelium, and mesenchymal derivatives. Subclones of fibroblastic phenotype, obtained from cultures of 1003 cells in serum-free defined medium to which serum had been readded at day 3, formed fibrosarcomas in most inoculated animals. However, neural derivatives obtained in defined medium did not form tumors (Darmon *et al.*, 1982b).

In the case of P19 cells, several routes of differentiation have also been obtained *in vitro* as a function of the culture conditions. In the presence of dimethylsulfoxide, aggregates of P19 cells differentiated into cardiac and skeletal muscle, but neurons and glial cells did not form (McBurney *et al.*, 1982). Recent studies of Edwards and McBurney (1983) have shown that the differentiated cell types formed by retinoic acid-treated aggregates were dependent on the concentration of the drug: cardiac muscle was predominant at 10^{-9} M, skeletal muscle was formed at 10^{-8} M, and neurons and astrocytes required an even higher concentration (10^{-7}–10^{-6} M) to appear.

Whether the modulators of differentiation active *in vitro* (serum factors, laminin, retinoic acid) are those which act *in vivo* remains to be determined. Also remaining to be found are the conditions (if any) which could make EC cells differentiate as widely *in vitro* as *in vivo*. The physiological significance of the various ways to obtain neuronal differentiation of EC cells *in vitro* is difficult to assess. Retinoic acid can substitute for the formation of aggregates in 1009 cells and for serum deprivation in 1003 cells. It is thus tempting to speculate that high cell densities or the depletion of serum inhibitors allow the cells to produce and/or accumulate inducers of differentiation such as retinoic acid. Moreover, the concentration of retinoic acid seems to be particularly important for the developmental fate of P19 cells. These experiments fit particularly well with those performed *in vivo* on the developing amphibian limb bud (Maden, 1982), which strongly suggest that during normal embryogenesis gradients of retinoids may play a role in cell determination.

REFERENCES

Adamson, E. D., 1976, Isoenzyme transitions of creatine phosphokinase, aldolase and phosphoglycerate mutase in differentiating mouse cells, *J. Embryol. Exp. Morphol.* **35**:355–367.

Artz, K., Dubois, P., Bennet, D., Condamine, H., Babinet, C., and Jacob, F., 1973, Surface antigens common to mouse cleavage embryos and primitive teratocarcinoma cells in culture, *Proc. Natl. Acad. Sci. USA* **70**:2988–2992.

Bignami, A., Raju, T., and Dahl, D., 1982, Localization of vimentin, the non-specific intermediate filament protein in embryonal glia and in early differentiating neurons. *Develop. Biol.* **91**:286–295.

Darmon, M. Y., 1982, Laminin provides a better substrate than fibronectin for attachment, growth and differentiation of 1003 embryonal carcinoma cells. *In Vitro* **18**:997–1003.

Darmon, M., and Serrero, G., 1983, Isolation of two different fibroblastic cell types from the embryonal carcinoma cell line 1003: Study of tumorigenic properties, surface antigens and differentiation responses to 5-azacytidine and dexamethasone. *Cold Spring Harbor Conf. Cell Prolif.* **10**:109–119.

Darmon, M., Bottenstein, J., and Sato, G., 1981a, Neural differentiation following culture of embryonal carcinoma cells in a serum-free defined medium, *Develop. Biol.* **85**:463–471.

Darmon, M., Serrero, G., Rizzino, A., and Sato, G., 1981b, Isolation of myoblastic, fibro-adipogenic and fibroblastic clonal cell lines from a common precursor and study of their hormonal requirements for growth and differentiation, *Exp. Cell Res.* **132**:313–327.

Darmon, M., Buc-Caron, M. H., Paulin, D., and Jacob, F., 1982a, Control by the extracellular environment of differentiation pathways in 1003 embryonal carcinoma cells: Study at the level of specific intermediate filaments, *EMBO J.* **1**:901–906.

Darmon, M., Stallcup, W., Pittman, Q. J., and Sato, G. H., 1982b, Control of differentiation pathways by the extracellular environment in an embryonal carcinoma cell line, *Cold Spring Harbor Conf. Cell Prolif.* **9**:997–1006.

Darmon, M., Stallcup, W. B., and Pittman, Q. J., 1982c, Induction of neural differentiation by serum deprivation in cultures of the embryonal carcinoma cell line 1003, *Exp. Cell Res.* **138**:73–78.

Darmon, M., Barret, A., Puymirat, J., and Faivre, A., 1982d, Cholinergic neurons and embryonic mesenchymal cells arise from the same population of precursor cells in cultures of embryonal carcinoma cells triggered to differentiate by serum-deprivation, *Biol. Cell.* **45**:10.

Eddé, B., Portier, M. M., Sahuquillo, C., Jeantet, C., and Gros, F., 1982, Changes in some cytoskeletal proteins during neuroblastoma cell differentiation, *Biochimie* **64**:141–151.

Eddé, B., Jakob, H., and Darmon, M., 1983, Two specific markers for neural differentiation of embryonal carcinoma cells. *EMBO J.* **2**:1473–1478.

Edwards, M. K. S., and McBurney, M. W., 1983, The concentration of retinoic acid determines the differentiated cell types formed by a teratocarcinoma cell line. *Develop. Biol.* **98**:187–191.

Fellous, M., Gunther, E., Kemler, R., Wiels, J., Berger, R., Guenet, J. L., Jakob, H., and Jacob, F., 1978, Association of the H-Y male antigen with β_2-microglobulin on human lymphoid and differentiated mouse teratocarcinoma cell lines. *J. Exp. Med.* **148**:58–70.

Jakob, H., Boon, T., Gaillard, J., Nicolas, J. F., and Jacob, F., 1973, Teratocarcinome de la souris: Isolement, culture et propriétés de cellules à potentialités multiples, *Ann. Microbiol. (Institut Pasteur)* **124B**:269–282.

Jones-Villeneuve, E. M. V., McBurney, M. W., Rogers, K. A., and Kalnins, V. I., 1982, Retinoic acid induces embryonal carcinoma cells to differentiate into neurons and glial cells. *J. Cell Biol.* **94**:253–262.

Kuff, E. L., and Fewell, J. W., 1980, Induction of neural-like cells and acetylcholinesterase activity in cultures of F9 teratocarcinoma treated with retinoic acid and dibutyryl cyclic adenosine monophosphate, *Develop. Biol.* **77**:103–115.

Liesi, P., Rechardt, L., and Wartiovaara, J., 1984, Nerve growth factor induces adrenergic neuronal differentiation in F9 teratocarcinoma cells, *Nature* **306**:265–276.

McBurney, M., 1976, Clonal lines of teratocarcinoma cells in vitro: Differentiation and cytogenetic characteristics, *J. Cell. Physiol.* **89**:441–456.

McBurney, M. W., Jones-Villeneuve, E. M. V., Edwards, M. K. S., and Anderson, P. J., 1982, Control of muscle and neuronal differentiation in a cultured embryonal carcinoma cell line, *Nature* **299**:165–167.

Maden, M., 1982, Vitamin A and pattern formation in the regenerating limb, *Nature* **295**:672–674.

Moura-Neto, V., Mallat, M., Jeantet, C., and Prochiantz, A., 1983, Microheterogeneity of tubulin proteins in neuronal and glial cells from the mouse brain in culture, *EMBO J.* **2**:1243–1248.

Muramatsu, T., Gachelin, G., Nicolas, J. F., Condamine, H., Jakob, H., and Jacob, F., 1978, Carbohydrate structure and cell differentiation: Unique properties of fucosyl-glycopeptides isolated from embryonal carcinoma cells, *Proc. Natl. Acad. Sci. USA* **75**:2315–2319.

Nicolas, J. F., Dubois, P., Jakob, H., Gaillard, J., and Jacob, F., 1975, Teratocarcinome de la souris: Differenciation en culture d'une lignée de cellules primitives à potentialités multiples, *Ann. Microbiol. (Institut Pasteur)* **126A**:3–22.

Nicolas, J. F., Avner, P., Gaillard, J., Guenet, J. L., Jakob, H., and Jacob, F., 1976, Cell lines derived from teratocarcinomas, *Cancer Res.* **36**:4224–4231.

O'Farrell, P. H., 1975, High resolution two dimensional electrophoresis of proteins. *J. Biol. Chem.* **250**:4007–4021.

Paulin, D., Jakob, H., Jacob, F., Weber, K., and Osborn, M., 1982, In vitro differentiation of mouse teratocarcinoma cells monitored by intermediate filament expression. *Differentiation* **22**:90–99.

Pfeiffer, S., Jakob, H., Mikoshiba, K., Dubois, P., Guenet, J. L., Nicolas, J. F., Gaillard, J., Chevance, L. G., and Jacob, F., 1981, Differentiation of a teratocarcinoma line: Preferential development of cholinergic neurons. *J. Cell Biol.* **88**:57–66.

Pierce, G. B., 1967, Teratocarcinoma: Model for a developmental concept of cancer, in: *Current Topics In Developmental Biology*, Volume 2 (A. Monroy and R. A. Mascona, eds.), Academic Press, New York, pp. 223–246.

Reiss, N. A., and Kaye, A. M., 1981, Identification of the major component of the estrogen-induced proteins as the BB isozymes of creatine kinase, *J. Biol. Chem.* **256**:5741–5749.

Rossant, J., and McBurney, M. W., 1982, The developmental potential of a euploid male teratocarcinoma cell line after blastocyst injection, *J. Embryol. Exp. Morphol.* **70**:99–112.

Sharp, G., Shaw, G., and Weber, K., 1982, Immunoelectronmicroscopical localization of the three neurofilament triplet proteins along neurofilaments of cultured dorsal root ganglion neurons, *Exp. Cell Res.* **137**:403–413.

Soreq, H., Safran, A., and Zisling, R., 1982, Variations in gene expression during development of the rat cerebellum, *Develop. Brain Res.* **3**:65–79.

Stallcup, W., 1981, The NG2 antigen, a putative lineage marker: Immunofluorescent localization in primary cultures of rat brain, *Develop. Biol.* **83**:154–165.

Stallcup, W., Arner, L., and Levine, J., 1981, Anti-N6, an antiserum that specifically binds to many types of neurons, *Soc. Neurosci. Abstr.* **7**:301.

Stevens, L. C., 1967, The biology of teratomas, *Adv. Morphol.* **6**:1–31.

Tapscott, S. J., Benett, G. S., and Holtzer, H., 1981, Neuronal precursor cells in the chick neural tube express neurofilament proteins, *Nature* **292**:836–838.

Vayssière, J. L., 1982, Contribution à l'étude de l'évolution des proteines cytosquelettiques et membranaires au cours de la neurogénèse, D.E.A. Université Paris VII, Paris.

II
Electrophysiology

10

Neuronal Development in Culture
Role of Electrical Activity

DOUGLAS E. BRENNEMAN and PHILLIP G. NELSON

1. INTRODUCTION

Analysis of the development of such a complex structure as the mammalian CNS obviously requires a variety of approaches in which different degrees of simplification and reductionism will be involved. It has been evident from the earliest experiments in cell culture that neural properties are expressed in culture and that application of this technique to appropriate questions could give highly instructive results. We wish to discuss one approach to a neurodevelopmental question which involves a relatively complex central neuronal preparation. Despite the complexity of our preparation, it departs significantly from the level of organization that characterizes intact neural structures and we note some of the substantial reservations that such departure entails. The difficulty in equating *in vitro* with *in vivo* phenomena must be addressed and we will point out some of the close parallels as well as the discrepancies.

The question we wish to address relates to the role of electrical activity in modulating or regulating neuronal survival and maturation.

DOUGLAS E. BRENNEMAN and PHILLIP G. NELSON • Laboratory of Developmental Neurobiology, National Institutes of Health, Bethesda, Maryland 20205.

A wealth of experimentation has been done *in vivo* on this question but some characteristics of cell culture would seem to lend themselves well to the study of such a problem. Neurons can be followed closely throughout development using biochemical, physiological, or morphological techniques. A variety of manipulations of the system can be performed readily and different neuronal combinations studied. We have felt that the analytical possibilities are considerable and that mammalian CNS cell cultures may be expected to express some of the developmental regulatory phenomena important for the intact system.

It is, perhaps, with respect to developmental problems, that some caution must be observed with regard to conclusions drawn from studies of "simplified" systems. The complex regulatory interactions that undoubtedly occur between cellular constituents in development may be altered in a partial system. Alternatively, and no less importantly, regulatory interactions important in an experimental preparation may have only limited significance in the intact nervous system. Nevertheless, the potential for control of parameters that effect development is best realized with culture techniques, where a single variable can be more readily isolated and studied.

2. METHODS OVERVIEW FOR DEVELOPMENTAL STUDIES

2.1. Cell Culture Techniques

The methods for culturing spinal cord from the fetal mouse have been described in detail and have been utilized successfully by numerous investigators. Briefly, the spinal cords are removed between days 12 and 14 of gestation and dissociated into isolated cells with mechanical and enzymatic techniques (Ransom *et al.*, 1977). The gestational age of the tissue is crucial to the success of the culture. A routine check of fetal limb development is done to confirm the age of the animal. For biochemical studies, the cells are plated in collagen-coated culture wells (2 cm^2). The trays of multiple wells provide a means of rapid and efficient processing of a large number of assays.

The methods of cell culture maintenance can have a marked influence on the effects of developmental experiments. Some of the details may appear trivial, but they represent potential problems of which investigators should be aware. Particularly in developmental studies, the volume of medium which is removed from the culture prior to the replenishment of culture nutrients may be crucial to the outcome of the experiment and the viability of the cells. In general, the amount of medium removed from the cultures should be kept to a minimum during the first 2 weeks in culture. The reason for this relates to the release of trophic substances during development which affect the survival and composition of the immature culture. The removal of these substances in an inconsistent manner during changes of medium can become a major source of experimental variation. The experimental control of the availability of these trophic substances is an advantage of the system, but this control must be scrupulously and deliberately maintained.

Another technical aspect which may affect developmental studies is the plating density of the culture inoculum. The density must be kept high enough to maintain cell viability but sufficiently low to allow the visualization of neuronal networks. It is a good practice to study any given experimental effect at several plating densities.

The composition and density of the background cells, over which the neurons grow, are also important to consider when assessing the response of the culture system. Support cells may contribute a significant portion of the trophic factors required for neuronal development (Banker, 1980; Varon et al., 1981). Antimitotic agents such as cytosine arabinoside, 2-fluorodeoxyuridine, or aminopterin are routinely added to the cultures to inhibit background cells from overgrowing the cultures. However, these agents may also contribute to the response of developing neurons by decreasing factors released from the support cells (Ishida and Deguchi, 1983).

A number of characteristics of the dissociated spinal cord culture system make it particularly useful for developmental studies. Since the variable of developmental age is intrinsic to these studies, it is desirable to have a large quantity of material from which statistical comparisons among age-related differences can be made. Through the use of multiwells, a large number of determinations can be made from a relatively small amount of starting tissue. Plating 200,000–300,000 cells per well affords adequate material for enzymatic and receptor binding studies. The reproducibility among wells and between experiments is high. Thus, one avoids the problems associated with variation between litters common to many developmental studies.

2.2. Analytical Probes

The ideal reduction of the nervous system might consist of obtaining homogeneous populations of neurons of a single type, e.g., cholinergic, GABAergic, etc. One could then study each isolated cell type or compare combinations of cell types for possible interactions. Since that ideal situation is not available, the objective has been to obtain specific probes of various neurochemical systems in order to assess development in culture. In addition to neurochemical-specific assays, one would also like to be able to monitor the overall state of the neuronal or background cell populations. Such requirements can be achieved to a considerable extent with the techniques to be described.

The most general and least sensitive of the culture assays for evaluating the effects of various experimental manipulations are total protein and DNA content. Although routinely conducted, their usefulness is limited since they reveal only the most drastic effects on developing neurons. Since background cells may be the most abundant cell type, these assays are usually an estimate of support cell response. One of the most revealing assays is direct counting of neuronal cell bodies under phase optics. When combined with autoradiography (Brenneman et al., 1983), it is a powerful measure of effects produced on a given type of neuron. The procedure of counting neurons according to a predetermined set of coordinates is, however, extremely time-consuming. Another major disadvantage is the uncertainty of identifying neurons from nonneuronal cells in immature cultures using morphological criteria. In addition, it is difficult to obtain accurate neuronal counts with highly aggregated cultures. However, cell counting is often essential to complement the observations made by biochemical methods.

The necessity of a neuronal assay which is rapid, easy to measure, and reliable is met in part by two markers, ^{125}I-labeled tetanus toxin fixation and ^{125}I-labeled scorpion toxin binding. The purification (Ledley et al., 1977) and iodination (Bolton and Hunter, 1973) of tetanus toxin have been described. It has been shown that cultured cells with neuronal morphology bind tetanus toxin and that minimal labeling of nonneuronal elements occurs (Dimpfel et al., 1975; Mirsky et al., 1978). Specific tetanus toxin fixation is detectable only in tissue containing certain gangliosides (Dimpfel et al., 1977). Tetanus toxin binds to the neuronal soma and processes and ^{125}I-labeled tetanus toxin binding has been used to study neuronal development in culture (Puymirat et al., 1982; Brenneman et al., 1983). A disadvantage of the tetanus toxin fixation assay is that the toxin apparently adheres to dead cells (Mirsky et al., 1978). Hence, in order to detect a decrease in toxin fixation, either extensive neurite withdrawal or loss of neurons from the culture must occur. ^{125}I-labeled scorpion toxin binding has also been used to estimate neuron-related changes (Berwald-Netter et al., 1981). Crude toxin (Leiurus quinquestriatus) was purified and iodinated as described by Catterall (1977a). The specificity of the probe resides in the high affinity of the toxin for the inactivation site of the voltage-dependent sodium channel (Catterall, 1977a). Excitable cells are specifically labeled at nanomolar concentrations of the scorpion toxin; nonspecific binding is determined with a 100-fold excess of unlabeled toxin. The site at which scorpion toxin binds is distinct from that which binds tetrodotoxin (Catterall, 1977b). The binding of scorpion toxin to neuronal membranes is dependent on membrane potential (Catterall, 1977a). This assay has rapid temporal resolution in that a response involving a loss of membrane potential produces a rapid decrease in scorpion toxin binding.

2.3 Neurochemical-Specific Assays

Two enzyme assays currently employed by us are choline acetyltransferase (CAT) and glutamic acid decarboxylase (GAD). These enzymes are markers for cholinergic and GABAergic neurons, respectively. Both of these assays are conducted *in situ* (Brenneman *et al.*, 1983). The cells are disrupted with a buffered Triton X-100 solution directly in the culture well. Radioactive substrate is added to the cell homogenate and the product is separated from reactant by appropriate ion-exchange chromatography. Details of the above assays can be found in the figure legends.

Another useful specific marker is high-affinity [^{3}H]-GABA uptake (Farb *et al.*, 1979; Neale *et al.*, 1983). This assay is performed on intact cells and can be done in the same well as the ^{125}I-labeled tetanus toxin fixation. Neuronal uptake of [^{3}H]-GABA is estimated from the difference between total uptake and that taken up in the presence of 1 mM diaminobutyric acid (DABA) (Iversen and Kelly, 1975). This blocker appears to be neuron-specific in some brain regions while in other areas the neuronal uptake blockade is not complete. The spinal cord falls into the latter category, particularly in cultures less than 1 week old. An alternative neuronal GABA uptake blocker is aminocyclohexane carboxylic acid (Bowery *et al.*, 1976). Glial uptake of [^{3}H]-GABA is estimated in a similar manner as indicated above with 1 mM β-alanine used as a specific blocker (Schon and Kelly, 1975).

Receptor binding studies can also be carried out with intact cells as long as certain precautions are taken. A common problem with receptor assays is the presence of endogenous ligands or inhibitors which affect the binding. If these cannot be satisfactorily removed, membrane preparations should be made for these studies. The development of benzodiazepine binding on intact cells has been explored in dissociated spinal cord (Sher, 1983) and cerebral cortical cultures (Sher and Schrier, 1982). Thorough washing of the cells is required for this determination, presumably to remove an endogenous substance which interferes with binding. Metabolism of the ligand is another potential problem with intact cell systems.

3. DESCRIPTION OF DEVELOPMENT

3.1. Morphology

The growth of neurons and the development of complex networks of neuronal processes have been described for the spinal cord culture system (Ransom et al., 1977). Impressive organizational changes occur during development in culture. The formation and continued modification of cellular networks is shown in Fig. 1. This series of photographs was taken of the same microscopic field during a period of 21 days in culture. The progression from single isolated cells to small aggregations of neurons with limited processes occurs within 24 hr of plating. Cells continue to migrate to form flattened aggregates through the sixth day in vitro. At this stage neuronal processes are dense, but consist of very thin strands in comparison to mature cultures. A marked change in morphological organization occurs between days 6 and 8 in culture. The aggregations become smaller, more spherical, and more phase-bright. The neurites become much thicker and give the appearance of cablelike structures consisting of multiple strands. After this major organizational development, the neuronal aggregates continue to exhibit changes in spatial relationships and in the degree of connectivity. Thus, the cells are a dynamic population which undergo diverse morphological changes during growth in culture. The spinal cord cultures can be maintained for long periods, commonly up to 3–4 months in vitro or even longer. For most developmental studies, parameters are stable or slowly declining after 1 month in vitro.

3.2. Electrophysiological Development

The electrophysiological characterization of cultured spinal cord neurons has been studied almost exclusively on cells older than 3 weeks. The small size of the neurons up to this stage has made conventional intracellular recording impractical. With the advent of the patch electrode, the developing neuron has become more accessible to physiological studies. The patch electrode, originally employed for recording current through single ionic channels (see Chapter 12), has been used for extracellular recording of developing neurons (Jackson et al., 1982). Cells as small as 5 μm can be monitored without penetration or injury.

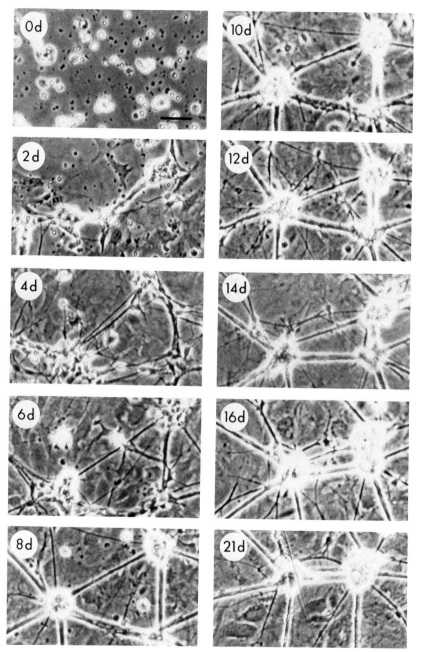

Figure 1. Development of dissociated spinal cord cultures. The same microscopic field was photographed during 3 weeks in culture. Numbers refer to the day in culture. Bar = 50 μm.

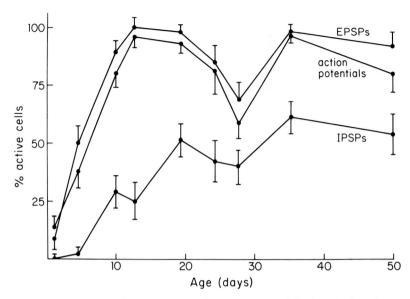

Figure 2. Development of various types of spontaneous activity in spinal cord neurons as measured by extracellular patch electrodes. Data were obtained from cells with a somal diameter greater than 10 μm. (From Jackson *et al.*, 1982.)

With this technique, the incidence of various types of spontaneous activity has been measured in cultured spinal cord neurons (Fig. 2). All neurons tested at 2 weeks in culture exhibited spontaneous excitatory postsynaptic potentials (EPSPs) and action potentials. Approximately 50% of the "mature" neurons had inhibitory postsynaptic potentials (IPSPs) and it appeared that this type of activity was somewhat slower in developing than the excitatory activity. Earlier studies (Tarrade and Crain, 1978) with spinal cord explants also indicated changes in electrical activity during development. A progressive shortening of both burst and cycle duration of phasic electrical activity was observed between days 4 and 21 in culture. The further physiological characterization of developing neurons *in vitro* represents an important area of study which is just beginning to be explored with new recording techniques.

3.3. Biochemical Development

The investigation of biochemical indices of CNS development has drawn wide interest. Application of cell culture to CNS development has also been utilized extensively (see Vernadakis and Arnold, 1980). The dissociated spinal cord neurons exhibit substantial biochemical de-

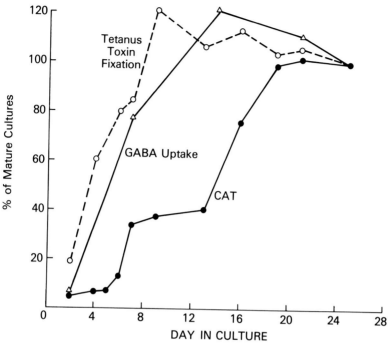

Figure 3. Development of choline acetyltransferase (CAT) activity, high-affinity GABA uptake, and ^{125}I-labeled tetanus toxin fixation in spinal cord cultures. High-affinity uptake of GABA was measured on intact cultures with 10^{-7} M [^{3}H]-GABA for 10 min. Neuronal GABA uptake was taken to be the difference in uptake in the presence and absence of 1 mM diaminobutyric acid. CAT activity was measured in cells which were disrupted in the culture well for 30 min with the following buffer: 50 mM KPO_4 (pH 6.8), 1 mM K-EDTA, 0.25% Triton X-100, and 0.2 M NaCl. The CAT reaction mixture contained 0.1 μCi [1-^{14}C]acetyl coenzyme A, 0.2 mM acetyl coenzyme A, 4 mM choline chloride, and 0.1 mM neostigmine bromide. Product was isolated by anion-exchange chromatography. Specificity of the reaction was estimated as the difference between the activity in the presence of 60 μM of the CAT inhibitor N-hydroxyethyl-4-(1-naphthylvinyl) pyridinium bromide (Cavallito et al., 1970). Tetanus toxin fixation was measured during 60-min incubations at 30°C with ^{125}I-labeled toxin (2 × 10^{-10} M; 100,000 cpm). Nonspecific fixation was determined by a 1-hr preincubation with 2 × 10^{-8} M unlabeled toxin in a parallel series of cultures.

velopment in tissue culture. The ontogenetic increase in several neuronal parameters is shown in Fig. 3. A comparision of CAT activity, high-affinity [^{3}H]-GABA uptake, and ^{125}I-labeled tetanus toxin fixation demonstrates the temporal diversity in biochemical maturation. For example, [^{3}H]-GABA uptake and ; ^{125}I-labeled tetanus toxin fixation show similar progressive increases as a function of age, whereas the devel-

opment of CAT activity suggests a biphasic pattern of cholinergic ontogenesis. This is significant since multiphasic patterns have been observed *in vivo* for the rat corpus striatum (Coyle and Yamamura, 1976),
spinal cord (Burt, 1975), and archicerebellum (Kasa *et al.*, 1982). The
chick spinal cord (Vernadakis, 1973) and brain (Werner *et al.*, 1971)
grown in culture also exhibit a phasic development. Studies of ciliary
ganglion (Nishi and Berg, 1981) and rabbit cerebrum (Hebb, 1956) have
not shown such a pattern. Direct comparisons of CAT activity have
indicated that cultured cells have less enzyme activity than the corresponding material *in vivo* (Meyer *et al.*, 1979). While a general conclusion
may be drawn that there are many features of CNS development which
are expressed in cell culture, the lesser activity of cultured cells suggests
that cell–cell interactions that are lost during dissociation are important
to the full development of the system. Nevertheless, the genetic expression of the temporal pattern of development appears fundamentally the
same.

4. ELECTRICAL ACTIVITY AND NEURONAL DEVELOPMENT

4.1. Overview

Electrical impulses have been suspected of having a role in neuronal
development for many years (Harris, 1981). Neuronal functions such as
synapse elimination (Benoit and Changeux, 1978; O'Brien *et al.*, 1978),
sprouting (Brown and Ironton, 1977), determination of neurotransmitter
type (Walicke *et al.*, 1977), synapse stabilization (Benoit and Changeux,
1975; Pittman and Oppenheim, 1979; Fishman and Nelson, 1981), and
neuronal survival (Bergey *et al.*, 1981); Oppenheim and Nunez, 1982)
are affected by alterations in bioelectric activity. Of particular interest
to the present discussion are studies which relate to neuronal survival
during development. Electrical blockade has been reported to increase
survival of motor neurons of the rat (Pittman and Oppenheim, 1979)
and neurons in the trochlear nucleus of the duck (Creazzo and Sohal,
1979), but to produce no change in the lumbar spinal motor neurons of
Xenopus (Olek and Edwards, 1980). A decrease in motor neuron survival
has been observed when neuromuscular activity is increased (Oppenheim and Nunez, 1982). Early studies with cultured spinal cord explants
and cerebral cortex indicated no significant detrimental effects after
blocking electrical activity during development (Crain *et al.*, 1968; Model
et al., 1971). Other studies suggest that altered or reduced electrical impulses may result in permanent loss of neuronal structure and function

if the perturbation occurs during a critical period during development. Sensory deprivation studies in visual (Wiesel and Hubel, 1963; Rothblat and Schwartz, 1979; Archer *et al.*, 1982), olfactory (Meisami and Mousavi, 1981), auditory (Parks, 1979), and somatosensory (Woolsey and Wann, 1976) systems have shown permanent loss of function. Studies with rat neocortical explants have shown that tetrodotoxin (TTX) produced substantial decreases in the number of synapses per unit area, fewer paired neuronal membrane thickenings, and a reduction in the nerve terminals with synaptic vesicles (Janka and Jones, 1982). Furthermore, studies with dissociated cortical cultures have shown that a low concentration of xylocaine produced 50% fewer synapses in these cultures and a decrease in the density of the neuronal networks (Romijn *et al.*, 1981). This decrement was reported to be a function of the type of horse serum added to the culture medium. Together, these studies indicate that some neuronal systems are vulnerable to the blockade of electrical activity during development.

Our interest has centered on the role of electrical activity in neuronal survival. Our working hypothesis is that some neuronal populations, or perhaps some types of neuronal networks, require impulse traffic in order to stabilize and survive during development. Since it is recognized that this impulse requirement may encompass restricted populations of neurons, the isolation of a vulnerable set of neurons into an experimentally accessible system has been a major goal. Having shown some of the developmental characteristics of the spinal cord culture system and described the various analytical probes used to assess the culture response, we will now examine the consequences of electrical blockade in developing cultures of the spinal cord.

4.2. Electrical Blockade and Neuronal Survival

The survival of cultured spinal cord neurons is decreased after electrical blockade with TTX, an agent which blocks voltage-dependent sodium channels. Initial studies (Bergey *et al.*, 1981) indicated that chronic (>1 month) application of TTX produced substantial loss of large spinal cord neurons (>30-μm soma diameter). Dorsal root ganglion (DRG) cell survival was not affected by TTX. This cell type-specific response is particularly interesting since all cultured spinal cord neurons exhibit spontaneous electrical activity, whereas DRG cells do not display such activity (Peacock *et al.*, 1973). Additional evidence for specificity of the TTX effect is suggested by [^{3}H]-GABA autoradiography experiments. Representative fields are shown in Fig. 4. No detectable changes were observed in the labeled cells, whereas there was a significant decrease

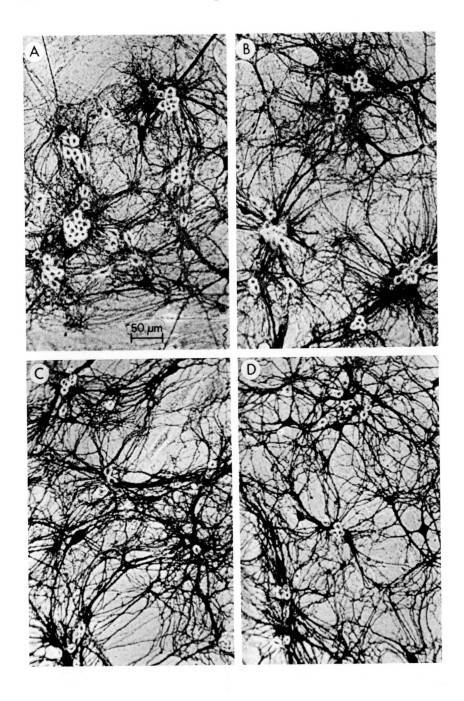

in unlabeled, phase-bright neurons. Cell counts revealed an approximately 25% decrease in total neurons after TTX treatment between days 2 and 14 in culture (Fig. 5). No change in the number of GABA-positive cells was observed. Culture response to TTX was also measured with the other probes described earlier. GABAergic indicators such as high-affinity [^{3}H]-GABA uptake and cell counts after [^{3}H]-GABA autoradiography confirm the lack of response for this class of neurons. In contrast, CAT activity and ^{125}I-labeled tetanus toxin fixation were decreased after TTX treatment between days 7 and 14 in culture. The tetanus assay indicates a significant loss of neuronal surface membrane and the CAT data demonstrate that cholinergic neurons are a population vulnerable to impulse blockade with TTX.

Other means of blocking electrical activity have been tested. Xylocaine, a local anesthetic, produces significant decreases in CAT activity and ^{125}I-labeled tetanus toxin fixation when applied during the second week in culture. High-affinity [^{3}H]-GABA uptake is not affected by this drug treatment. Chronic exposure (3 weeks) to 10 mM Mg^{2+}, which greatly reduces synaptic activity, produces decreases in neuronal surface as measured by the tetanus toxin assay.

The effect of cell plating density was also investigated (Fig. 6). Nonlinearity was observed between initial plating density and ^{125}I-labeled tetanus toxin fixation. These experiments indicated that TTX-mediated decrements in toxin fixation only occurred at subsaturating plating densities. This finding illustrates the need for conducting a given experiment at a variety of plating densities. Another cell density-dependent effect which relates to the vulnerability of neurons to electrical blockade is treatment with 2-fluorodeoxyuridine (FDU). At plating densities greater than 7.5 × 10^5, deletion of FDU treatment results in no observable decrease in ^{125}I-labeled tetanus toxin fixation after TTX treatment. At low plating densities, TTX-mediated decreases in tetanus fixation are detected regardless of the absence or presence of FDU. If one assumes no neuronal division in these cultures, these observations suggest that background cells may be contributing an activity-independent trophic substance which alters the response of neurons to electrical blockade.

←——————————————————————————

Figure 4. Phase-contrast micrographs of 2-week-old cultures after [^{3}H]-GABA autoradiography. (A, B) Control cultures. Neuronal counts of similar preparations indicate that 12–15% of total neurons are labeled by [^{3}H]-GABA uptake. (C, D) Cultures chronically exposed to 1 μM tetrodotoxin. The total number of neurons per culture is reduced by 25% from controls. The number of neurons labeled by [^{3}H]-GABA uptake is unchanged, whereas the number of nonlabeled neurons is decreased. Furthermore, it appears that ^{3}H-GABA-labeled neurites in tetrodotoxin-exposed cultures do not show the tight organization around aggregates that is seen in control cultures. (From Brenneman et al., 1983.)

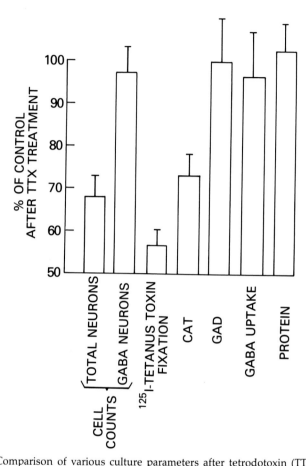

Figure 5. Comparison of various culture parameters after tetrodotoxin (TTX) treatment between days 7 and 14 in culture. ^{125}I-labeled tetanus toxin fixation, choline acetyltransferase (CAT), and [^{3}H]-GABA uptake were assayed as described in Fig. 3. Neuronal cell counts were made directly on the stage of an inverted phase-contrast microscope at a magnification of 160×. Labeled ([^{3}H]-GABA autoradiography) and nonlabeled neurons were counted in 130 regularly spaced fields (each 0.12 mm^2) at predetermined locations on the culture dish. Glutamic acid decarboxylase (GAD) was measured in the culture well after disruption of the cells with the following buffer: 0.25% Triton X-100, 50 mM KH$_2$PO$_4$, 0.5 mM 2-aminoethylisothiouronium bromide hydrobromide, and 0.1 mM pyridoxal phosphate. The reaction was initiated by the addition of 8 mM [^{3}H]glutamate. Product was isolated by ion-exchange chromatography. GAD activity was determined by subtracting the activity measured in the presence of 2 mM aminooxyacetic acid from the total activity. Error bars are S.E.M. (Data from Brenneman et al., 1983.)

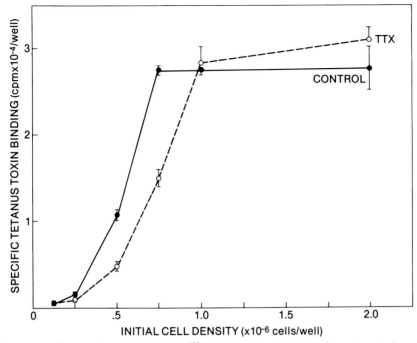

Figure 6. Effect of plating density on ^{125}I-labeled tetanus toxin fixation in spinal cord cultures. Control cultures (○) and TTX-treated cultures (●) were compared 2 weeks after plating. TTX application was during days 7–14 in culture. Each value is the mean ± S.E.M. of nine determinations. (From Brenneman *et al.*, 1983.)

If the density of these background cells is low, either by inhibition of cell division or by reduction in the number plated, the neurons become more vulnerable to impulse blockade.

Neuronal survival is central to the activity-dependent effects we have observed with TTX. During the course of normal development *in vivo*, almost all neural tissue exhibits a significant loss of neurons (Hamburger and Levi-Montalcini, 1949; Nurcombe *et al.*, 1981; Lance-Jones, 1982). Characteristics of normally occurring neuronal death during development are given in Table I. These characteristics share a number of common points with those observed for cell death after electrical blockade in culture. First, both involve a substantial proportion of neurons. It is not uncommon to observe a 25–50% decrease in the total number of neurons. The target dependence *in vivo* has been shown by supernumerary and extirpated limb experiments which indicate the marked influence of target tissue on neuronal survival. TTX treatment in culture

Table I. Characteristics of Neuronal Cell Death during Vertebrate Development

Characteristic	References
Quantitatively significant: 30–80% die	Cowan and Wenger (1967), Harris (1969), Landmesser and Pilar (1974), Hamburger (1975)
Target-dependent	Hamburger and Levi-Montalcini (1949), Cowan and Wenger (1967), Prestige (1967), Hollyday and Hamburger (1976)
Critical period of vulnerability	Landmesser and Pilar (1974), Hamburger (1975), Chu-Wang and Oppenheim (1978), Oppenheim and Majors-Willard (1978)
Stochastic event	Hollyday and Hamburger (1976), Narayanan and Narayanan (1978)
Activity-dependent	Creazzo and Sohal (1979), Pittman and Oppenheim (1979), Oppenheim and Nunez (1982)
Trophic factor involvement	Nishi and Berg (1979), Hamburger *et al.* (1981)

functionally disrupts the relationship between neurons and the other neurons which they innervate. The existence of a critical period during which neurons are particularly vulnerable is also common to both, although the exact time at which this occurs may differ. Whether neuronal death in both cases is a probabilistic event and not one that is predetermined is a point of some conjecture. An interesting difference in response is shown in comparing the activity-dependence of these two observations. Treatment with botulinum toxin or curare at the neuromuscular junction results in an increase in motor neuron survival (Pittman and Oppenheim, 1978); it should be noted that electrical activity within the spinal cord is not eliminated by this procedure. In contrast, the spinal cord neurons in culture exhibit a decreased survival during electrical blockade. There are a number of potential explanations for this apparent discrepancy. It may be that the synaptic contacts at the neuromuscular junction and some CNS connections are fundamentally different and are under differing control mechanisms which become apparent after electrical blockade. A second possibility is that the culture system has been manipulated to express an event which is uncharacteristic of events which occur *in vivo*. For example, the supply of trophic factors might influence the survival response in cell culture either because of a reduction of such factors during medium replenishment or perhaps a decreased survival of support cells which produce trophic factors. Our working hypothesis is that some central synapses, perhaps like those involved in sensory information processing, behave like the cell culture system and hence require electrical traffic to stabilize connections and neuronal populations.

4.3. Critical Developmental Periods

The unique vulnerability of developing organisms to environmental changes has long been recognized on the basis of nutritional and toxicological evidence (Winick et al., 1972; Dobbing et al., 1971; Scott et al., 1974) Drugs and malnutritional states which produce no permanent effect on adults may be devastating to the fetus. This vulnerability can be described as a constellation of critical periods during which a particular organ or component of an organ system is most susceptible to perturbation. Periods of rapid growth and differentiation often have been correlated with these vulnerable periods. The identification of critical periods and the developmental events responsible for their occurrence is an important area in developmental neurobiology. We have used cell culture to investigate the existence of such critical periods in neuronal development.

The onset and duration of a developmental period during which neuronal survival is dependent on electrical activity were delineated. A variety of probes were used to investigate this problem, not only to define the critical period, but also to evaluate the relative temporal resolution and sensitivity of the various assays. The response of spinal cord neurons after electrical blockade with TTX was examined at various stages of development. The effect of chronic and 1-week exposures to TTX is shown in Fig. 7. With ^{125}I-labeled tetanus toxin fixation, a sensitive period was identified between days 7 and 21 in culture. ^{125}I-labeled scorpion toxin was also used to evaluate the spinal cord cultures after TTX treatment (Fig. 8). A direct comparison with ^{125}I-labeled tetanus toxin fixation revealed that the scorpion toxin indicated a neuronal change with TTX exposure during the first week in culture while the tetanus toxin assay did not. This difference was attributed to the delay in response intrinsic to the tetanus toxin assay (Brenneman et al., 1983). This delay (24 hr) was too long to capture the TTX-mediated decreases during the first week in culture. The delay was not a significant factor during the second week in culture because the entire week was within the critical period. The insensitivity of total culture protein to neuron-specific changes is also evident in Fig. 7.

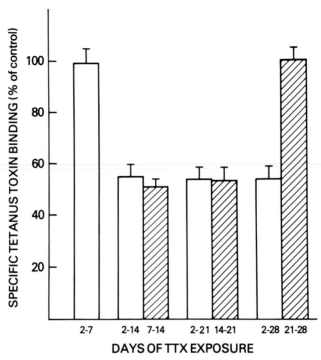

Figure 7. Specific ^{125}I-labeled tetanus toxin fixation in spinal cord cultures after TTX application at weekly intervals (striped bars) and after chronic exposure (open bars). Each value is the mean of 12 determinations from 3 dissections. The error bar represents S.E.M. (From Brenneman *et al.*, 1983.)

Of primary interest to us was the delineation of the onset of the critical period and its correlation with other developmental events. CAT activity was used based on the reasoning that events leading to compromised neurons may initially decrease function before progressing to cell death. CAT is a specific marker of cholinergic neurons and an important enzyme in neurotransmitter synthesis. TTX was added 24 hr prior to testing for changes in activity. This was done daily until a significant change in activity was found. A sharp developmental onset was observed on day 7 in culture (Fig. 9). This abrupt and selective change in CAT activity is evidence that a specific process, not just nonspecific cell death, is activity-related. Several interesting events coincide with the beginning of the critical period. First, a significant increase in the organizational pattern of neuronal aggregates and the size of neuronal

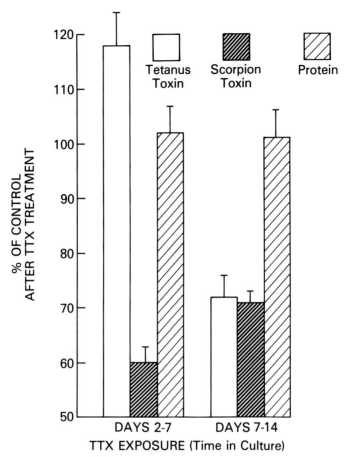

Figure 8. Comparisons of ^{125}I-labeled tetanus toxin fixation, ^{125}I-labeled scorpion toxin binding, and culture protein after TTX treatment during the first and second week in culture. The tetanus toxin fixation was conducted as described in Fig. 3. Binding was measured with 10 nM ^{125}I-labeled scorpion toxin after 1-hr incubations at 37°C. Specific binding was defined as the difference in total binding minus binding in the presence of a 100-fold excess of unlabeled scorpion toxin. Each value is the mean of 8–12 determinations ± S.E.M.

processes occurs between days 6 and 8 in culture (Fig. 1). In addition, day 7 marks the start of a major developmental increase in CAT activity. Both of these observations indicate a period of rapid neuronal growth and change on day 7. It is also of interest that day 7 in culture corresponds to day 20 of gestation, just before birth is to occur.

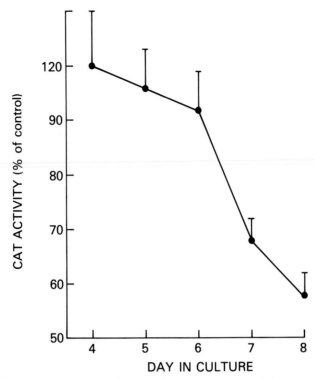

Figure 9. Developmental onset of TTX-mediated decreases in choline acetyltransferase activity in spinal cord cultures. TTX was applied 24 hr prior to measurement of enzyme activity. Each value is the mean ± S.E.M. of four to six determinations. (Redrawn from Brenneman *et al.*, 1983.)

4.4. Trophic Factors

The influence of target tissue on neuronal maturation and function has been recognized. The existence of releasable substances from target tissue which could mediate these effects has been hypothesized widely. With the discovery of nerve growth factor (NGF) (Levi-Montalcini and Hamburger, 1951), the search for other neuronotrophic factors has greatly increased and now represents a major area of research. Several reviews of progress in this area are available (Varon and Adler, 1981; Berg, 1982). Of particular relevance to the present discussion is the occurrence of survival factors. Examples of survival factors which have been reported include those for ciliary ganglia (Nishi and Berg, 1979; Bonyhady *et al.*, 1980), retinal ganglia (Nurcombe and Bennett, 1981),

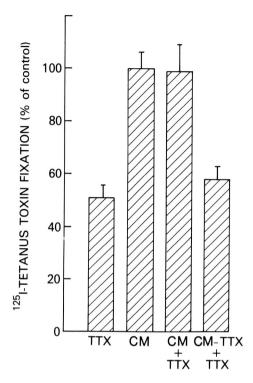

Figure 10. Effect of conditioned medium (CM) on TTX-mediated decreases in ^{125}I-labeled tetanus toxin fixation. The following conditions were studied. TTX group: spinal cord cultures were exposed to 1 μm TTX from days 10 to 14 in culture; CM group: CM obtained from day 0–5 cultures was added to cultures from days 10 to 14; CM + TTX group: CM obtained from day 0–5 was applied during days 10–14 to other cultures along with 1 μm TTX; CM–TTX + TTX group: CM was obtained from day 0–5 cultures to which 10^{-7} M TTX had been added during the collection period. The CM obtained during electrical blockade was added to cultures between days 10 and 14. TTX (9×10^{-7} M) was added to the CM–TTX conditioned medium during the testing period. The CM in all cases comprised 50% of the culture medium. Each value is the mean of six to eight determinations from two experiments.

sympathetic ganglia (Edgar *et al.*, 1981; Belford and Rush, 1983), and DRG (Barde *et al.*, 1980).

The influence of trophic substances in the activity-dependent survival of spinal cord neurons in culture has also been suspected (Brenneman *et al.*, 1984). The hypothesis is that electrical activity is obligatory at certain stages in development because the release of trophic factors is associated with impulse traffic. When electrical activity is blocked, the concentration of these vital factors is reduced and some neuronal populations do not survive. Evidence for trophic activity which affects neuronal survival during electrical blockade is presented in Fig. 10. The source of the trophic substances is conditioned medium (CM), i.e., normal nutrient medium which has bathed the cultured cells for an extended period. CM was collected from untreated cultures during the first 5 days in culture, before the beginning of the critical period. When TTX was added to this CM and applied to older cultures (during their sensitive period), the neuronal decrements associated with TTX treatment were not observed. This is an excellent example of a culture manipulation that permits an analysis of a process that is difficult to define *in vivo*. Since the critical period, as measured by tetanus fixation, appears to have limited duration, one might speculate that the particular trophic substance which affects neuronal survival in spinal cord may be developmentally produced and released. That is, the survival factor would be in limited supply during a period in which synapse stabilization and neuronal death are occurring. To test this hypothesis, CM was collected during 3- to 5-day intervals within the course of development. This CM was applied to cultures treated with TTX during the critical period. It was found that media obtained between days 7 and 21 in culture had no "protective" properties for the TTX-mediated decreases in neuronal survival. This evidence supports the existence of a survival factor(s) which is released within developmental constraints.

The role of electrical activity in the release of trophic materials is not known. To our knowledge, no one has demonstrated the release of trophic substances during electrical stimulation. Evidence which is compatible with a relationship between electrical activity and release of trophic factors is shown in Fig. 10. Since essentially all cultured spinal cord neurons are electrically active, the blockade of this activity may decrease the release and availability of survival factors. To test this idea, the electrical activity of cultures was blocked during the CM collection period. CM did not have survival trophic activity as measured with ^{125}I-labeled tetanus toxin fixation (Fig. 10). The lack of response could not be attributed to neuronal cell death during the collection period because this collection time preceded the critical period of susceptibility.

5. SUMMARY

It is clear from the data that cholinergic development in these cultures is dependent to a substantial degree on the presence in the culture medium of constituents ("cholinotropins") produced by cells in the cultures. Both the supply and the requirement for this material appear to be dependent on the developmental stage and the state of electrical activity of the cultures; some activity-independent production of a cholinotropin also exists and the amount produced depends on the density of the cultures. Cholinotropin appears to be produced at a rate that is influenced strongly by electrical activity. From days 7 to 21, production of cholinotropin is relatively low whereas the requirement is high. We have found that CM from active cultures of this age does not reverse TTX effects on sensitive cultures. The result is that this day 7–21 period is a "sensitive period" during which cholinergic development is partic-

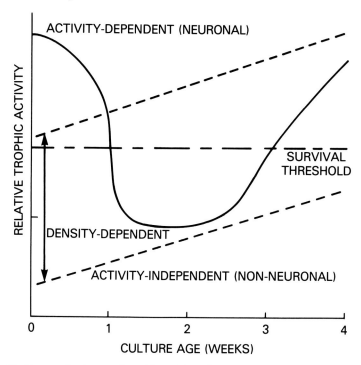

Figure 11. Proposed scheme of trophic activity effects in spinal cord cultures during development. See text for explanation.

ularly responsive to environmental influences such as electrical activity. As the cultures mature, cholinotropin production increases and the requirement probably also changes.

Model Scheme

The observations concerning the neuronal survival and electrical activity in spinal cord cultures have been incorporated into the model shown in Fig. 11. The purpose of this model is to account for all cell culture data and represent a hypothesis for future experimentation. Essential features of this model include the following:

1. There is a critical period in development during which electrical blockade can decrease neuronal survival.
2. The critical period represents a time during which there is a limited supply of activity-dependent trophic factor.

3. The trophic factor which affects neuronal survival during electrical blockade is released within developmental time constraints.
4. There are also activity-independent survival factors which are released from background cells. The availability of these substances is markedly dependent on the number of background cells. At high plating densities, the activity-independent factors dominate and mask activity-dependent processes.

We feel that the use of neural cell cultures allows an experimental approach to defining and analyzing some of the important processes involved in nervous system development. Ambiguities related to possible discrepancies between the culture and the intact CNS must be kept in mind. Our working assumption is, however, that regulatory phenomena shown to be important *in vitro* will have a significant role also in the developing CNS.

ACKNOWLEDGMENTS

We wish to thank Linda Bowers for assistance with the photography and Sandra Fitzgerald for expert technical assistance in culture maintenance.

REFERENCES

Archer, S. M., Dubin, M. W., and Stark, L. A., 1982, Abnormal development of kitten retino-geniculate connectivity in the absence of action potentials, *Science* **217**:743–745.

Banker, G. A., 1980, Trophic interactions between astroglial cells and hippocampal neurons in culture, *Science* **146**:610–619.

Barde, Y.-A., Edgar, D., and Thoenen, H., 1980, Sensory neurons in culture: Changing requirements for survival factors during embryonic development, *Proc. Natl. Acad. Sci. USA* **77**:1199–1203.

Belford, D. A., and Rush, R. A., 1983, A survival factor for sympathetic neurons from avian smooth muscle, *Develop. Brain Res.* **6**:304–377.

Benoit, P., and Changeux, J.-P., 1975, Consequences of tenotomy on the evolution of multiinnervation in developing rat soleus muscle, *Brain Res.* **99**:354–358.

Benoit, P., and Changeux, J.-P., 1978, Consequences of blocking the nerve with a local anaesthetic on the evolution of multi-inervation at the regenerating neuromuscular junction of the rat, *Brain Res.* **149**:89–96.

Berg, D. K., 1982, Cell death in neuronal development: Regulation by trophic factor, in: *Neuronal Development* (N. C. Spitzer, ed.), Plenum Press, New York, pp. 297–331.

Bergey, G. K., Fitzgerald, S. C., Schrier, B. K., and Nelson, P. G., 1981, Neuronal maturation in mammalian cell cultures is dependent on spontaneous electrical activity, *Brain Res.* **207**:49–58.

Berwald-Netter, Y., Martin-Moutot, N., Koulakoff, A., and Couraud, F., 1981, Na^+-channel-associated scorpion toxin receptor sites as probes for neuronal evolution *in vivo* and *in vitro*, *Proc. Natl. Acad. Sci. USA* **78**:1245–1249.

Bolton, A. E., and Hunter, W. M., 1973, The labelling of proteins to high specific radioactivities by conjugation to a ^{125}I-containing acylating agent, *Biochem. J.* **133**:529–539.

Bonyhady, R. E., Hendry, I. A., Hill, C. E., and McLennan, I., 1980, Characterization of a cardiac muscle factor required for the survival of cultured parasympathetic neurons, *Neurosci. Lett.* **18**:197–201.

Bowery, N. G., Jones, G. P., and Neal, M. J., 1976, Selective inhibition of neuronal uptake by cis-1,3-aminocyclohexane carboxylic acid, *Nature* **264**:281–284.

Brenneman, D. E., Neale, E. A., Habig, W. H., Bowers, L. M., and Nelson, P. G., 1983, Developmental and neurochemical specificity of neuronal deficits produced by electrical impulse blockade in dissociated spinal cord cultures, *Develop. Brain Res.* **9**:13–27.

Brenneman, D. E., Fitzgerald, S., and Nelson, P. G., 1984, Interaction between trophic action and electrical activity in spinal cord cultures, *Develop. Brain Res.* **15**:211–217.

Brown, M. C., and Ironton, R., 1977, Motor neurone sprouting induced by prolonged tetrodotoxin block of nerve action potentials, *Nature* **265**:459–461.

Burt, A. M., 1975, Choline acetyltransferase and acetylcholinesterase in the developing rat spinal cord, *Exp. Neurol.* **47**:173–180.

Catterall, W. A., 1977a, Membrane potential-dependent binding of scorpion toxin to the action potential sodium ionophore: Studies with a toxin derivative prepared by lactoperoxidase-catalyzed iodination. *J. Biol. Chem.* **252**:8660–8668.

Catterall, W. A., 1977b, Activation of the action potential Na^+ ionophore by neurotoxins: An allosteric model, *J. Biol. Chem.* **252**:8669–8676.

Cavallito, C. J., Yun, H. S., Kaplan, T., Smith, J. C., and Foldes, F. F., 1970, Choline acetyltransferase inhibitors: Dimensional and substituent effects among styrylpyridine analogs, *J. Med. Chem.* **13**:221–224.

Chu-Wang, I.-W., and Oppenheim, R. W., 1978, Cell death of motoneurons in the chick embryo spinal cord. I. A light and electron microscopic study of naturally occurring and induced cell loss during development, *J. Comp. Neurol.* **177**:33–58.

Cowan, W. M., and Wenger, E., 1967, Cell loss in the trochlear nucleus of the chick during normal development and after radical extirpation of the optic vesicle, *J. Exp. Zool.* **164**:267–280.

Coyle, J. T., and Yamamura, H. I., 1976, Neurochemical aspects of the ontogenesis of cholinergic neurons in the rat brain. *Brain Res.* **118**:429–440.

Crain, S. M., Bornstein, M. B., and Peterson, E. R., 1968, Maturation of cultured embryonic CNS tissue during chronic exposure to agents which prevent bioelectric activity, *Brain Res.* **8**:363–372.

Creazzo, T. L., and Sohal, G. S., 1979, Effects of chronic injections of α-bungarotoxin on embryonic cell death, *Exp. Neurol.* **66**:135–145.

Dimpfel, W., Neale, J. H., and Habermann, E., 1975, ^{125}I-labelled tetanus toxin as a neuronal marker in tissue cultures derived from embryonic CNS, *Naunyn-Schmiedeberg's Arch. Pharmacol.* **290**:329–333.

Dimpfel, W., Huang, R. T. C., and Habermann, E., 1977, Gangliosides in nervous tissue cultures and binding of ^{125}I-labelled tetanus toxin, a neuronal marker, *J. Neurochem.* **29**:329–334.

Dobbing, J., Hopewell, J. W., and Lynch, A., 1971, Vulnerability of developing brain. VII. Permanent deficit of neurons in cerebral and cerebellar cortex following early mild undernutrition, *Exp. Neurol.* **32**:439–447.

Edgar, D., Barde, Y.-A., and Thoenen, H., 1981, Subpopulations of cultured chick sympathetic neurons differ in their requirements for survival factors, *Nature* **289**:294–295.

Farb, D. H., Berg, D. K., and Fischbach, G. D., 1979, Uptake and release of [³H] γ-aminobutyric acid by embryonic spinal cord neurons in dissociated cell culture, *J. Cell Biol.* **80:**651–661.

Fishman, M. C., and Nelson, P. G., 1981, Depolarization-induced synaptic plasticity at cholinergic synapses in tissue culture, *J. Neurosci.* **1:**1043:1051.

Hamburger, V., 1975, Cell death in the development of the lateral motor column of the chick embryo, *J. Comp. Neurol.* **160:**535–546.

Hamburger, V., and Levi-Montalcini, R., 1949, Proliferation, differentiation and degeneration in the spinal ganglia of the chick embryo under normal and experimental conditions. *J. Exp. Zool.* **111:**457–501.

Hamburger, V., Brunso-Bechtold, J. K., and Yip, J. W., 1981, Neuronal death in the spinal ganglia of the chick embryo and its reduction by nerve growth factor, *J. Neurosci.* **1:**60–71.

Harris, A. E., 1969, Differentiation and degeneration in the motor horn of foetal mouse, *J. Morphol.* **129:**281–305.

Harris, W. A., 1981, Neural activity and development, *Annu. Rev. Physiol.* **43:**689–710.

Hebb, C. O., 1956, Choline acetylase in the developing nervous system of the rabbit and guinea pig, *J. Physiol.* **133:**566–570.

Hollyday, M., and Hamburger, V., 1976, Reduction of the naturally occurring motor neuron loss by enlargement of the periphery, *J. Comp. Neurol.* **170:**311–320.

Ishida, I., and Deguchi, T., 1983, Regulation of choline acetyltransferase in primary cell cultures of spinal cord by neurotransmitter 1-norepinephrine, *Develop. Brain Res.* **7:**13–23.

Iverson, L. L., and Kelly, J. S., 1975, Uptake and metabolism of γ-aminobutyric acid by neurons and glial cells, *Biochem. Pharmacol.* **124:**933–938.

Jackson, M. B., Lecar, H., Brenneman, D. E., Fitzgerald, S., and Nelson, P. G., 1982, Electrical development in spinal cord cell culture, *J. Neurosci.* **2:**1052–1061.

Janka, Z., and Jones, D. G., 1982, Junctions in rat neocortical explants cultured in TTX-, GABA-, and Mg^{++} environments, *Brain Res. Bull.* **8:**273–278.

Kasa, P., Bansaghy, K., Rakonczay, Z., and Gulya, K., 1982, Postnatal development of the acetylcholine system in different parts of the rat cerebellum, *J. Neurochem.* **39:**1726–1732.

Lance-Jones, C., 1982, Motoneuron cell death in the developing lumbar spinal cord of the mouse, *Develop. Brain Res.* **4:**473–479.

Landmesser, L., and Pilar, G., 1974, Synaptic transmission and cell death during normal ganglionic development, *J. Physiol.* **241:**737–749.

Ledley, G. D., Lee, G., Kohn, L. D., Habig, W. H., and Hardegree, M. C., 1977, Tetanus toxin interaction with thyroid plasma membranes: Implications for structure and function of tetanus toxin receptors and potential pathophysiological significance, *J. Biol. Chem.* **252:**4049–4055.

Levi-Montalcini, R., and Hamburger, V., 1951, Selective growth-stimulating effects of mouse salivary glands on the sympathetic system of mammals, *J. Exp. Zool.* **116:**321–362.

Meisami, E., and Mousavi, R., 1981, Lasting effects of early olfactory deprivation on the growth, DNA, RNA, and protein content, and Na-K-ATPase and AChE activity of the rat olfactory bulb, *Develop. Brain Res.* **2:**217–229.

Meyer, T., Burkart, W., and Jockusch, H., 1979, Choline acetyltransferase induction in cultured neurons: Dissociated spinal cord cells are dependent on muscle cells, organotypic explants are not, *Neurosci. Lett.* **11:**59–62.

Mirsky, R., Wendon, L. M. B., Black, P., Stolkin, C., and Bray, D., 1978, Tetanus toxin: A cell surface marker for neurones in culture, *Brain Res.* **148:**251–259.

Model, P. G., Bornstein, M. B., Crain, S. M., and Pappas, G. D., 1971, An electron microscopic study of the development of synapses in cultured fetal mouse cerebrum continuously exposed to xylocaine, *J. Cell Biol.* **49:**362–371.

Narayanan, C. H., and Narayanan, Y., 1978, Neuronal adjustments in developing nuclear centers of the chick embryo following transplantation of an additional optic primordium, *J. Embryol. Exp. Morphol.* **44:**53–70.

Neale, E. A., Oertel, W. H., Bowers, L. M., and Weise, V. K., 1983, Glutamate decarboxylase immunoreactivity and γ-[³H]-aminobutyric acid accumulation within the same neurons in dissociated cell cultures of cerebral cortex, *J. Neurosci.* **3:**376–382.

Nishi, R., and Berg, D. K., 1979, Survival and development of ciliary ganglion neurons in cell culture, *Nature* **277:**232–234.

Nishi, R., and Berg, D. K., 1981, Effects of high K⁺ concentrations on the growth and development of ciliary ganglion neurons in cell culture, *Develop. Biol.* **87:**301–307.

Nurcombe, V., and Bennett, M. R., 1981, Embryonic chick retinal ganglion cells identified *in vitro*: Their survival is dependent on a factor from the optic tectum, *Exp. Brain Res.* **44:**249–258.

Nurcombe, V., McGrath, P. A., and Bennett, M. R., 1981, Postnatal death of motor neurons during the development of the brachial spinal cord of the rat, *Neurosci. Lett.* **27:**249–254.

O'Brien, R. A. D., Östberg, A. J. C., and Vrbová, G., 1978, Observations on the elimination of polyneuronal innervation in developing mammalian skeletal muscle, *J. Physiol.* **282:**571–582.

Olek, A. J., and Edwards, C., 1980, Effects of anesthetic treatment on motor neuron death in *Xenopus*, *Brain Res.*. **191:**483–488.

Oppenheim, R. W., and Majors-Willard, C., 1978, Neuronal cell death in the brachial spinal cord of the chick is unrelated to the loss of polyneuronal innervation in wing muscle, *Brain Res.* **154:**148–152.

Oppenheim, R. W., and Nunez, R., 1982, Electrical stimulation of hindlimb increases neuronal cell death in chick embryo, *Nature* **295:**57–59.

Parks, T. N., 1979, Afferent influences on the development of the brain stem auditory nuclei of the chicken: Otocyst ablation, *J. Comp. Neurol.* **183:**665–678.

Peacock, J. H., Nelson, P. G., and Goldstone, M. W., 1973, Electrophysiologic study of cultured neurons dissociated from spinal cords and dorsal root ganglia of fetal mice, *Develop. Biol.* **30:**137–152.

Pittman, R., and Oppenheim, R. W., 1978, Neuromuscular blockade increases motoneurone survival during normal cell death in the chick embryo, *Nature* **271:**364–366.

Pittman, R., and Oppenheim, R. W., 1979, Cell death of motoneurons in the chick embryo spinal cord. IV. Evidence that a functional neuromuscular interaction is involved in the regulation of naturally occurring cell death and the stabilization of synapses, *J. Comp. Neurol.* **187:**425–446.

Prestige, M. C., 1967, The control of cell number in the lumbar ventral horn during the development of *Xenopus laevis* tadpoles, *J. Embryol. Exp. Morphol.* **18:**359–387.

Puymirat, J., Faivre-Bauman, A., Bizzini, B., and Tixier-Vidal, A., 1982, Prenatal and postnatal ontogenesis of neurotransmitter-synthetizing enzymes and [¹²⁵I] tetanus toxin binding capacity in the mouse hypothalamus, *Develop. Brain Res.* **3:**199–206.

Ransom, B. R., Neale, E., Henkart, M., Bullock, P. N., and Nelson, P. G., 1977, Mouse spinal cord in cell culture. I. Morphology and intrinsic neuronal electrophysiologic properties, *J. Neurophysiol.* **40:**1132–1150.

Romijn, H. J., Mud, M. T., Habets, A. M. M. C., and Wolters, P. S., 1981, A quantitative electron microscopic study on synapse formation in dissociated fetal rat cerebral cortex *in vitro*, *Develop. Brain Res.* **1:**591–605.

Rothblat, L. A., and Schwartz, M. L., 1979, The effect of monocular deprivation on dendritic spines in visual cortex of young and adult rats: Evidence for a sensitive period, *Brain Res.* **161**:156–161.

Schon, F., and Kelly, J. S., 1975, Selective uptake of (^{3}H)β-alanine by glia: Association with the glial uptake system for GABA, *Brain Res.* **86**:243–257.

Scott, J. P., Stewart, J. M., and DeGhett, V. J., 1974, Critical periods in the organization of systems, *Develop. Psychobiol.* **7**:489–513.

Sher, P. K., 1983, Development and differentiation of the benzodiazepine receptor in cultures of fetal mouse spinal cord, *Develop. Brain Res.* **7**:343–348.

Sher, P. K., and Schrier, B. K., 1982, Benzodiazepine receptor development in cultures of fetal mouse cerebral cortex mimics its development *in vivo*, *Develop. Neurosci.* **5**:263–270.

Tarrade, T., and Crain, S. M., 1978, Regional localization of patterned spontaneous discharges during maturation in culture of fetal mouse medulla and spinal cord explants, *Dev. Neurosci.* **1**:119–132.

Varon, S., and Adler, R., 1981, Trophic and specifying factors directed to neuronal cells, in: *Advances in Cellular Neurobiology*, Volume 2 (S. Fedoroff and L. Hertz, eds.), Academic Press, New York, pp. 115–163.

Varon, S., Skaper, S. D., and Manthorpe, M., 1981, Trophic activities for dorsal root and sympathetic ganglionic neurons in media conditioned by Schwann and other peripheral cells, *Develop. Brain Res.* **1**:73–87.

Vernadakis, A., 1973, Comparative studies of neurotransmitter substances in the maturing and aging central nervous system of the chicken, *Prog. Brain Res.* **40**:231–243.

Vernadakis, A., and Arnold, E. B., 1980, Age-related changes in neuronal and glial enzyme activities, in: *Advances in Cellular Neurobiology*, Volume 1 (S. Fedoroff and L. Hertz, eds.), Academic Press, New York, pp. 229–283.

Walicke, P. A., Campenot, R. B., and Patterson, P. H., 1977, Determination of transmitter function by neuronal activity, *Proc. Natl. Acad. Sci. USA* **74**:5767–5771.

Werner, I., Peterson, G. R., and Shuster, L., 1971, Choline acetyltransferase and acetylcholinesterase in cultured brain cells from chick embryos, *J. Neurochem.* **18**:141–151.

Wiesel, T. N., and Hubel, D. H., 1963, Effects of visual deprivation on morphology and physiology of cells in the cat's lateral geniculate body, *J. Neurophysiol.* **26**:978–993.

Winick, M., Rosso, P., and Brasel, J. A., 1972, Malnutrition and cellular growth in the brain: Existence of critical periods, in: *Lipids, Malnutrition, and the Developing Brain*, Associated Scientific Publishers, Amsterdam, pp. 199–206.

Woolsey, T. A., and Wann, J. R., 1976, Areal changes in mouse cortical barrels following vibrissal damage at different postnatal ages, *J. Comp. Neurol.* **170**:53–66.

11

Electrophysiological Studies of Cultured Mammalian CNS Neurons

THOMAS G. SMITH, JR., and JEFFERY L. BARKER

1. INTRODUCTION

Neurophysiology is an important area of neuroscience that is concerned in large part with two of the most important functions of neurons and neuronal networks, namely the membrane excitability of the individual elements and the process of intercellular communication of "information" into and throughout the CNS. Neurophysiology is often divided into two broad areas of investigation. One involves quantitative analysis of the basic membrane mechanisms underlying the generation of electrical and chemical signals. The other involves studies into how neuronal messages are communicated in the CNS. The complexity inherent in the vertebrate CNS has made it difficult to study the details underlying the excitable membrane properties and the various modes of intercellular signaling. The complexity of the vertebrate CNS has been reduced to monolayer simplicity through the innovative efforts of many investigators, including and especially Dr. Phillip Nelson and colleagues at the

THOMAS G. SMITH, JR., and JEFFERY L. BARKER • Laboratory of Neurophysiology, National Institute of Neurological and Communicative Disorders and Stroke, National Institutes of Health, Bethesda, Maryland 20205.

National Institutes of Health, who have developed methods for culturing neurons from the embryonic CNS.

The monolayer character of the culture allows ready accessibility to a variety of electrophysiological assay techniques. Such techniques are difficult-to-impossible to apply in an intact vertebrate CNS. The purpose of this chapter is to demonstrate the utility of cultured CNS neurons for studying excitable membrane mechansims and intercellular signals but not to dwell on the results of the actual investigations undertaken. Those results, as well as most of the methodological details, can be found in the referenced papers.

2. METHODS OVERVIEW

2.1. Mechanical Requirements

Because of the relatively small size of the cell bodies of cultured CNS neurons (10–40 μm), where intracellular recordings are generally made, it is absolutely essential to have a recording table that is effectively isolated from the environmental vibrations that would otherwise perturb the stability of the recording. This almost always requires the use of an air-suspension table (Fig. 1). In addition, precisely controllable and drift-free micromanipulators are necessary. Finally, to realize the need for clear visibility at relatively high magnification (250–400×), a microscope employing phase-contrast, Hoffman modulation, or Nomarski optics is required. The microscope should preferably have a fixed stage and focusable optics so that the position of the microelectrodes with respect to the stage is constant. Figure 1 illustrates a phase-contrast optical system used in many laboratories.

The stage of the microscope has to be modified to hold the culture dish containing the cells under investigation, the bath electrodes, and other components. Figure 2 shows the stage employed in our laboratory. This stage also allows for rapid changes in the extracellular medium. It is a three-compartment system, with the culture dish as the central compartment. The input and output wells are connected to the central compartment via fluid-containing, glass U-tubes (not shown). Flow rates are adjusted to ensure a constant-level bath. Also shown in Fig. 2 are two recording electrodes on the right; the two electrodes on the left are connected to a pressure-ejection system for the controlled delivery of neuroactive chemicals and drugs (Smith and Cunningham, 1983). A Faraday cage is necessary to reduce ambient electrical noise. We have found it advantageous to construct the cage around, rather than on the table, so

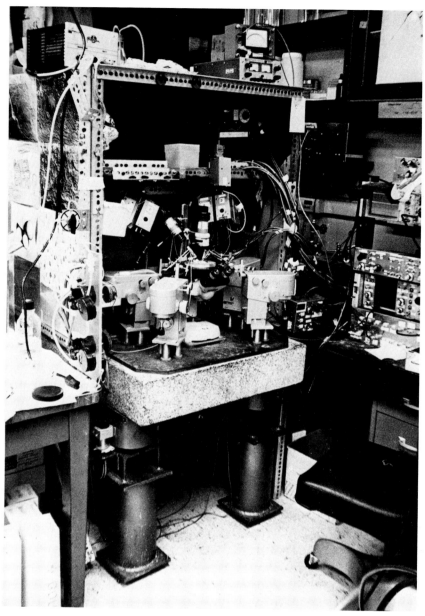

Figure 1. Equipment for electrophysiological studies of mammalian CNS neurons with intracellular recordings. Note that micromanipulators, microscope, and other components are joined to a metal plate on the top of a granite block, with magnets to increase mechanical stability. The Faraday cage is mounted on the floor around an air-suspension table. All components not on the table (electronics, pressure control, iontophoresis unit, and others) are mounted onto the cage and the only connection to the table is with microelectrodes.

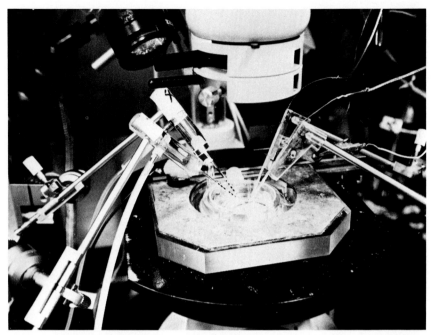

Figure 2. A close-up view of the chamber to hold a culture dish. The chamber is mounted on an inverted phase-contrast microscope. The two microelectrodes on the right are for intracellular recordings; the two on the left are for pressure-ejection of neuroactive compounds onto the extracellular surface of the neuron under study.

that accidental perturbations of the cage do not disturb the recordings (Fig. 1). All input amplifiers and the final stages of stimulus electronics are mounted on the cage so that the only direct physical contacts between the tabletop and the environment are the connections to the electrodes and the air balloons of the table.

With these arrangements hours-long recordings with one or two intracellular microelectrodes are practically routine, thus allowing extensive investigation of the excitability of individual neurons. Such long-term recordings are next-to-impossible even with a single intracellular microelectrode in an intact vertebrate CNS.

2.2. Electronic Requirements

For simple membrane potential measurements with microelectrodes, conventional electronics with high-impedance, head-stage amplifiers and a Wheatstone bridge are sufficient for accurate recording of potentials during the passage of intracellular current through a single microelectrode. Voltage control, or "clamping" with two microelectrodes, requires the use of special electronics owing to the frequency response characteristics of the CNS cells, the high-resistance microelectrodes, and the feedback circuits involved in voltage clamping (for details consult Smith *et al.*, 1980, 1981).

While there is nothing unique about the microelectrodes used to study vertebrate CNS neurons grown in culture, fine, precisely shaped tips are a prerequisite to developing adequate signal-to-noise ratio. A variety of microelectrode pullers are now available (Brown-Flaming, Campden Instruments, and others) whose heat and pull parameters can be controlled well enough to fashion the necessary fine-tipped microelectrodes.

In the remainder of this chapter we will illustrate several kinds of electrophysiological experiments that can be conducted using monolayer cultures of CNS neurons. Complete details regarding the electrophysiological data to be reviewed can be obtained by consulting the original references.

3. MEMBRANE EXCITABILITY

Conventional intracellular recordings from phase-bright CNS-neurons maintained in dissociated cell culture reveal that cells which stain for the presence of the neuron-specific enzyme, neuron-specific enolase, are invariably electrically and chemically excitable (Schmechel *et al.*, 1980). If a physiological saline is used as the recording medium, most neurons cultured from the spinal cord display spontaneous synaptic and electrical activity (Fig. 3). Close application of Mg^{2+} ions, which depress neurotransmitter release at many synaptic sites, attenuates the spontaneous synaptic activity characteristically present in cultured monolayers (Fig. 3A). In this way neurotransmitter-evoked responses can be isolated for detailed study. In a similar manner, delivery of tetrodotoxin, which blocks voltage-gated Na^+ conductances in a wide variety of membranes, eliminates most, if not all, of the ambient synaptic and electrical activity, leaving chemically excitable membrane properties in relative isolation (Figs. 3B, C). Isolation of individual cells from others in the same culture with elevated Mg^{2+} and/or TTX thus allows detailed study of chemical and electrical forms of membrane excitability.

3.1. Chemical Excitability

Nelson and colleagues have used cultures quite effectively to investigate synaptic transmissions at the presynaptic level (Fig. 4) (Ransom

Thomas G. Smith, Jr., and Jeffery L. Barker

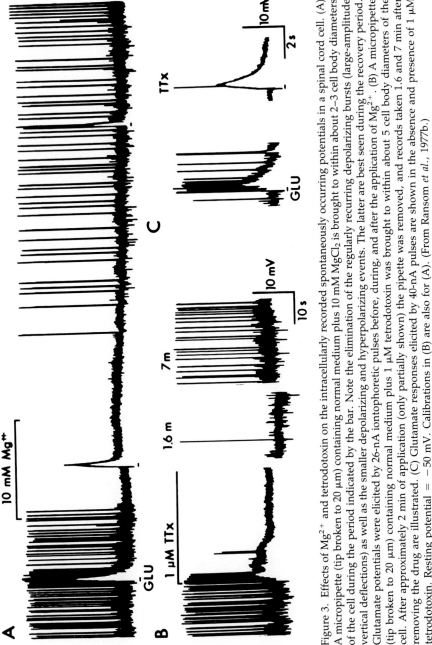

Figure 3. Effects of Mg^{2+} and tetrodotoxin on the intracellularly recorded spontaneously occurring potentials in a spinal cord cell. (A) A micropipette (tip broken to 20 μm) containing normal medium plus 10 mM $MgCl_2$ is brought to within about 2–3 cell body diameters of the cell during the period indicated by the bar. Note the elimination of the regularly recurring depolarizing bursts (large-amplitude vertical deflections) as well as the smaller depolarizing and hyperpolarizing events. The latter are best seen during the recovery period. Glutamate potentials were elicited by 26-nA iontophoretic pulses before, during, and after the application of Mg^{2+}. (B) A micropipette (tip broken to 20 μm) containing normal medium plus 1 μM tetrodotoxin was brought to within about 5 cell body diameters of the cell. After approximately 2 min of application (only partially shown) the pipette was removed, and records taken 1.6 and 7 min after removing the drug are illustrated. (C) Glutamate responses elicited by 40-nA pulses are shown in the absence and presence of 1 μM tetrodotoxin. Resting potential = −50 mV. Calibrations in (B) are also for (A). (From Ransom et al., 1977b.)

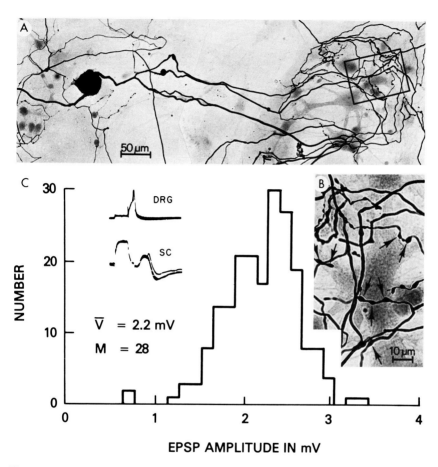

Figure 4. Morphological and physiological features of a dorsal root ganglion cell (DRG) to spinal cord cell (SC) excitatory synapse. (A) Photomicrograph of a horseradish perox-idase-labeled DRG neuron which, when stimulated, produced synaptic responses in a nearby SC neuron. ×240. (B) High-power photomicrography showing individual boutons (some indicated by arrows) on an SC neuron. The total number of boutons contacting the SC neuron was about 36. ×800. (C) The peak of the early monosynaptic excitatory component of the synaptic response in the SC cell was detected; this peak amplitude for a series of evoked excitatory postsynaptic potentials (EPSPs) is plotted in the amplitude histogram. Three data runs were performed with this connection with a resultant average quantal content (*m*) value of 35. Inset to the lower figure shows simultaneous recordings from DRG and SC neurons. The calibration pulse early on the traces represents 5 mV and 2 msec. (From Neale *et al.*, 1983.)

et al., 1977a,b,c); Nelson *et al.*, 1983; Neale *et al.*, 1983). They have combined classical statistical techniques applied at many peripheral synapses with contemporary morphological methods to analyze the physiology and anatomy of synaptic transmissions between various pairs of sensory and spinal cord neurons. Their results indicate that, as at peripheral synapses, the amplitude of the postsynaptic potential reflects release of quantized amounts of neurotransmitter. Furthermore, the number of quanta corresponds closely to the number of investing presynaptic terminals, as if fluctuations in the amplitude of the postsynaptic signal result from fluctuations in the number of active transmitting terminals, each of which releases a quantum of neurotransmitter substance. The success of this strategy suggests that the advent of identified pairs of CNS neurons in culture should permit relatively precise study of specific synaptic signals.

Postsynaptic pharmacology and physiology of the inhibitory and excitatory actions of putative neurotransmitters have received extensive study, the aim being to identify the underlying molecular mechanisms and to correlate these with the naturally occurring synaptic signals. Virtually all cells cultured from the embryonic vertebrate spinal cord respond to pharmacologic applications of GABA (Barker and Ransom, 1978). As shown in Fig. 5, the applications can be made sufficiently discrete that a nonuniform distribution of GABA-evoked responses can be demonstrated. The ionic mechanism underlying the hyperpolarizing response to GABA commonly seen at the level of the cell body has been identified by a series of ion substitution experiments, which can usually be carried out without much difficulty. The GABA-evoked response involves Cl^- ions (Barker and Ransom, 1978).

The elementary mechanisms underlying the Cl^- conductance response have been studied using a mathematical protocol first applied by Katz and Miledi (1972) to cholinergic responses elicited in muscle membranes. Katz and Miledi hypothesized that the cholinergic excitation resulted from the summed activities of many microscopic conductance steps, each about the same value but of variable duration. Thus, they analyzed the "noise" associated with cholinergic responses as if it really reflected a complex biological signal. Their estimates of the elementary electrical properties of cholinergically activated conductances have been confirmed and extended to many other agonist responses generated in other excitable membranes. Sustained applications of GABA to neurons under voltage clamp evoke current responses, which, like cholinergic responses, are invariably associated with excess "noise," or membrane current variance (Fig. 6). The increase in variance is directly proportional to the amplitude of the current response, as if

GABA

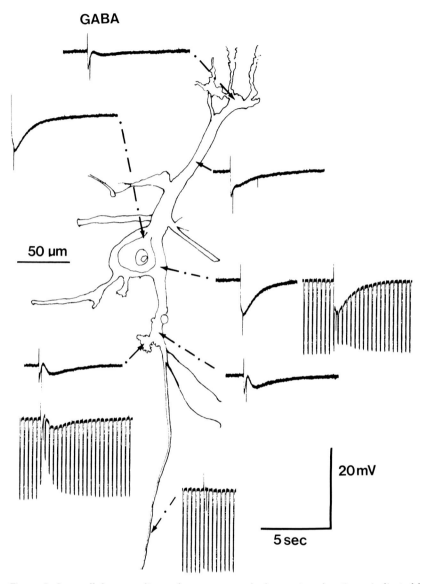

50 µm

20 mV

5 sec

Figure 5. Intracellular recordings of responses evoked at various locations, indicated by arrows, of extracellularly applied GABA in spinal cord neurons grown in culture. In some traces, constant-current pulses are applied which decrease in amplitude during the GABA-evoked responses, indicating that the response is due to an increase in membrane conductance.

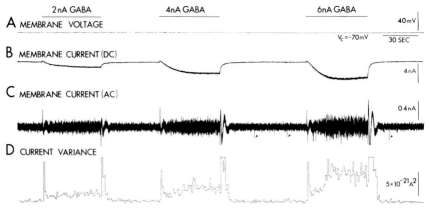

Figure 6. GABA-evoked noise in a spinal cord neuron. (A) Membrane potential or voltage; (B) low-gain, DC recording of membrane current; (C) high-gain AC recording of membrane current; (D) variance of membrane current. The record shows an increase in iontophoretically applied GABA during the bars above. An increase in membrane current noise or fluctuations (B and C: increases in baseline thickness) and in current variance (D: upward deflections) occurs. Also, noise and variance amplitude increase with increased GABA current. All calibrations are shown on the right.

the responses reflected the summed activities of increasing numbers of similarly sized unitary conductance steps. Spectral analysis of the fluctuations in membrane current induced by GABA shows that, as expected from the rather simple model originally outlined by Katz and Miledi, the spectrum can be reasonably well-fitted by a single Lorentzian equation (Fig. 7). Using fluctuation analysis it has been possible to estimate the electrical properties of the unitary conductance events activated by GABA and other neutral amino acid neurotransmitters (Barker *et al.*, 1982). The results show that, on average, each neurotransmitter activates a unique set of electrical properties. If these pharmacological observations have any physiological relevance, then the inhibitory, Cl^--dependent postsynaptic actions generated physiologically by different neutral amino acids may well be different.

More recently, "patch-clamp" recordings of the individual Cl^- ion channels activated by GABA have been used to confirm and extend the observations and estimates made using fluctuation analysis (see Chapter 12 for details regarding patch-clamp assays). The results show that, as predicted, the neutral amino acid transmitters GABA and glycine gate unitary Cl^- conductances in a manner consistent with predictions from quantitative analysis of fluctuations in the activities of thousands of individual ion channels (Jackson *et al.*, 1982; Hamill *et al.*, 1983). A second,

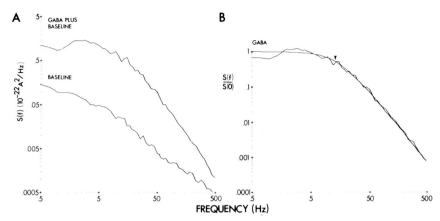

Figure 7. Spectral analysis of GABA-induced fluctuations in membrane current. (A) The normalized spectrum of fluctuations in membrane current obtained at the level of the resting membrane potential before delivery of GABA ("baseline") shows that power declines monotonically with increasing frequency. After application of GABA sufficient to sustain a current response of several nanoamperes, the power in the spectrum is greater at all frequencies sampled relative to that derived from analysis of baseline fluctuations ("GABA plus baseline"). (B) The spectrum calculated from the difference between the spectrum obtained before and during the GABA-induced response is closely fit by a Lorentzian equation. The corner-frequency, f_c (marked by an arrowhead), is 12.7 Hz, corresponding to an estimated channel lifetime of 12.5 msec. (From Barker et al., 1982.)

more rapid phase of conductance activity has also been detected at the microscopic level, but it accounts for less than 10% of the conductance response.

The pharmacological observations on neutral amino acid-evoked responses and quantitative analysis of their underlying molecular mechanism indicate that these putative neurotransmitters act in a manner quite similar to cholinergically operated cation conductances in muscle membranes. In fact, the kinetics of conductances pharmacologically activated in muscle membranes are sufficiently similar to the time course of the synaptically elaborated conductance responses that there is reason to consider using the pharmacological data to identify specific neurotransmitters at other synapses. Cultured hippocampal neurons, like spinal cord neurons, manifest both excitatory and inhibitory synaptic conductances (Segal, 1983). The inhibitory synaptic events are sufficiently frequent that, when pairs of cells in synaptic contact are studied, about half of the signals are hyperpolarizing and invert in polarity at the same potential as Cl^--dependent responses evoked by GABA (Fig. 8) (Segal and Barker, 1984). Quantitative analysis of the synaptically

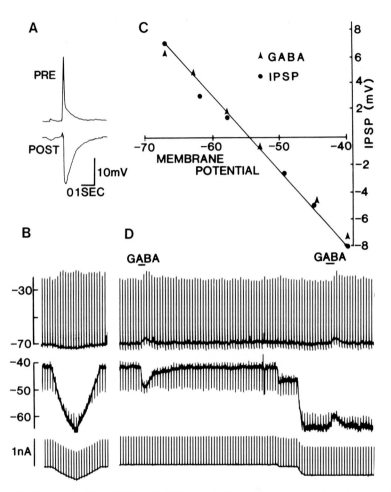

Figure 8. Hyperpolarizing IPSPs and GABA-evoked responses reverse in polarity at the same potential. The presynaptic cell was recorded with a KCl-filled microelectrode while the postsynaptic cell was recorded with a KAc-filled microelectrode. (A) Depolarizing current injected in the presynaptic neuron triggers an action potential, which is followed immediately by an IPSP in the postsynaptic element. (B) Polarization of the postsynaptic cell from −42 mV to −64 mV reverses the IPSPs and GABA-induced responses in polarity (D). (C) A plot of synaptic and pharmacologic response amplitudes as a function of potential shows that the reversal for both events is about −55 mV. (Modified from Segal and Barker, 1984.)

activated Cl^- conductance can be achieved by applying the two-electrode voltage-clamp technique to the postsynaptic element while stimulating the presynaptic cell. Since three simultaneous, high-fidelity penetrations of two cultured neurons are difficult, one can resort to chemical rather than electrical stimulation using brief pulses of the excitatory neurotransmitter glutamate applied to the cell body of the presynaptic neuron (schematically diagrammed in Fig. 9A2). The brief pulses transiently depolarize the presynaptic cell, triggering a series of action potentials, which propagate to the terminals to trigger neurotransmitter release. In this way synaptic signals can be studied at a relatively quantitative level in culture neurons.

Voltage-clamp analysis of postsynaptic Cl^--dependent currents recorded in cultured hippocampal neurons shows that the currents rise rapidly and then decay as a single exponential (Fig. 9) whose time constant, on average, is similar to that estimated for the average duration of the unitary conductance evoked by GABA. Furthermore, clinically important drugs that modulate pharmacologic responses to GABA alter the synaptic currents in a parallel fashion. Fluctuation analysis of the drug-mediated modulation of GABA-evoked responses suggests that all of the modulation can be accounted for by effects on the kinetics of unitary conductances (Study and Barker, 1982; Barker *et al.*, 1983). The synaptic currents are modulated by the same drugs in a manner consistent with these actions. This parallelism leads to the conclusion that the synaptic currents are likely to be mediated by GABA. If this is true, then by knowing the average value of the unitary conductance activated by GABA, one can estimate that between 1500 and 2000 elementary steps sum to generate the peak of the synaptically induced conductance. The exponential distribution in the durations of all the microscopic steps describes the exponential time course of synaptic current decay. These results indicate that monolayer cultures of CNS neurons are a useful preparation to study excitability of the postmembrane and that pharmacologically operated conductances may serve as useful reference for identifying physiologically activated signals at certain synapses.

3.2. Electrical Excitability

Electrical forms of membrane excitability have been studied in many different preparations since the pioneering investigations of Hodgkin and Huxley in the squid giant axon. By electrical excitability is meant the gating of ion conductance mechanisms by changes in the membrane potential of the cell. The action potential first analyzed by Hodgkin and Huxley at the squid giant axon some 35 years ago is comprised of the

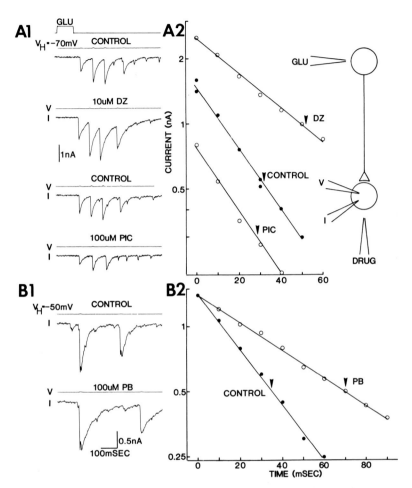

Figure 9. Clinically important drugs modulate IPSPs evoked in rat hippocampal neurons. The experimental arrangements are schematized to the right of panel A2. Current (I) and voltage (V) electrodes were placed in a postsynaptic element and 100 µM glutamate (GLU) was applied by pressure to the cell body of a presynaptic cell. Clinically important drugs were delivered by pressure in the vicinity of the postsynaptic neuron, which was held at −70 mV in (S) and at −50 mV in (B). Under control conditions glutamate applied presynaptically triggers a series of nanoampere-sized postsynaptic currents (PSCs), whose time constant of decay is about 30 msec (arrowhead). In (A) diazepam (DZ) enhances PSC amplitude to over 2 nA and prolongs PSC time constant to about 50 msec, while picrotoxin (PIC) decreases PSC amplitude without affecting PSC time constant. (B) Pentobarbital (PB) increases PSC time constant without changing PSC amplitude. (Modified from Segal and Barker, 1984.)

commonest known electrically gated conductances. Since their initial observations, many other forms of electrical excitability have been discovered in a variety of invertebrate and peripheral vertebrate membranes. Although these conductances have not been completely characterized, it is already clear that they can serve to shape the pattern of action potential activity. Most of these ionic conductances have also been identified in neurons cultures from spinal and supraspinal regions of the embryonic mammalian CNS.

Figure 10 shows one of these electrically gated conductances when it is activated under current-clamp recording conditions. With the cell held at a resting level of membrane potential and current steps of increasing intensity injected, it is evident that the resulting voltage responses are more complex when depolarizing currents are applied than when hyperpolarizing stimuli are delivered. By plotting the voltage responses as a function of injected current, one can readily see that for depolarizing currents the current–voltage (I–V) relationships developed for early (10 msec) and late times (40 msec) during the current injections are decidedly different. At 10 msec the depolarizing voltage responses are much less than would have been expected had the I–V relationship observed for hyperpolarizing stimuli been extrapolated to depolarized levels. This type of transient rectification is alleviated in a selective manner by application of 4-aminopyridine (Segal *et al.*, 1984). Although some rectification is evident at 40 msec, it is not altered by the drug. This later-developing rectification is in fact blocked by Ca^{2+} conductance antagonists.

Under voltage-clamp an outwardly directly current response can be triggered over the same range of membrane potential as rectification occurs under current-clamp (Fig. 11A). Furthermore, the current response is markedly attenuated by the same concentration of 4-aminopyridine that blocks the transient rectification (Fig. 11A). By applying classic voltage-clamp protocols, one involving conditioning the cell at different holding potentials, then stepping to the same depolarized level, the other involving holding the cell at a hyperpolarized level, then commanding to different depolarized levels, it is possible to describe the "inactivation" and "activation" characteristics of this transient outward current (Fig. 11B1). From this type of analysis it becomes clear that the activation of the conductance and the resulting current response require a relatively hyperpolarized cell, that the more depolarized the cell, the less will this conductance be activatable. Finally, a semilogarithmic plot of the outward current decay reveals a simple time constant of about 12 msec (Fig. 11B2). Ion substitution experiments, in combination with another classic voltage-clamp protocol, which includes ac-

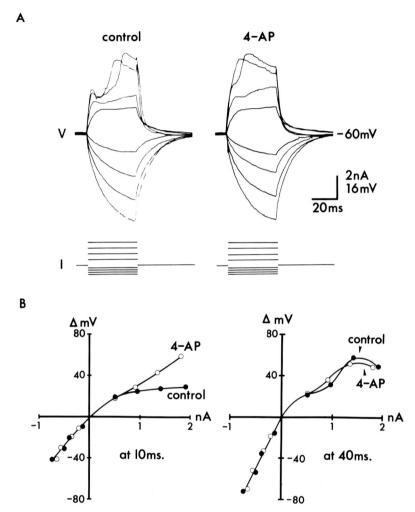

Figure 10. Electrically excitable membrane properties in a cultured spinal neuron. The cell was bathed in tetraethylammonium and tetrodotoxin (to block ubiquitous Na$^+$ and K$^+$ conductances) and current-clamped with KCl-filled microelectrodes. A series of 40-msec current steps was injected to hyperpolarize and depolarize the cell. (A) Voltage responses in the hyperpolarizing direction appear as relatively simple exponentials under control conditions and in the presence of 4-aminopyridine (4-AP). Responses in the depolarizing direction are more complex and include sags or droops, the earlier of which is effectively eliminated by 4-AP. (B) Plots of membrane potential changes as a function of injected current at 10 and 40 msec after current injections reveal linear relationships in the hyperpolarizing range of potential that remain unchanged in 4-AP. Obvious rectification in the depolarizing direction at 10-msec times is blocked by 4-AP, while rectification at 40 msec remains essentially unchanged. (Modified from Barker *et al.*, 1984.)

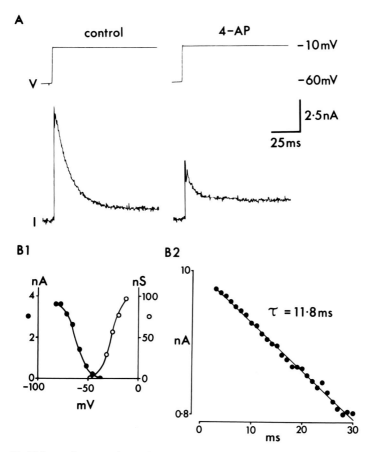

Figure 11. Voltage-clamp analysis of transient rectification in a cultured spinal neuron. The same cell illustrated in Fig. 10 was voltage-clamped at −60 mV. (A) Stepping the cell from −60 to −10 mV triggers a transient outward current response that is markedly attenuated by 4-AP. (B1) Conditioning the cell at different holding potentials and stepping to −10 mV (●) shows that the maximum amplitude is evoked when the cell is held at about −90 mV, which is the threshold for inactivation. Holding the cell at −90 mV and stepping to various potentials (○) shows that outward current becomes detectable at about −50 mV, which is the threshold for activation. (B2) The transient current decays with a time constant of about 12 msec. (Modified from Barker *et al.*, 1984.)

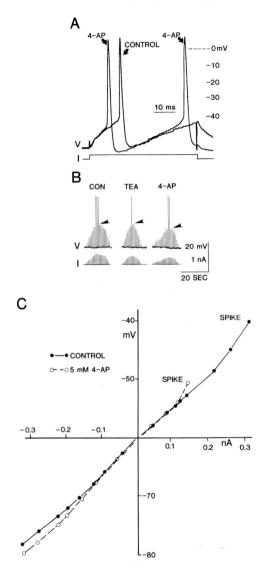

Figure 12. Functional role of transient rectification studied with 4-AP in a cultured spinal neuron. (A) The cell was current-clamped to −60 mV (V) and identical depolarizing current steps (I) were applied under control conditions and in the presence of 4-AP. 4-AP lowers the threshold for single and repetitive action potential activity but does not change their duration afterhyperpolarization amplitude. (B) A series of depolarizing current stimuli were applied under control conditions and in the presence of tetraethylammonium ions (TEA) or 4-AP. The arrowheads mark the threshold for a single action potential, which is lowered by 4-AP, but not TEA. (C) Current–voltage (I–V) plots of voltage responses to

tivation of the conductance followed by commands to a wide range of potentials, have led to the conclusion that the transient conductance involves primarily, if not exclusively, K^+ ions.

This transient K^+ conductance is similar to that originally described in invertebrate ganglia and since observed in a wide variety of excitable membranes. It is expressed in the majority of cultured neurons studied thus far. Its functional role in the excitability of cultured spinal cord and hippocampal neurons has been studied by assessing action potential generation in the absence or presence of 4-aminopyridine (Fig. 12). The results indicate that 4-aminopyridine facilitates the generation of action potentials, so that in its presence action potential threshold is closer to the resting potential and more action potentials occur for the same amount of depolarizing current. There is little or no change in other parameters of action potential generation or in passive properties of the cell in the presence of 4-aminopyridine. These results indicate that the electrically excitable properties of cultures CNS neurons can be studied as well as chemical excitability at a relatively quantitative level of resolution.

4. CONCLUSION

In this chapter we have briefly reviewed several types of electrophysiological studies into the chemically and electrically excitable membrane properties expressed *in vitro*. It is clear from these strategies that different types of chemical and electrical excitability survive *in vitro* and that a quantitative level of analysis can be achieved. The results obtained thus far indicate that the excitable properties of cultured CNS neurons are superficially similar to those described in invertebrate and peripheral vertebrate membranes. Further progress in understanding the roles of these excitable membrane properties and of the types of synaptic signals communicated between cultured neurons will come when more precise identification of the individual cells can be made. At present, the experiment control and accessibility of dissociated cultures of CNS cells are compromised to a degree by the lack of knowledge concerning the natural development and differentiation of the phenotypic properties expressed by functionally distinct neurons. Thus, the development of

50-msec current stimuli under control conditions and in the presence of 4-AP, which lowers the threshold for a spike without changing the I–V relations in the hyperpolarizing quadrant. (Modified from Segal *et al.*, 1984.)

methods both to identify specific cells in heterogeneous cultures and to isolate specific subpopulations is a prerequisite to understanding which types of CNS cells have what excitable membrane mechanisms and why.

REFERENCES

Barker, J. L., and Ransom, B. R., 1978, Amino acid pharmacology of mammalian central neurones grown in tissue culture, *J. Physiol.* **280:**331–354.

Barker, J. L., McBurney, R. N., and MacDonald, J. F., 1982, Fluctuation analysis of neutral amino acid responses in cultured mouse spinal neurons, *J. Physiol.* **322:**365–387.

Barker, J. L., McBurney, R. N., and Mathers, D. A., 1983, Convulsant-induced depression of amino acid responses in cultured mouse spinal neurons studied under voltage clamp, *Br. J. Pharmacol.* **80:**619–629.

Barker, J., Dufy, B., Owen, D. G., and Segal, M., 1984, Excitable membrane properties of cultured central nervous system neurons and clonal pituitary cells, *Cold Spring Harbor Symp. Quant. Biol.* **48:**259–268.

Hamill, O. P., Bormann, J., and Sakmann, B., 1983, Activation of multiple conductance state chloride channels in spinal neurones by glycine and GABA, *Nature* **305:**805–808.

Jackson, M. B., Lecar, H., Mathers, D. A., and Barker, J. L., 1982, Single channel currents activated by GABA, muscimol, and ($-$)pentobarbital in cultured mouse spinal neurons, *J. Neurosci.* **2:**889–894.

Katz, B., and Miledi, R., 1972, The statistical nature of acetylcholine potential and its molecular components, *J. Physiol.* **224:**665–699.

Neale, E. A., Nelson, P. G., Macdonald, R. L., Christian, C. N., and Bowers, L. M., 1983, Synaptic transmission between mammalian central neurons in cell culture. III. Morpho-physiologic correlates of quantal synaptic transmission. *J. Neurophysiol.* **49:**1459–1468.

Nelson, P. G., Marshall, K. D., Pun, R. Y. K., Christian, C. N., Sheriff, W. H., Jr., Macdonald, R. L., and Neale, E. A., 1983, Synaptic interactions between mammalian central neurons in cell culture. II. Quantal analysis of EPSPs, *J. Neurophysiol.* **49:**1442–1458.

Ransom, B. R., Neale, E., Henkart, M., Bullock, P. N., and Nelson, P. G., 1977a, Mouse spinal cord in cell culture. I. Morphology and intrinsic neuronal electrophysiological properties, *J. Neurophysiol.* **40:**1132–1150.

Ransom, B. R., Christian, C. N., Bullock, P. N., and Nelson, P. G., 1977b, Mouse spinal cord in cell culture. II. Synaptic activity and circuit behavior, *J. Neurophysiol.* **40:**1151–1162.

Schmechel, D. E., Brightman, M. S., and Barker, J. L., 1980, Localization of neuron-specific enolase in mouse spinal neurons grown in tissue culture, *Brain Res.* **181:**391–400.

Segal, M., 1983, Rat hippocampal neurons in culture: Responses to electrical and chemical stimuli, *J. Neurophysiol.* **50:**1249–1264.

Segal, M., and Barker, J. L., 1984, Rat hippocampal neurons in culture: Voltage clamp analysis of inhibitory synaptic connections. *J. Neurophysiol.*, **52:**469–487.

Segal, M., Rogawski, M. A., and Barker, J. L., 1984, A transient K^+ conductance regulates the excitability of cultured hippocampal and spinal neurons. *J. Neurosci.* **4:**604–09.

Smith, T. G., Jr., and Cunningham, M., 1983, A pressure ejection system for the focal application of neuroactive substances from micropipettes, *Med. Biol. Eng. Comp.* **21:**138–144.

Smith, T. G., Barker, J. L., Smith, B. M., and Colburn, T. R., 1980, Voltage clamping with microelectrodes, *J. Neurosci. Methods* **3**:105–128.

Smith, T. G., Jr., Barker, J. L., Smith, B. M., and Colburn, T. R., 1981, Voltage clamp techniques applied to cultured skeletal muscle and spinal neurons, in: *Excitable Cells in Tissue Culture* (P. G. Nelson and M. Liberman, eds.), Plenum Press, New York, pp. 111–136.

Study, R. E., and Barker, J. L., 1982, Cellular mechanisms of benzodiazepine action in the central nervous sytem. *J. Am. Med. Assoc.* **247**:2147–2151.

12

What We Have Learned from Patch Recordings of Cultured Cells

LI-YEN MAE HUANG

1. INTRODUCTION

Dissociated neural cell cultures have been used as model systems to study a host of questions in neurobiology such as regulation of cell differentiation, interactions between cells, mechanisms of morphogenesis and synaptogenesis. Because culture systems are experimentally accessible to anatomical, biochemical, and pharmacological techniques, they provide the investigator with a great deal of information as well as the opportunity to correlate the knowledge obtained from various techniques. Until recently, these advantages of culture systems had not been exploited in studies of the gating properties of ion channels in the excitable membrane. The main reason is that cultured neuronal cells are usually quite small (<30 μm in diameter). Conventional voltage-clamp techniques, which have been used so successfully in nonmammalian preparations, such as squid axon and frog node, cannot be employed as effectively in cultured systems. Membrane potentials in cultured cells are commonly measured with microelectrodes. The tip resistance of microelectrodes used in these cells is usually high, ranging from 10 to 100

LI-YEN MAE HUANG • Marine Biomedical Institute and Department of Physiology and Biophysics, University of Texas Medical Branch, Galveston, Texas 77550.

MΩ. This results in poor time resolution of the microelectrode voltage clamp. Moreover, electrode penetration often inflicts cell injury, and the ion composition of the cell interior cannot be controlled with this technique. Thus, electrophysiologists were reluctant to choose cultured cells as their preparations despite the successes of some research groups (Moolenaar and Spector, 1977, 1978; Nathan and DeHaan, 1979; Ebihara *et al.*, 1980).

In 1976, Neher and Sakmann introduced the patch-clamp method to record the opening and closing of individual acetylcholine (ACh)-activated channels in the extrajunctional membrane of denervated frog muscle fibers. Gating properties of single-membrane channels have been directly studied in artificial bilayers doped with channel-forming substances (Bean *et al.*, 1969; Ehrenstein *et al.*, 1974; reviewed by Ehrenstein and Lecar, 1977) and have been extensively extracted from noise analysis of postjunctional synapses, axonal membranes, and node of Ranvier (Katz and Miledi, 1972; Anderson and Stevens, 1973; Sachs and Lecar, 1973; Conti *et al.*, 1975, 1976; Fishman *et al.*, 1975). The direct observations of the conductance change of single channels in biological membranes was nevertheless an exciting development. The impact of the patch-clamp technique in neurophysiology was not completely felt until it was later discovered that an extremely tight seal can be formed between the pipette glass and the cell membrane (Horn and Patlak, 1980; Hamill *et al.*, 1981). This finding has made patch-clamp a simpler method and more importantly has completely changed the role of cultured cells in membrane research. Since cultured cells can be made free of surface coating and readily give good seals, they have become popular preparations for neurophysiologists.

In this review, I will summarize the results of some of the studies on various aspects of neuronal functions using patch-clamp techniques and cultured cells. The purpose is to illustrate the versatility of such approaches. Since the topics and results are chosen to emphasize these points, the review is neither exhaustive nor does justice to many important results obtained from other preparations using various biochemical and electrophysiological techniques. Interested readers on certain topics mentioned here are encouraged to refer to articles that deal with these subjects in detail.

2. PATCH-CLAMP TECHNIQUE

In recent years, electrophysiologists have searched for alternatives to microelectrodes for measuring the membrane potential in small neurons or heart cells. Kostyuk *et al.* (1975) and Lee *et al.* (1978, 1980) have developed internal dialysis techniques to study the ionic current in molluscan neurons. A polyethylene tubing or glass pipette with a tip opening of about 5–10 μm is pressed against the cell membrane. After a tight seal is formed (seal resistance <1 GΩ) between electrodes and membrane, a needle is used to rupture the membrane. Internal dialysis is accomplished by using a V-shaped electrode or by inserting perfusion tubing down to the electrode tip. The low resistance of the current electrode and pipette electrode (<1 MΩ) greatly speeds the clamping of cells. The internal ion compositions can be reasonably controlled. The technique can be used effectively to voltage-clamp medium to large cells (30–100 μm in diameter) with a current flow of less than 20 nA (Kostyuk and Krishtal, 1977; Lee *et al.*, 1978; Byerly and Hagiwara, 1982; Huang *et al.*, 1982). The moderate pipette–cell membrane seal limits its usefulness in recording from small cells (<20 μm in diameter).

About the same time, Neher and Sakmann (1976) used a pipette of much smaller opening (<1 μm in diameter) placed against the membrane to obseve current flow through single ACh channels. During the next few years in those studies of biological single channels, the seals between the membrane and the pipette were in the range of 50 MΩ (Neher and Sakmann, 1976; Neher *et al.*, 1978; Neher and Steinbach, 1978; Nelson and Sachs, 1979; Jackson and Lecar, 1979; Sakmann *et al.*, 1980; Cull-Candy *et al.*, 1981). This technique was subsequently modified and substantially improved (Horn and Patlak, 1980; Hamill *et al.*, 1981). By keeping the pipette glass clean and applying suction to the interior of the electrode, an extremely tight seal (seal resistance >10 GΩ) between glass pipette and membrane is obtained. The "giga seal" of the patch electrode reduces the current leakage through the seal and total background noise (rms noise = 0.15 pA at 1 kHz bandwidth) to such a low level that current flowing through the individual channels can be clearly resolved (cell-attached patch recording). Moreover, the giga seal is mechanically stable, allowing a number of clever manipulations (Fig. 1) (Hamill *et al.*, 1981). After the cell pipette forms a giga seal with the membrane, a patch of membrane can be torn away without destroying the seal. When the patch is excised without first rupturing the membrane, the cytoplasmic side of the membrane is facing the bath (inside-out patch). If the cell membrane is ruptured first, the pipette is then drawn away from the cell. The patch of membrane that sealed across the pipette tip will have its extracellular side facing the bath solution (outside-out patch; Fig. 1). In these two cases, the single-channel events can be studied in a cell-free environment. The ion compositions facing both sides of the membrane are known. The content of bathing solutions

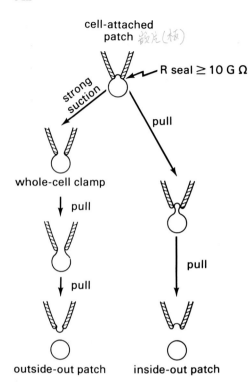

cell-attached
patch 敗片(板)

R seal ≥ 10 G Ω

strong suction

pull

whole-cell clamp

pull

pull

pull

pull

outside-out patch   inside-out patch

Figure 1. Different recording configurations of a patch clamp. Cell-attached patch: after the electrode forms a tight seal with a cell, the membrane patch stays intact on the cells. Inside-out patch: as the electrode is withdrawn from the cell, a patch of membrane is excised; the cytoplasmic side of the membrane faces the bath. Whole-cell clamp: after the formation of a giga seal, the membrane patch underneath the pipette is ruptured by strong suction; the patch pipette is then used as an internal electrode to control the membrane potential of the entire cell. Outside-out patch: when the electrode is withdrawn after the cell membrane is ruptured, a membrane patch is sealed over a pipette tip; the extracellular side of the membrane now faces the bath.

can be modified, and drugs, proteins, second messengers, or other molecules can be introduced to the cytoplasmic side (for the inside-out patch) or to the extracellular side (for the outside-out patch) of the membrane during the course of an experiment. On the other hand, if the pipette is left attached to the cells after the rupturing of the membrane, the patch pipette can be used as an internal electrode to record membrane current of the whole cell (whole-cell clamp; Fig. 1). The relatively low resistance of the patch electrode and the tight seal formation allow voltage-clamping of small cells (diameter <20 μm) with good speed (50–200 μsec time constant) (Marty and Neher, 1983). This technique offers the unique opportunity to study a variety of cells which are too small to employ the conventional voltage-clamp method and to analyze the membrane properties at the single-channel level under a variety of experimental conditions. The technical details of the patch-clamp method have been described extensively in the original paper by Hamill et al. (1981) and a number of other articles (Corey and Stevens, 1983; Marty and Neher, 1983; Sakmann and Neher, 1983; Sigworth, 1983; Corey, 1983).

To improve the efficiency of solution change in this system, Cull-Candy *et al.* (1981) and Yellen (1982) have introduced ways to rapidly exchange the solution inside or outside of the patch electrode. Cull-Candy *et al.* (1981) use a micromanipulator to insert a multibarrel perfusion pipette into the patch electrode. The tip of the perfusion pipette is positioned within 100 μm of the tip of the patch electrode. A hypodermic needle is cemented at the back of the perfusion pipette. When air pressure is applied to the hypodermic needle, the solution inside the patch electrode can be changed within 10 sec. Thus, one can change solutions both inside and outside of the patch electrode simultaneously during an experiment. Yellen (1982), on the other hand, has designed a way to rapidly change the solution outside the patch electrode. He places several large-tipped glass pipettes in the bath. Different solutions are flowing continuously out of these pipettes. The patch electrode is brought to the mouth of the glass pipettes, and the solution change can be accomplished in seconds. When another solution is desired, the patch electrode is moved to the opening of another pipette. Solutions can be changed swiftly back and forth by simply moving patch pipettes among the openings of the glass pipettes. These manipulations are very useful in studying the selectivities of an ion channel where many solution changes are often needed.

3. ANALYSIS OF SINGLE-CHANNEL RECORDS

In order to probe the function of the channel protein underlying many cellular processes, we often ask the following questions: Is one type of channel responsible for the phenomenon observed? What is the conductance of these channels? What ions do these channels select? How do the channels switch between open or closed states? Is this channel gating regulated by membrane potential or by certain neurotransmitters? Do ions, cAMP, or hormones modulate the gating processes? This information is obtainable from the analysis of single-channel records.

The single-channel activities are often recorded under a stationary condition where the membrane potential is held at a constant level. For each record one can first estimate the amplitude of the channel (Colquhoun and Sigworth, 1983). The distribution of amplitude, in most cases, can be fitted with a Gaussian curve (Fig. 2). This is expected when the channel activities observed are contributed by channels that open for variable intervals. If the amplitude distribution shows more than one peak, this indicates either that several independent populations of chan-

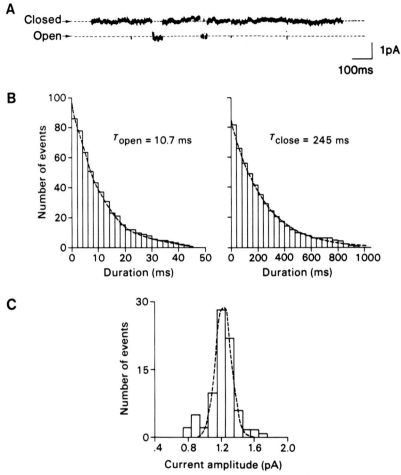

Figure 2. Example of a batrachotoxin-activated Na$^+$ channel from neuroblastoma NG108-15 showing the records and analysis of single-channel recording. (A) Single-channel current recorded from a cell-attached patch at −96 mV; downward deflections indicate channel opening. (B) Cumulative open time and closed time histograms. Dashed lines are the best fit for a simple exponential. In this case, the mean open time was $\tau_{open} = 1/\alpha = 10.7$ msec, and the mean closed time was $\tau_{closed} = 1/\beta = 245$ msec. (C) Amplitude histograms; dashed line is the Gaussian distribution fit of the experimental data. The mean current was 1.25 pA.

nel are active simultaneously or that one of the channels has multiple conductance states. From the single-channel current versus voltage relations, we can determine the conductance of the channel and its dependence on voltage.

Second, one can determine from the single-channel record the duration of channels staying in the open or in the closed conformation. Since the channels are open and closed at random at steady state, a stochastic process is used to describe the gating behavior of the channel (Colquhoun and Hawkes, 1981, 1983). It is often assumed that the probability of transition from one state to another is a Markov process. Namely, the future stochastic behavior of a channel depends solely on the present state of the channel, not on how the channel reaches this state. When various kinetic schemes are employed to give a more quantitative description of the process, the Markov assumption implies that at constant membrane potential and temperature, the rate constants between states are constant, i.e., independent of time. In order to illustrate the basic idea underlying gating properties of the channel, we will consider a very simple example. Let us assume that there is only one channel in the patch of membrane to avoid the complexity in determining the lifetimes of open channels from overlapping events. The channel has only two conductance states: open or closed. The transition between these two states is voltage-dependent. This can be described by the following kinetic scheme where the rate constants are α for channel closing and β for channel opening, respectively:

$$\text{closed} \underset{\alpha}{\overset{\beta}{\rightleftharpoons}} \text{open}$$

In probabilistic terms, rate constants measure the probabilities of a channel opening or closing in unit time. A channel in the closed conformation has to go through a large number of trials before it can overcome the energy barrier to open the channel. If this is the case, the probability of the channel being in a closed state can be described by a Poisson distribution function which gives mean closed time ($\tau_{closed} = 1/\beta$). The same reasoning is applied for mean open time ($\tau_{open} = 1/\alpha$). From histograms or cumulative histograms of open time and closed time which are obtained from measuring the duration of open channel and closed channel, we can find the transition rate of α and β between two states (Fig. 2).

From the values of α and β we can further estimate the fraction of time channels spend in the open or closed state. If we assume that voltage-dependence of the conductance arises from the transition be-

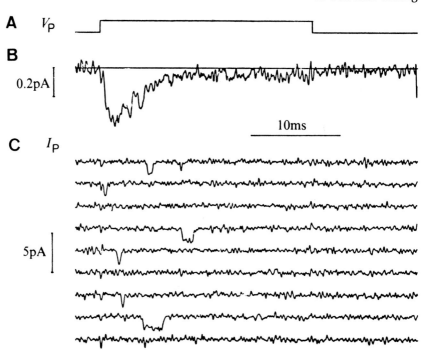

Figure 3. Single Na$^+$ channel current from cultured myotube observed by Sigworth and Neher (1980). (A) The pulse protocol: a 10 mV depolarized membrane potential was applied to the membrane patch at 1 sec intervals. (B) Average of 300 of such current records shown in (C). Leakage and capacitance current was subtracted in each case. (C) Nine successive current records obtained from such depolarizations shown in (A). The downward deflection indicates the inward current. The mean channel current was -1.6 pA and the mean open time was 0.7 msec. (From Sigworth and Neher, 1980.)

tween closing and opening of the channel, involving motion of charged groups or dipoles across the membrane, the slope of the fraction open time versus voltage curve gives the number of electronic charges required to move across the membrane in order to open one channel.

The single-channel activities can also be measured under a nonstationary condition where many depolarized voltage pulses of fixed magnitude are repeatedly applied to the membranes. Summing many of these individual responses together, an average current record can be reconstructed (Fig. 3) (Sigworth and Neher, 1980; Horn et al., 1981; Aldrich et al., 1983). This current is similar to the macroscopic current observed in a voltage-clamp experiment if there are no interactions among the channels. The average current represents then the probability that a channel is open at various times. Besides the parameters obtainable as described under stationary conditions, additional information can be extracted from the ensemble of single-channel records with the nonstationary protocols. For example, one can measure the first latency which is the duration between the onset of depolarizing pulses and the first channel opening. By comparing the temporal distribution of the average current and the first latency distribution, one can decide how many first opening events contribute, for example, to the declining phase of the current and thus determine the contribution of channel activation in that part of the current (Horn *et al.*, 1981; Aldrich *et al.*, 1983). It is sometimes of interest to determine how the condition of the channel prior to test pulse determines the channel behavior during the pulse. One can perform a double-pulse experiment and determine whether the channel opening during prepulse affects the average probability of channel opening during the test pulse (Fig. 4) (Aldrich and Stevens, 1983; Aldrich and Yellen, 1983). From the above information, we can understand in more detail the interaction between activation and inactivation of the channel directly, which is inferred from the voltage-clamp method.

4. STUDIES OF ION CHANNELS

Ion channels are generally divided into two classes: those neurotransmitter-activated channels that are responsible for the generation of a postsynaptic potential, such as the ACh-activated channel at the end plate, gaba-activated Cl^- channels, and glutamate-activated Na channels; and those voltage-sensitive channels that are responsible for the generation of an action potential such as the Na^+ channel, Ca^2 -activated K^+ channel, and Ca^{2+} channel. Some of these channels will be discussed below.

4.1. ACh-Activated Channel

After ACh molecules are released from a nerve terminal, they diffuse across the synaptic cleft and bind to the ACh receptors in the postsynaptic membrane. This leads to the opening of ion channels and depolarization of the membrane. The chemical signal delivered from the nerve ending is then transduced into electrical activity at the neuromuscular junction. The kinetic properties of these channels were studied in detail in neuromuscular function using conventional voltage-clamp (Magleby and Stevens, 1972) and noise analyses (Katz and Miledi, 1970, 1972; Anderson and Stevens, 1973). Anderson and Stevens (1973) ana-

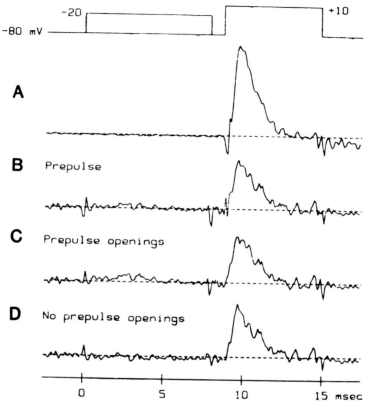

Figure 4. Average of single Na^+ channel records from a cell-attached patch on a cultured neuroblastoma N1E-115 cell. The pulse protocol contains a 6 msec voltage step from -80 mV to $+10$ mV relative to the cell resting potential without (A) or with (B–D) an 8 msec prepulse to -20 mV. (A) Ensemble average of the probability of a channel being open (p_o) during a test pulse without a prepulse. (B) Ensemble average of p_o during the same test pulse preceded by a prepulse. Note the p_o here is smaller than in (A) because the inactivation occurs during the prepulse. (C) Average of all the records in (B) that have openings during the prepulse. (D) Average of all the records in (B) that have no openings during the prepulse. Note the p_o are the same in both (C) and (D). (From Aldrich and Yellen, 1983.) With permission of Plenum Press.

lyzed the current fluctuation of ACh-activated channels under voltage-clamp conditions and found that the covariance function of the fluctuation was a single exponential function. The time constant of this function is identical to the decay time constant of an end-plate current following a voltage step (Magleby and Stevens, 1972). They assumed that an ACh-activated channel can exist in only two states, open or closed, and suggested that ACh molecules can be present in the neuromuscular junction for only a very brief period of time before they are hydrolyzed by acetylcholinesterase. Thus, the binding of the ACh molecule to its channel protein is rapid compared to the conformational changes between the open and the closed state of the channel. The latter is then the rate-limiting step of the channel activation. Under these model assumptions, the time constants measured by the noise and voltage-clamp experiments are direct measures of the mean open time of the channel. It was later found that two ACh molecules are required to open one channel (Adams, 1975; Dionne et al., 1978).

Studies of single ACh channels have revealed several interesting behaviors. Taking advantage of the better resolution of the patch-clamp method, Colquhoun and Sakmann (1981, 1983) found that opening of the ACh channel was much more complex than was first suggested. At low agonist concentrations where desensitization is negligible, the opening of the ACh channel occurs in a burst which is separated by a relatively long closed period. The distribution of the open-channel durations cannot be described by a single exponential function. A sum of two exponentials, a short- and a long-duration component, is required to fit the data. Thus, an ACh channel has two open states. They further suggested that a channel with only one agonist bound to it can open, which results in the short opening of the channel. Recently, Sine and Steinbach (1984) studied cultured BC_3Hl cells and found that these brief openings do not become less abundant with increasing agonist concentration. Thus, the brief opening is probably not contributed by an open channel with a single ligand.

During each burst, the open channel closes and then opens in rapid succession before it enters into the long closed period (Fig. 5) (Colquhoun and Sakmann, 1981). This has been termed the "Nachschlag" phenomenon (Fig. 6). These flickering activities of channels have been found subsequently in other types of channels and seem to be a common feature of ion channels (Cull-Candy et al., 1981; Barrett et al., 1982). A more complex model has emerged from analysis of experimental results (Dionne and Leibowitz, 1982; Colquhoun and Sakmann, 1983; Jackson et al., 1983; Sine and Steinbach, 1984):

$$2A + R \rightleftharpoons A + A_1R \rightleftharpoons A_2R \underset{\alpha}{\overset{\beta}{\rightleftharpoons}} A_2R^*$$
$$\updownarrow$$
$$A_1R^*(?)$$

Here, A represents the agonist molecule; R is the receptor; A_1R, A_2R are the closed channels with one or two agonists bound to it; A_1R^*, A_2R^*

A

B

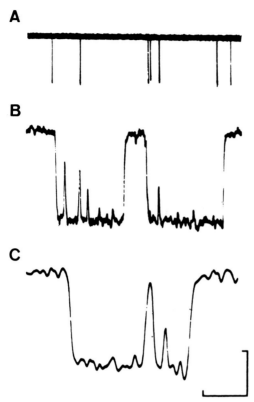

C

Figure 5. Burst activities of ACh channels. Inward current is plotted as a downward deflection. (A) The low-frequency events are shown in slow time scale. Calibration bars: 4 pA, 1 sec. (B) Several brief closures which interrupted an open channel are shown in an expanded scale. Calibration bars: 2 pA, 10 msec. (C) Another group of three openings is shown in even faster time scale. Calibration bar: 2 pA, 2 msec. Partial closings may represent brief but complete closures of the channel if the frequency response of the system is not limited. (From Colquhoun and Sakmann, 1981.)

are the corresponding open channels; α, β, k_1, k_{-1}, k_2, and k_{-2} are rate constants between the states. In order to explain the data, the channel opening rate β has to be very fast compared with the closing rate α. β should also be comparable to k_{-2}. The channel then has to open rather quickly before the agonist can dissociate from the receptor. Once the channel is open, it can switch back and forth between states A_2R and A_2R^* several times. The channel then enters into the long closed state upon dissociation of the agonist.

In addition to having distinct kinetic states, ACh-activated channels also have several different conductance states (Hamill and Sakmann, 1981; Hamill, 1983) (Fig. 7). At low temperature (8°C), ACh-activated channels of cultured rat muscle have three conductance states (10, 25, 35 pS). Over 60% of the total channel openings have a conductance state of 25 pS; the 35 pS conductance state makes up the other 36% of channel openings; and the 10 pS state is rarely observed (<1%). Multiple con-

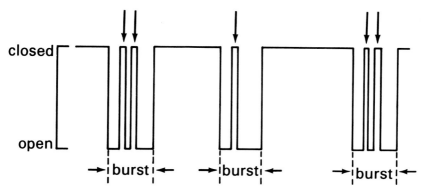

Figure 6. Definition of a burst—a group of openings that is separated by a long closed time. The arrows indicate the brief closure within the burst. This is termed the "Nachschlag" phenomenon.

ductance states were also observed in cultured chick muscle cells, both above and below room temperature, and in the cloned cell line BC_3H1 (Chabala et al., 1982; Auerbach and Sachs, 1983; Sachs, 1983). The physiological significance of these substates has not been determined. However, these observations do change the simple view that open channels can have only one conductance state.

When the ACh-activated channel was recorded under the condition where the background noise was extremely low, the current record during the open channel period was noiser than the record during the closed channel period (Sigworth, 1982). The noise spectrum computed from the record has a time constant of 0.5 msec. Since the channel is opening and closing at a much slower time scale (50 msec), this open channel noise may actually be fluctuations of channel conductance resulting from the structural dynamics of the channel. This excess noise in the open channel has also been observed in the subconductance state of chick muscle cells (Auerbach and Sachs, 1983).

4.2. Sodium Channel

Ion channels play a central role in membrane excitability. Their ion-selective properties and the ability of fast switching (gating) between open and closed conformations in response to voltage changes endow the membrane with steep voltage-dependent permeability. This characteristic property allows the neuronal or muscle cells to generate action potentials upon stimulation.

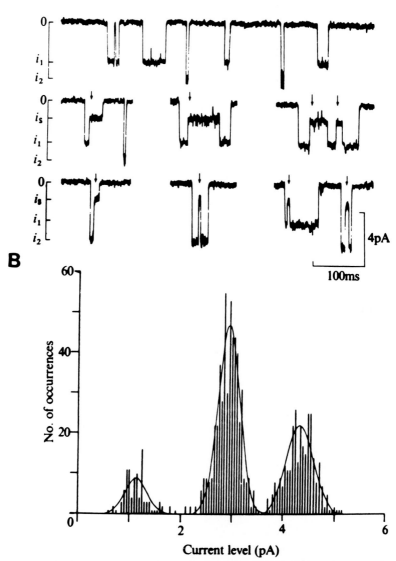

A

B

Figure 7. Subconductance state of an ACh channel from cultured muscle cells. (A) Three conductance states: $i_s = 10$ pS, $i_1 = 25$ pS, $i_2 = 35$ pS. Arrow indicates the occurrence of 10 pS substate. (B) The amplitude histogram for the patch described in (A). There are three different current levels. The curves are the Gaussian fit of the experimental data. The mean values are 1.1, 2.9, and 4.3 pA (data were obtained at 8°C in 2 μM ACh and at −70 mV). (From Hamill and Sakmann, 1981.)

Na$^+$ channels are responsible for the fast depolarizing phase of the action potential in most mature excitable cells. These channels open and then close when the membrane potential is stepped from resting to a constant depolarized level. Hodgkin and Huxley (1952) assumed that Na$^+$ channels can be in one of three functional states: resting, open, or inactivated. The rapid increase of Na$^+$ current is identified as the activation process and the slow decline of Na$^+$ current as the inactivation process. One of the assumptions of their model is that activation and inactivation of Na$^+$ channels are two independent processes. This assumption has been disputed by several detailed voltage-clamp and gating current experiments (Goldman, 1976; Armstrong, 1981; French and Horn, 1983). It is now generally believed that the inactivation and activation processes are coupled.

The studies on single Na$^+$ channels have further revised our understanding of the gating of Na$^+$ channels. Single Na$^+$ channels have been recorded in cultured myotubes (Sigworth and Neher, 1980; Horn *et al.*, 1981; Patlak and Horn, 1982), neuroblastoma cells (Quandt and Narahashi, 1982; Aldrich and Stevens, 1983; Aldrich *et al.*, 1983; Huang *et al.*, 1984; Yamamoto *et al.*, 1984), and pituitary cells (Horn *et al.*, 1984). In these preparations, the activation and inactivation processes overlap significantly in time (Horn *et al.*, 1981; Patlak and Horn, 1982; Aldrich *et al.*, 1983). When the average Na$^+$ current is compared with the distribution of first latency of a channel during a depolarizing pulse, many channels are found to open for the first time during the inactivation of Na$^+$ current. The rate of activation has a slow component (Patlak and Horn, 1982; Aldrich *et al.*, 1983). Its magnitude is comparable to the rate of decay of Na$^+$ current. Thus, the activation process of the Na$^+$ channel contributes both the rising phase and the declining phase of Na$^+$ current, contrary to the Hodgkin and Huxley (1952) interpretation of activation and inactivation processes.

Aldrich *et al.* (1983) described the activation and inactivation of Na$^+$ channels using a three-state fate model. They assumed that the channel can be in resting, open, or inactivated states, and considered only the time-independent transition between these states. Since the inactivated channel is rarely reopened, they also assumed that the channel can only open once during each depolarization. According to this model, the probability that open channels go to the inactivated state is larger than 0.8. The rate of inactivation derived from the analysis is fast and relatively voltage-independent. Thus, most open Na$^+$ channels are closed by going to the inactivated state rather than back to the resting state. This result is consistent with the finding that the lifetime of the open state is markedly increased when the inactivation is removed by treatment with N-bromoacetamide (Patlak and Horn, 1982; Horn et al., 1984) or batrachotoxin (Quandt and Narahashi, 1982; Huang et al., 1984). Under these conditions, the channel lifetime is mainly determined by the closing rate of an open channel and is not affected by the process of inactivation.

Horn et al. (1981) have shown that the resting Na^+ channel can enter the inactivated state directly without being opened first. Aldrich and Stevens (1983) and Aldrich and Yellen (1983) clearly confirmed this by measuring the probability of a channel being open (p_o) during a test pulse which is preceded by a -20 mV prepulse (Fig. 4). Identical p_o values were obtained from the records with prepulse opening and without prepulse opening. Both p_o values are smaller than the probabilities measured during the test pulse when a prepulse is not applied. This observation suggests that there is a significant inactivation process occurring during prepulse. Its occurrence does not depend on whether there is any channel opening during the prepulse. Thus a resting channel does not have to open before it can inactivate. When the membrane potential is stepped from -90 mV to -20 mV, a substantial percentage of the resting channels (50%) are found to transfer into the inactivated state directly without ever going through the open state.

Questions still remain on the voltage-dependence of Na^+ inactivation. The inactivation rate of Na^+ channels in N1E-115 neuroblastoma cells is voltage-independent (Aldrich et al., 1983), in agreement with the results of gating experiments (Bezanilla and Armstrong, 1977; Armstrong, 1981). However, Vandenberg and Horn (1984) estimated the rate constant from a five-state (three closed, one open, one inactivated) model using the maximum likelihood method (Horn and Lange, 1983) and found that the rate of inactivation in GH3 cells increases with depolarization. The reason for this discrepancy is not clear at the moment.

4.3. Calcium-Activated Potassium Channel

An increase in K^+ conductance is involved in many physiological functions, such as generation of action potentials in neurons (Hodgkin and Huxley, 1952), pacemaker activities of neurons and cardiac cells (Isenberg, 1977; Gorman et al., 1981), secretion (Putney, 1979), and the response of photoreceptors to light (Bolsover, 1981). The voltage-activated K^+ channels and the Ca^{2+}-activated K^+ ($K^+_{(Ca)}$) channels are two general classes of K^+ channels that are responsible for the K^+ current increase. Despite the presence of $K^+_{(Ca)}$ channels in a wide variety of tissues, the analysis of these channels has been hampered by the strong

Ca^{2+}-buffering capacity of the cytoplasm. Patch recordings have led to intensive studies of $K^+_{(Ca)}$ channels (Lux *et al.*, 1981; Marty, 1981; Barrett *et al.*, 1982; Wong *et al.*, 1982). The main reason is that the patch-clamp method allows the ion concentration of either side of the membrane to be controlled. This is especially appealing for the studies of $K^+_{(Ca)}$ channels because their activation depends not only on membrane potential but also on the intracellular Ca^{2+} concentration ($[Ca^{2+}]_i$). The conductance of this channel in many preparations is quite large (>100 pS). The size of the conductance and the ubiquitous presence of the channel make their detection relatively easy.

Detailed information on the $K^+_{(Ca)}$ channels is now available from cultured adrenal chromaffin cells (Marty, 1981), muscle cells (Barrett *et al.*, 1982), and cloned anterior pituitary cells (Wong *et al.*, 1982). In these systems, the $K^+_{(Ca)}$ channels open for a longer time and display more burst activities when the $[Ca^{2+}]_i$ is raised. The frequency and duration of the single $K^+_{(Ca)}$ channel are a sensitive function of $[Ca^+]_i$. The activities of this channel, on the other hand, are not affected by Ca^{2+} at the extracellular surface of the membrane. Since the fraction of time the channel is open is a sigmoidal function of $[Ca^{2+}]_i$, it is suggested that two or more intracellular Ca^{2+} ions are required to open a $K^+_{(Ca)}$ channel. At a given $[Ca^{2+}]_i$, the probability of the channel opening is increased with depolarization. As the $[Ca^{2+}]_i$ is increased, the channel opening probability versus voltage curve shifts toward the hyperpolarized direction. In other words, channels can be activated at a more hyperpolarized potential. This explains the previous observation that $K^+_{(Ca)}$ conductance is voltage-independent in the depolarized region when a large amount of Ca^{2+} is injected into the cells (Meech, 1976).

Similar to the ACh-activated channel, the $K^+_{(Ca)}$ channel in muscle cells has multiple conductance states (200 and 88 pS) (Barrett *et al.*, 1982). The 88-pS open channel appears occasionally. It comprises only 0.1% of the total channel open time. Furthermore, two exponentials are needed to fit the open time distribution of large conductance states. It was suggested that there are at least three open states for the K^+ channels. Thus, the kinetic behavior of this channel is rather complex.

Latorre *et al.* (1982) have studied $K^+_{(Ca)}$ channels in reconstituted transverse tubular membrane and found that this channel is very selective for K^+ over other cations even though their conductance is very large (>100 pS). Latorre and Miller (1983) suggested that $K^+_{(Ca)}$ channels have a large opening and a very narrow as well as short selectivity region.

4.4. Calcium Channel

Ca^{2+} channels which regulate the Ca^{2+} influx across the membrane play very important roles in many cellular functions such as secretion, muscle contraction, and control of K$^+$ permeability. Ca^{2+} channels are often difficult to study because their channel properties are labile and vary with different preparations (Hagiwara and Byerly, 1981; Tsien, 1983). The patch-clamp method has made it possible to study the single Ca^{2+} channel and provide new information on its activation and inactivation properties.

Single Ca^{2+} channel current is very small at the physiological Ca^{2+} concentration. For example, in adrenal chromaffin cells unitary channel current calculated from fluctuation analysis is 0.025 pA in a 1 mM external Ca^{2+} solution for a membrane potential where the inward Ca^{2+} current is at a maximum (Fenwick et al., 1982). This current amplitude is too small to be recorded by the patch electrode. Thus, single Ca^{2+} current is commonly studied in elevated external Ca^{2+} or Ba^{2+} solutions.

The single Ca^{2+} channel has only two conductance levels, open and closed (Fenwick et al., 1982; Hagiwara and Ohmori, 1982; Reuter et al., 1982). The open Ca^{2+} channel shows a great deal of burst activity. Ca^{2+} channels turn on at a membrane potential around -40 to -30 mV. The rising phase of Ca^{2+} current has a sigmoidal time course. Thus, the activation of Ca^{2+} channels is not a first-order process, which is in agreement with studies of molluscan neurons (Kostyuk and Krishtal, 1977; Byerly and Hagiwara, 1982) and heart cells (Lee and Tsien, 1983). An open time histogram can be fitted with a single exponential. The closed time histogram has at least two components. The slow component corresponds to the intervals between the bursts and the fast component corresponds to the gaps within the burst. Fenwick et al. (1982) used a three-state kinetic scheme to describe the activation of the Ca^{2+} channel:

$$\text{closed}_1 \underset{k_{-1}}{\overset{k_1}{\rightleftharpoons}} \text{closed}_2 \underset{k_{-2}}{\overset{k_2}{\rightleftharpoons}} \text{open}$$

where k_1, k_2, k_{-1}, k_{-2} are rate constants between the states. At -5 mV and in 95 mM external Ba^{2+}, k_1 is much slower than the other three rate constants and is the rate-limiting step for the activation.

In both GH3 and adrenal chromaffin cells (Hagiwara and Ohmori, 1982; Fenwick et al., 1982), the Ca^{2+} channel has shown very little genuine voltage-dependent inactivation. Most of the decline in Ca^{2+} current during a depolarizing pulse can be attributed to an irreversible elimination of Ca^{2+} channels available for activation during the course of experiments. This is quite different from some other excitable cell systems, such as *Helix* (Brown *et al.*, 1981) and cardiac cells (Marban and Tsien, 1981), which have shown both Ca^{2+}-dependent and voltage-dependent inactivation. Tillotson (1979) and Brehm *et al.* (1980) suggested that accumulation of intracellular Ca^{2+} reduces the Ca^{2+} conductance, thus producing the inactivation of Ca^{2+} current. The mechanism underlying the Ca^{2+}-dependent inactivation is not quite understood. In those two preparations mentioned, inactivation of Ca^{2+} current can also be produced by membrane depolarization analogous to the inactivation found in the Na^+ channel.

4.5. Discovery of New Ion Channels

Several new species of channels have been discovered with the patch clamp. For example, a Ca^{2+}-activated nonselective cation channel was found in cardiac cells (Colquhoun *et al.*, 1981) and neuroblastoma cells (Yellen, 1982). A large voltage activated anion channel was observed in cultured muscle cells (Blatz and Magleby, 1983). The functional significance of these channels has not been determined.

Two new types of channels that may have considerable functional significance were found in non-cultured systems. Novel serotonin-sensitive K^+ channels were observed in *Aplysia* sensory neurons (Siegelbaum *et al.*, 1982). These channels open at most of the physiological range of the membrane potential, including the resting level (Siegelbaum *et al.*, 1982; Camardo and Siegelbaum, 1983). They are closed by bath-applied serotonin, a neurotransmitter which has an important role in presynaptic facilitation (Castellucci and Kandel, 1976; Klein *et al.*, 1982). Another new type of channel was identified in dissociated pancreatic acinar cells. These channels are activated by the neurotransmitter ACh or the hormone cholecystokinin, two substances that stimulate the pancreatic acinar cells to secrete digestive enzymes and NaCl-rich fluid (Maruyama and Petersen, 1982a,b).

As shown in the above discussion, the studies of various single channels not only deepen our understanding of channel properties but also help us to find new channels which are difficult to identify with macroscopic ion current measurements, but are important to cell functions and physiology.

5. ACTION OF NEUROHORMONES

5.1. Effect of Epinephrine

Recent studies of the action of neurotransmitters indicate that many of them do not activate channels directly; instead, they modulate the gating of ion channels by affecting the concentration of intracellular second messengers such as cAMP. β-Adrenergic agonists, epinephrine and norepinephrine, which modulate the Ca^{2+} channel in cardiac cells, are one example of such neurotransmitters. Epinephrine was found to increase the inflow of Ca^{2+} current and thus prolong the plateau phase of the cardiac action potential (Reuter, 1967; Vassort et al., 1969; Reuter and Scholz, 1977). Because the β-adrenergic response can be mimicked by direct injection of cAMP, or cAMP-dependent protein kinase, and is inhibited by injection of the regulatory subunit of the kinase (Trautwein et al., 1982; Osterrieder et al., 1982; Cacheline et al., 1983; Reuter, 1983), the modulation of Ca^{2+} channels by β-adrenergic agonists is thought to be mediated by cAMP and protein phosphorylation. The sequence of events involved can be expressed as follows:

β-adrenergic agents + β-receptor → activation of adenylate cyclase
→ increase of cAMP → protein phosphorylation
→ change in Ca^{2+} channel properties → increase of I_{Ca}

Since epinephrine increases only the maximal conductance of Ca^{2+} channels and does not change the time course and reversal potential of Ca^{2+} current, it was suggested that the effect of Ca^{2+} channel phosphorylation is to increase the number of functional Ca^{2+} channels (Reuter and Scholz, 1977). As discussed previously, single-channel recording can unambiguously determine the conductance and the probability of a channel staying in the open or closed state. The hypothesis was tested in cultured cardiac cells (Reuter et al., 1982; Cacheline et al., 1983). When cells were treated with the β-agonist isoproterenol or β-bromo-cAMP, the single Ca^{2+} channel current remained unchanged, but the probability of the channel being open increased. Quantitative kinetic analyses of the data indicate that the increase in the probability is caused primarily by shortening the closed interval between the bursts, and less importantly by lengthening the average duration of an open channel. Although the experiments have not ruled out that Ca^{2+} channel phosphorylation can increase the number of channels, the observation that epinephrine increases open channel probability is an interesting and surprising one.

5.2. Effect of Thyrotropin-Releasing Hormone

Secretory activities of anterior pituitary cells are controlled by releasing hormones which are produced by and released from the neurons in the hypothalamus and then carried to their target cells through the

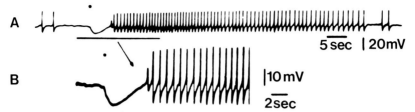

Figure 8. Effect of TRH on the membrane potential of GH3 cells. (A) When 5 μM TRH was applied externally to the cells (indicated by the dot), the membrane was transiently hyperpolarized and produced a long-lasting spike generation. (B) The underlined part of the record is shown in expanded scale. (From Ozawa and Kimura, 1979.)

hypothalamic portal system (Tixier-Vidal and Gourdji, 1981). The actions of these releasing hormones are often studied in the clonal pituitary cell lines GH3 and GH3/B6 because of the homogeneity of the cell populations. These cells are spontaneously electrically active. The action potential displays a positive overshoot and a prominent afterpotential (Biales *et al.*, 1977; Dufy *et al.*, 1979; Ozawa and Kimura, 1979). Since these action potentials persist in the presence of tetrodotoxin or in the absence of Na^+ and can be reduced by the calcium blocker D600, it was suggested that the Ca^{2+} channel is responsible for most of the spike activities of pituitary cells (Douglas and Taraskevitch, 1977). When thyrotropin-releasing hormone (TRH) is injected in the vicinity of the cell membrane, it transiently hyperpolarizes the membrane and after several seconds delay, a train of action potentials is elicited. This spiking activity could last up to as long as 10 min (Dufy *et al.*, 1979; Ozawa and Kimura, 1979; Ozawa, 1981) (Fig. 8).

TRH stimulates the release of prolactin. This process is partially dependent on the Ca^{2+} concentration in the incubation medium. The acute prolactin release can be completely blocked by the Ca^{2+} antagonist Co^{2+} and partially blocked by organic Ca^{2+} antagonists such as nifedipine and verapamil (Tan and Tashjian, 1984). The release can also be stimulated by elevated external K^+ concentration, the response of which requires the presence of extracellular Ca^{2+}. These observations lead to the proposal that Ca^{2+} entry during the TRH-elicited action potential stimulates the release of prolactin. However, this concept of stimulus-release coupling is not entirely consistent with observations that TRH causes a large increase in $^{45}Ca^{2+}$ efflux but has no measurable effect on the influx of $^{45}Ca^{2+}$ (Williams, 1976; Geras *et al.*, 1982). An alternative hypothesis suggests that TRH mobilizes the Ca^{2+} from intracellular stores which leads to the transient increase of cytosal Ca^{2+} concentration and to the release of prolactin (Gershengorn and Thaw, 1983). This idea has gained some support from the patch-clamp studies of the TRH effect on membrane current (Ritchie, 1983). Whole-cell recording of GH3 cells showed that TRH hyperpolarized the membrane potential by activating $K^+_{(Ca)}$ channels. Since the activation of $K^+_{(Ca)}$ current persists in Ca^{2+}-free solution, or when the voltage-dependent Ca^{2+} channel is completely blocked by cadmium chloride, the source of Ca^{2+} for the activation of $K^+_{(Ca)}$ must be intracellular (Ritchie, 1983).

Preliminary studies showed that TRH also decreased voltage-dependent K^+ current and slowed the activation of this current (Dubinsky and Oxford, 1984). The role of the ion channel in the release mechanism is not quite clear at present. It remains to be established whether the effect of TRH on voltage-dependent K^+ channels indeed results in repetitive firing of action potentials and whether there is a link between Ca^{2+} entry during the regenerative action potential and maintenance of internal stores of calcium.

6. NEUROTRANSMITTER RELEASE

6.1. Growth Cone

The membrane patch can also be used as a probe to study neurotransmitter release at the nerve terminal or synapse. In a number of in vitro and in vivo systems, the exploring growth cone can have functional synaptic transmission with the muscle cells minutes after the formation of the synapse between the nerve and the muscle (Cohen, 1980; Kidokoro and Yeh, 1982). It is of interest to know whether the growth cones have acquired the ability to release the appropriate neurotransmitter before or after contacting their target cells. Hume et al. (1983) and Young and Poo (1983) designed a bioassay to test this. They pulled from the cultured myotube an outside-out patch of membrane containing a high density of ACh receptors and placed it close to a growth cone of either an embryonic chick ciliary ganglion neuron or an isolated Xenopus embryonic neuron. The rate and location of ACh release can then be studied by monitoring activities of ACh channels in the patch pipette. In both systems, a large increase of channel events was observed as the patch electrode approached the growth cone in the absence of target cells. Thus, the growth cones had already obtained the machinery and the neurotransmitter prior to contacting the target cells. In a Xenopus neuron, the growth cones release ACh spontaneously (Young and Poo, 1983), whereas growth cones of ciliary ganglion neurons release ACh only after the cell bodies of the neurons are repetitively stimulated (Hume et al., 1983). This approach is very useful in studying the properties of growth cones during development and their relationship to target cells during synaptogenesis. This imaginative use of an excised patch of membrane illustrates another potential of this technique.

6.2. Exocytosis

The chromaffin cells of the mammalian adrenal medulla are derived from the neural crest. They respond to cholinergic preganglionic sympathetic stimuli and secrete catecholamines into the bloodstream. They have many of the characteristics of sympathetic neuronal postganglionic cells. They have a resting membrane potential of -50 to -80 mV and are capable of generating all-or-none action potentials (Biales et al., 1976). ACh depolarizes chromaffin cells, triggers action potentials, and stimulates the release of catecholamines (Douglas et al., 1967; Douglas, 1975). It was suggested that ACh increases the influx of Na^+ and possibly Ca^{2+}. The Ca^{2+} entry, in turn, triggers the secretion of catecholamines. It is assumed that release of the content of chromaffin granules is brought about by exocytosis. This process involves fusion of the secretory granules with the plasma membrane and release of the contents into the extracellular medium (Abrahams and Holtzman, 1973; Baker and Knight, 1981).

Taking advantage of the fact that small cells can be voltage-clamped with a patch electrode, Neher and Marty (1982) studied the mechanism of exocytosis. If exocytosis were the result of a vesicle fusing to the plasma membrane, the area of this membrane should increase with the process. Since membrane capacitance is proportional to the area of the membrane, it can be used as the parameter to determine the increase of membrane area resulting from the fusion of the granules and plasma membranes. The method designed can detect capacitance changes of 0.4×10^{-15} F which is sufficiently sensitive to resolve membrane areal changes resulting from the fusion of single vesicles with a diameter of 0.12 μm (Neher and Marty, 1982). Electron microscopic observation indicates that the diameter of catecholamine-containing granules ranges from 0.1 to 0.4 μm (Fenwick et al., 1978; Unisicker et al., 1980); and the small and large electron-lucent vacuoles formed after endocytosis have a diameter of 0.08 μm (Benedeczky and Smith, 1972) and 0.2–1 μm (Baker and Knight, 1981), respectively. Thus, if vesicle fusion is not numerous, one can observe a step increase or decrease of membrane capacitance which corresponds to fusion or budding of single vesicles on the inner face of the membrane. When the extracellular Ca^{2+} concentration was maintained at 0.2 μM, the spontaneous increase or decrease of capacitance step expected from exocytosis or endocytosis was observed (Neher and Marty, 1982). The frequency of the step change of capacitance was increased when Ca^{2+} influx was enhanced by activating Ca^{2+} channels with a short depolarizing voltage pulse. A large step decrease of capacitance (20–80 × 10^{-15} F) occurs seconds after extensive stimulation. These capacitance changes were not observed when internal Ca^{2+} was maintained at a low level (10 nM). This measurement gave physiological evidence that vesicle fusion accompanied the exocytosis and suggested the role of Ca^{2+} in the fusion process. Since the change in cell capacitance can be abolished by the potent calmodulin inhibitor trifluoperazine, this suggests that the effect of Ca^{2+} is mediated by the calcium-binding protein calmodulin (Clapham and Neher, 1984).

7. AGGREGATION OF CHANNEL PROTEINS

Transport proteins or channel proteins are often distributed unevenly in the membrane. The mobility of these proteins is sometimes restricted. For example, electron microscope autoradiographic studies of α-bungarotoxin binding sites have shown that the acetylcholine receptor (AChR) is closely packed at the crest of the junctional fold (30,000 sites/μm²) (Hartzell and Fambrough, 1973; Axelrod et al., 1976; Land et al., 1977). The density of AChR decreases rapidly to less than 1200 per μm² at the bottom of the fold 1 μm away. The AChR aggregates, once formed, are extremely stable. The degradation of junctional AChR has a half-life of 10 days (Weiberg et al., 1981). The distribution of AChR is tied closely to the development of the cells. During the initial developmental stage, AChR are distributed uniformly along the myotubes; as the nerve makes synaptic contact with the myotubes, AChR assemble to form aggregates. The size of the aggregates at the junctional region increases and the density of the extrajunctional receptors steadily decreases with development (Bevan and Steinbach, 1977). In cultured myotubes, neurites can also induce the clustering of AChR at the synaptic regions (Anderson et al., 1977; Frank and Fishbach, 1979). It is suggested that a trophic substance which is secreted from nerve terminals induces the aggregation of AChR (Podleski et al., 1978; Jessell et al., 1979; Bauer et al., 1981). This hypothesis received further support when the same sequence of events was observed in uninnervated cultured rat muscle after its exposure to embryonic brain extract (Olek et al., 1983).

It has long been known that action potentials in vertebrate motor neurons originate at the axon hillock, the initial segment of axon emerging from the cell body, and not from the cell body itself (Coombs et al., 1957; Fuortes et al., 1957). Dodge and Cooley (1973) have suggested that Na^+ channel density is highest at the axon hillock and declines sharply toward the cell body and dendrite. Differences of Na^+ channel densities between cell body and neurite have also been observed in cultured neural cells by autoradiographic studies of iodinated scorpion toxin binding sites (Catterall, 1981). The binding activities drop sevenfold from neurite to cell body within 10 μm. Using mild osmotic shock, Chiu and Ritchie (1980, 1981) exposed the channels underneath the myelin sheath and found that the number of Na^+ channels in the internode region was about 250 times less than at the nodal region of rabbit nerve. The distribution of the Ca^{2+} channel is also not uniform. The Ca^{2+} channel tends to concentrate within the presynaptic nerve terminal (Katz and Miledi, 1969). Over 90% of the Ca^{2+} channels in vertebrate skeletal muscle cells are located in the transverse tubular membrane. The density of these Ca^{2+} channels is about 4 times that of the Ca^{2+} channel in the plasma membrane (Almers and Stirling, 1984). Thus, the aggregation of ion channels is a common occurrence in biological membranes.

The aggregation of channels can be studied by measuring current flow from a localized patch of membrane. Using a similar circuit design of single-channel recording. Stühmer and Almers (1982) and Smith et al. (1982) have recorded current from a membrane patch (5–20 μm) containing a few hundred channels. Since the seal resistance is quite low (<2 MΩ), the measurement errors introduced by the series resistance of the electrode and the leakage current across the seal are compensated electronically (Stühmer et al., 1983) or are eliminated by using a concentric pipette (Roberts and Almers, 1984). Comparing the current flow from axonal and somatic patches, Smith et al., (1982) found that the density of Na^+ channels in the soma of both *Aplysia* neurons and cultured spinal cord neurons is, at most, 10–20% of the channel density in the axon. They suggested that the Na^+ channel density in the soma may be too low to generate an action potential. Thus, soma membrane is probably passive and serves as the return pathway for spike current initiated in the axons.

Stühmer and Almers (1982) studied the lateral distribution of Na^+ channels in the sarcolemma of frog skeletal muscle and detected a two- to fivefold variation in Na^+ current amplitude over a distance of 10–30 μm. They further used the patch pipette as a light guide to pass ultraviolet light and destroyed the ion channels in the pipette. The rate of recovery of ion current after destruction of the channel can be used as an index of the mobility of the channels. When this technique was used in frog skeletal muscle, the mobility of Na^+ channels was rather low.

Although most of the studies were done on intact cells, culture systems are good models for studying the distribution of channel proteins. Combining the biochemical, anatomical, and patch-clamp techniques, we can start to tackle some fascinating questions: How do other nonrandomized distributions of channel proteins affect the function of cells? How is the aggregation of channels maintained?

8. SUMMARY

The advent of the giga-seal patch-clamp technique has generated a great deal of excitement among membrane physiologists. The method has provided investigators with a powerful tool to study the properties of small cells effectively, to observe the behavior of individual ion channels with high resolution, and to control the solution content on both sides of the membrane with ease. Because of their clean membrane surface, cultured cells are especially suitable for patch-clamp recordings. Cultured cells provide numerous cell types, accessibility to many biochemical and anatomical manipulations, and the possibility of obtaining homogeneous cell populations. The combination of patch technique and cell cultures gives membrane physiologists unusual freedom to choose electrophysiological problems rather than being limited to a few technically manageable preparations. In a short 5 years, we have benefited handsomely with such approaches as described here.

We have, however, to be keenly aware of the limitation of culture systems. The properties of cultured cells vary with their stage of cell development, origin, culture environment, and the time in culture. Whenever a culture preparation is chosen, one of the first considerations has to be whether the *in vivo* phenomenon we are interested in is faithfully reflected in the cultured cells. This determination is by no means easy. Nevertheless, efforts should be made to demonstrate whether the particular properties studied in cultured cells are similar to those found *in vivo* and whether the responses to experimental manipulations *in vitro* resemble those observed in intact systems. Only by frequent evaluation and validation can we use these two versatile techniques and make rapid progress in understanding many fascinating phenomena in neurobiology.

ACKNOWLEDGMENTS

The author wishes to thank Drs. G. Ehrenstein, N. Moran, A. Ritchie, and T. Smith for their comments. The support of National Institutes of Health Grants NS-19352 and NS-31599 is acknowledged.

REFERENCES

Abrahams, S. J., and Holtzman, E., 1973, Secretion and endocytosis in insulin-stimulated rat adrenal medulla cells, *J. Cell Biol.* **56**:540–558.

Adams, P. R., 1975, An analysis of the dose–response curve at voltage clamped frog endplates, *Pfluegers Arch.* **360**:145–153.

Aldrich, R. W., and Stevens, C. F., 1983, Inactivation of open and closed sodium channel determined separately, *Cold Spring Harbor Symp. Quant. Biol.* **48**:147–153.

Aldrich, R. W., and Yellen, G., 1983, Analysis of nonstationary channel kinetics, in: *Single-Channel Recording* (B. Sakmann and E. Neher, eds.), Plenum Press, New York, pp. 287–300.

Aldrich, R. W., Corey, D. P., and Stevens, C. F., 1983, A reinterpretation of mammalian sodium channel gating based on single channel recording, *Nature* 306:436–441.

Almers, W., and Stirling, C., 1984, Distribution of transport proteins over animal cell membranes. *J. Membr. Biol.* **77**:169–186.

Anderson, C. R., and Stevens, C. F., 1973, Voltage clamp analysis of acetylcholine produced by end-plate current fluctuation at frog neuromuscular junction, *J. Physiol.* **235**:655–691.

Anderson, M. J., Cohen, M. W., and Zoryehta, E., 1977, Effect of innervation on the distribution of acetylcholine receptors on cultured muscle cells, *J. Physiol.* **268**:731–746.

Armstrong, C. M., 1981, Sodium channels and gating currents, *Physiol. Rev.* **61**:644–683.

Auerbach, A., and Sachs, F., 1983, Flickering of a nicotinic ion channel to a subconductance state, *Biophys. J.* **42**:1–10.

Axelrod, D., Ravdin, P., Koppel, D. E., Schlessiges, J., Webb, W. W., Elso, E. L., and Podleski, T. R., 1976, Lateral motion of fluorescently labelled acetylcholine receptors in membranes of developing muscle fibers, *Proc. Natl. Acad. Sci. USA* **73**:4594–4598.

Baker, P. F., and Knight, D. E., 1981, Calcium control of exocytosis and endocytosis in bovine adrenal medullary cells, *Philos. Trans. R. Soc. London Ser. B* **296**:83–103.

Barrett, J. N., Magleby, K. L., and Pallotta, B. S., 1982, Properties of single calcium-activated potassium channels in cultured rat muscle, *J. Physiol.* **331**:211–230.

Bauer, H. C., Daniels, M. P., Pudimat, P. A., Jacques, L., Sugiyama, H., and Christian, C. N., 1981, Characterization and partial purification of a neuronal factor which increases acetylcholine receptor aggregation on cultured muscle cells, *Brain Res.* **209**:395–404.

Bean, R. C., Shepherd, W. C., Chan, H., and Eichner, J., 1969, Discrete conductance fluctuations in lipid bilayer protein membrane, *J. Gen. Physiol.* **53**:741–757.

Benedeczky, I., and Smith, A. D., 1972, Ultrastructural studies on the adrenal medulla of golden hamster: Origin and fate of secretory granules, *Z. Zellforsch. Mikrosk. Anat.* **124**:367–386.

Bevan, S., and Steinbach, J. H., 1977, The distribution of α-bungarotoxin binding sites on mammalian skeletal muscle developing *in vivo, J. Physiol.* **267:**195–213.

Bezanilla, F., and Armstrong, C. M., 1977, Inactivation of Na channel, *J. Gen. Physiol.* **70:**549–566.

Biales, B., Dichter, M., and Tischler, A., 1976, Electrical excitability of cultured adrenal chromaffin cells, *J. Physiol.* **262:**743–753.

Biales, B., Dichter, M. A., and Tischler, A., 1977, Sodium and calcium action potential in pituitary cells, *Nature* **267:**172–174.

Blatz, A. L., and Magleby, K. L., 1983, Single voltage-dependent chloride-selective channels of large conductance in cultured rat muscle, *Biophys. J.* **43:**237–241.

Bolsover, S. R., 1981, Calcium dependent potassium current in barnacle photoreceptor, *J. Gen. Physiol.* **78:**617–636.

Brehm, P., Eckert, R., and Tillotson, D., 1980, Calcium-mediated inactivation of calcium current in paramecium, *J. Physiol.* **306:**193–203.

Brown, A. M., Morimoto, K., Tsuda, Y., and Wilson, D. L., 1981, Ca current-dependent and voltage-dependent inactivation of Ca channels in *Helix aspersa, J. Physiol.* **320:**193–218.

Byerly, L., and Hagiwara, S., 1982, Calcium currents in internally perfused nerve cell bodies of *Limnea stagnalis, J. Physiol.* **322:**503–528.

Cacheline, A. B., dePeyer, J. E., Kokubun, S., and Reuter, H., 1983, Ca^{2+} channel modulation by 8-bromocyclic AMP in cultured heart cells, *Nature* **304:**462–464.

Camardo, J. S., and Siegelbaum, S. A., 1983, Single-channel analysis in *Aplysia* neurons: A specific K^+ channel is modulated by serotonin and cyclic AMP, in: *Single-Channel Recording* (B. Sakmann and E. Neher, eds.), Plenum Press, New York, pp. 409–422.

Castellucci, V., and Kandel, E. R., 1976, Presynaptic facilitation as a mechanism for behavioral sensitization in *Aplysia, Science* **194:**1176–1178.

Catterall, W. A., 1981, Localization of sodium channels in cultured neural cells, *J. Neurosci.* **1:**777–783.

Chabala, L. D., Lester, H. A., and Sheridan, R. E., 1982, Single channel currents from cholinergic receptors in cultured muscle, *Soc. Neurosci. Abstr.* **8:**498.

Chiu, S. Y., and Ritchie, J. M., 1980, Potassium channels in nodal and internodal axonal membrane of mammalian myelinated fibres, *Nature* **284:**170–171.

Chiu, S. Y., and Ritchie, J. M., 1981, Evidence for the presence of potassium channels in the paranodal region of acutely demyelinated mammalian single nerve fibers, *J. Physiol.* **313:**415–437.

Clapham, D., and Neher, E., 1984, Changes in cell capacitance used to measure exocytosis are prevented by the calmodulin inhibitor, trifluoperazine, *Biophys. J.* **45:**395a.

Cohen, S. A., 1980, Early nerve–muscle synapses *in vitro* release transmitter over post-synaptic membrane having low acetylcholine sensitivity, *Proc. Natl. Acad. Sci. USA* **77:**644–648.

Colquhoun, D., and Hawkes, A. G., 1981, On the stochastic properties of single ion channels, *Proc. R. Soc. London Ser. B* **211:**205–235.

Colquhoun, D., and Hawkes, A. G., 1983, The principles of the stochastic interpretation of ion-channel mechanisms, in: *Single-Channel Recording* (B. Sakmann and E. Neher, eds.), Plenum Press, New York, pp. 135–176.

Colquhoun, D., and Sakmann, B., 1981, Fluctuations in the microsecond time range of the current through single acetylcholine receptor ion channels, *Nature* **294:**464–466.

Colquhoun, D., and Sakmann, B., 1983, Bursts of openings in transmitter-activated ion channels, in: *Single-Channel Recording* (B. Sakmann and E. Neher, eds.), Plenum Press, New York, pp. 345–364.

Colquhoun, D., and Sigworth, T. J., 1983, Fitting and statistical analysis of single channel recordings, in: *Single-Channel Recording* (B. Sakmann and E. Neher, eds.), Plenum Press, New York, pp. 191–263.

Colquhoun, D., Neher, E., Reuter, H., and Stevens, C. F., 1981, Inward current channels activated by intracellular Ca in cultured cardiac cells, *Nature* **294**:752–754.

Conti, F., DeFlice, L. J., and Wanke, E., 1975, Potassium and sodium ion current noise in the membrane of the squid giant axon, *J. Physiol.* **248**:45–82.

Conti, F., Hille, B., Neumcke, B., Nonner, W., and Stampfli, R., 1976, Measurement of the conductance of the sodium channel from current fluctuations at the node of Ranvier, *J. Physiol.* **262**:699–727.

Coombs, J. S., Curtis, D. R., and Eccles, J. C., 1957, The generation of impulses in motoneurones, *J. Physiol.* **139**:232–249.

Corey, D. P., 1983, Patch clamp: Current excitement in membrane physiology, *Neurosci. Comment.* **1**:99–110.

Corey, D. P., and Stevens, C. F., 1983, Science and technology of patch recording electrodes, in: *Single-Channel Recording* (B. Sakmann and E. Neher, eds.), Plenum Press, New York, pp. 53–68.

Cull-Candy, S. G., Miledi, R., and Parker, I., 1981, Single glutamate-activated channels recorded from locust muscle fibers with perfused patch clamp electrodes, *J. Physiol.* **321**:195–210.

Dionne, V. E., and Leibowitz, M. D., 1982, Acetylcholine receptor kinetics: A description from single-channel currents at snake neuromuscular junctions, *Biophys. J.* **39**:253–261.

Dionne, V. E., Steinbach, J. H., and Stevens, C. F., 1978, An analysis of the dose–response relationship at voltage-clamped frog neuromuscular junctions, *J. Physiol.* **281**:421–444.

Dodge, F. A., and Cooley, J. W., 1973, Action potential of the motorneuron, *IBM J. Res. Develop.* **17**(3):219–229.

Douglas, W., 1975, Secrotomotor control of adrenal medullary secretion: Synaptic membrane and ion events in stimulus–secretion coupling, in: *Handbook of Physiology*, Section 7, Volume 6 (H. Blaschko, G. Sayers, and A. D. Smith, eds.), American Physiological Society, Washington D.C., pp. 367–388.

Douglas, W. W., and Taraskevitch, P. S., 1977, Action potential (probably calcium spikes) in normal and adenomatous cells of the anterior pituitary and the stimulant effect of thyrotropin releasing hormone, *J. Physiol.* **272**:41–43.

Douglas, W., Kanno, T., and Sampson, S., 1967, Effects of acetylcholine and other medullary secretagogues and antagonists on the membrane potential of adrenal chromaffin cells: An analysis employing techniques of tissue culture, *J. Physiol.* **188**:107–120.

Dubinsky, J. M., and Oxford, G. S., 1984, Effects of TRH on membrane potassium current in clonal pituitary tumor cells, *Biophys. J.* **45**:143a.

Dufy, B., Vincent, J.-D., Fleury, H., Du Pasquier, P., Gourdji, D., and Tixier-Vidal, A., 1979, Membrane effects of thyrotropin-releasing hormone and estrogen shown by intracellular recording from pituitary cells, *Science* **204**:590–611.

Ebihara, L., Shigeto, N., Lieberman, M., and Johnson, E. A., 1980, The initial inward current in spherical clusters of chick embryonic heart cells, *J. Gen. Physiol.* **75**:437–456.

Ehrenstein, G., and Lecar, H., 1977, Electrically gated ionic channels in lipid bilayers, *Q. Rev. Biophys.* **10**:1–34.

Ehrenstein, G., Blumenthal, R., Latone, R., and Lecar, H., 1974, Kinetics of the opening and closing of individual excitability inducing material channels in a lipid bilayer, *J. Gen. Physiol.* **63**:707–721.

Fenwick, E. M., Fajdiga, P. B., Howe, N. B. S., and Livett, B. G., 1978, Functional and morphological characterization of isolated bovine adrenal medullary cells, *J. Cell Biol.* **76:**12–30.

Fenwick, E. M., Marty, A., and Neher, E., 1982, Sodium and calcium channels in bovine chromaffin cells, *J. Physiol.* **331:**599–635.

Fishman, H. M., Moore, L. E., and Poussart, D. J. M., 1975, Potassium-ion conduction noise in squid axon membrane, *J. Membr. Biol.* **24:**305–328.

Frank, E., and Fishbach, G. D., 1979, Early events in neuromuscular junction formation in vitro: Induction of acetylcholine receptor clusters in the postsynaptic membrane and morphology of newly formed synapses, *J. Cell Biol.* **83:**143–158.

French, R. J., and Horn, R., 1983, Sodium channel gating: Models, mimics and modifiers, *Annu. Rev. Biophys. Bioeng.* **12:**319–356.

Fuortes, M. G. F., Frank, K., and Becker, M. C., 1957, Steps in the production of moto-neuron spikes, *J. Gen. Physiol.* **40:**735–752.

Geras, E., Rebecchi, M. J., and Gershengorn, M. C., 1982, Evidence that stimulation of thyrotropin and prolactin secretion by thyrotropin-releasing hormone occur via different calcium-mediated mechanisms: Studies with verapamil, *Endocrinology* **110:**901–906.

Gershengorn, M. C., and Thaw, C., 1983, Calcium influx is not required for TRH to elevate free cytoplasmic calcium in GH3 cells, *Endocrinology* **113:**1522–1524.

Goldman, L., 1976, Kinetics of channel gating in excitable membrane, *Q. Rev. Biophys.* **9:**491–526.

Gorman, A. L. F., Hermann, A., and Thomas, M. V., 1981, Intracellular calcium and the control of neural pacemaker activity, *Fed. Proc.* **40:**2233–2239.

Hagiwara, S., and Byerly, L., 1981, Calcium channel, *Annu. Rev. Neurosci.* **4:**69–125.

Hagiwara, S., and Ohmori, H., 1982, Studies of calcium channels in rat clonal pituitary cells with patch electrode voltage clamp, *J. Physiol.* **331:**231–252.

Hamill, O. P., 1983, Membrane ion channels, in: *Topics in Molecular Pharmacology* (A. S. V. Bergen and G. C. K. Roberts, eds.), Elsevier Science Publishers, New York, pp. 182–205.

Hamill, O. P., and Sakmann, B., 1981, Multiple conductance states of single acetylcholine receptor channels in embryonic muscle cells, *Nature* **294:**462–464.

Hamill, O. P., Marty, A., Neher, E., Sakmann, B., and Sigworth, F. J., 1981, Improved patch-clamp techniques for high-resolution current recording from cells and cell-free membrane patches, *Pfluegers Arch.* **391:**85–100.

Hartzell, H., and Fambrough, D. M., 1973, Acetylcholine receptor production and incorporation into membrane of developing muscle fibers, *Develop. Biol.* **30:**153–165.

Hodgkin, A. L., and Huxley, A. F., 1952, A quantitative description of membrane current and its application to conduction and excitation in nerve, *J. Physiol.* **116:**497–506.

Horn, R., and Lange, K., 1983, Estimating kinetic constants from single channel data, *Biophys. J.* **43:**207–223.

Horn, R., and Patlak, J., 1980, Single channel currents from excised patches of muscle membrane, *Proc. Natl. Acad. Sci. USA* **77:**6930–6934.

Horn, R., Patlak, J., and Stevens, C. F., 1981, Sodium channels need not open before they inactivate, *Nature* **291:**426–427.

Horn, R., Vandenberg, C. A., and Lange, K., 1984, Statistical analysis of single sodium channels: Effects of N-bromoacetamide, *Biophys. J.* **45:**323–335.

Huang, L.-Y.M., Moran, N., and Ehrenstein, G., 1982, Batrachotoxin modifies the gating kinetics of sodium channels in internally perfused neuroblastoma cells, *Proc. Natl. Acad. Sci. USA* **79:**2082–2085.

Huang, L.-Y.M., Moran, N., and Ehrenstein, G., 1984, Gating kinetics of batrachotoxin-modified sodium channels in neuroblastoma cells determined from single-channel measurements, *Biophys. J.* **45:**313–322.

Hume, R. I., Role. L. W., and Fischbach, G. D., 1983, Acetylcholine release from growth cones detected with patches of acetylcholine receptor-rich membranes, *Nature* **305:**632–634.

Isenberg, G., 1977, Cardiac Purkinje fibres: Ca^{2+} controls the potassium permeability via the conductance components g_{k1} and g_{k2}, *Pfluegers Arch.* **371:**77–85.

Jackson, M. B., and Lecar, H., 1979, Single postsynaptic channel currents in tissue cultured muscle, *Nature* **282:**863–864.

Jackson, M. B., Wong, B. S., Morris, C. E., Lecar, H., and Christian, C. N., 1983, Successive openings of the same acetylcholine receptor channel are correlated in open time, *Biophys. J.* **42:**109–114.

Jessell, T. M., Siegel, R. E., and Fischbach, G. D., 1979, Induction of acetylcholine receptors on cultured skeletal muscle by a factor extracted from brain and spinal cord, *Proc. Natl. Acad. Sci. USA* **76:**5397–5401.

Katz, B., and Miledi, R., 1969, Tetrodotoxin-resistant electric activity in presynaptic terminals, *J. Physiol.* **203:**459–487.

Katz, B., and Miledi, R., 1970, Membrane noise produced by acetylcholine, *Nature* **226:**962–963.

Katz, B., and Miledi, R., 1972, The statistical nature of the acetylcholine potential and its molecular components, *J. Physiol.* **224:**665–699.

Kidokoro, Y., and Yeh, E., 1982, Initial synaptic transmission at the growth cone in *Xenopus* nerve–muscle cultures, *Proc. Natl. Acad. Sci. USA* **79:**6727–6731.

Klein, M., Comardo, J. S., and Kandel, E. R., 1982, Serotonin modulates a specific potassium current in the sensory neurons that show presynaptic facilitation in *Aplysia*, *Proc. Natl. Acad. Sci. USA* **79:**5713–5717.

Kostyuk, P. G., and Krishtal, D. A., 1977, Separation of sodium and calcium currents in the somatic membrane of mollusc neurons, *J. Physiol.* **270:**545–568.

Kostyuk, P. G., Krishtal, D. A., and Pidoplichko, V. I., 1975, Effect of internal fluoride and phosphate on membrane currents during intracellular dialysis of nerve cells, *Nature* **257:**691–693.

Land, B. R., Podleski, T. R., Salpeter, E. E., and Salpeter, M. M., 1977, Acetylcholine receptor distribution on myotubes in culture correlated to acetylcholine sensitivity, *J. Physiol.* **269:**155–176.

Latorre, R., and Miller, C., 1983, Conductance and selectivity in potassium channel, *J. Membr. Biol.* **71:**11–30.

Latorre, R., Vergara, C., and Hildago, C., 1982, Reconstitution in planar lipid bilayers of Ca dependent K channel from transverse tubule membrane isolated from rabbit skeletal muscle, *Proc. Natl. Acad. Sci. USA* **79:**805–809.

Lee, K. S., Akaike, N., and Brown, A. M., 1978, Properties of internal perfused voltage-clamped, isolated nerve cell bodies, *J. Gen. Physiol.* **71:**489–507.

Lee, K. S., Akaike, N., and Brown, A. M., 1980, The suction pipette method for internal perfusion and voltage clamp in small excitable cells, *J. Neurosci. Methods* **2:**58–78.

Lee, K. S. and Tsien, R. W., 1983, Mechanism of calcium channel blockade by verapamil, D600, diltiazem and nitrendipine in single dialysed heart cells. *Nature* **302:**790–794.

Lux, H. D., Neher, E., and Marty, A., 1981, Single channel activity associated with the calcium dependent outward current in *Helix pomatia*, *Pfluegers Arch.* **389:**293–295.

Magleby, K. L., and Stevens, C. F., 1972, A quantitative description of end-plate currents, *J. Physiol.* **223**:173–197.

Marban, E., and Tsien, R. W., 1981, Is the slow inward calcium current of heart muscle inactivated by calcium?, *Biophys. J.* **33**:143a.

Marty, A., 1981, Ca-dependent K channels with large unitary conductance in chromaffin cell membranes, *Nature* **291**:497–500.

Marty, A., and Neher, E., 1983, Tight-seal whole-cell recording, in: *Single-Channel Recording* (B. Sakmann and E. Neher, eds.), Plenum Press, New York, pp. 107–122.

Maruyama, Y., and Petersen, O. H., 1982a, Single channel currents in isolated patches of plasma membrane from basal surface of pancreatic acini, *Nature* **299**:159–161.

Maruyama, Y., and Petersen, O. H., 1982b, Cholecystokinin activation of single channel currents is mediated by internal messenger in pancreatic acinar cells, *Nature* **300**:61–63.

Meech, R. W., 1976, The sensitivity of *Helix aspersa* neurones to injected calcium ions, *J. Physiol.* **237**:259–277.

Moolenaar, W. H., and Spector, I., 1977, Membrane currents examined under voltage clamp in cultured neuroblastoma cells, *Science* **196**:331–333.

Moolenaar, W. H., and Spector, I., 1978, Ion currents in cultured mouse neuroblastoma cells under voltage clamp conditions, *J. Physiol.* **278**:265–286.

Nathan, R., and DeHaan, R., 1979, Voltage clamp analysis of embryonic heart cell aggregates, *J. Gen. Physiol.* **73**:175–178.

Neher, E., and Marty, A., 1982, Discrete changes of cell membrane capacitance observed under conditions of enhanced secretion in bovine adrenal chromaffin cells, *Proc. Natl. Acad. Sci. USA* **79**:6712–6716.

Neher, E., and Sakmann, B., 1976, Single-channel currents recorded from membrane of denervated frog muscle fibres, *Nature* **260**:779–802.

Neher, E., and Steinbach, J. H., 1978, Local anesthetics transiently block currents through single acetylcholine-receptor channels, *J. Physiol.* **277**:153–176.

Neher, E., Sakmann, B., and Steinbach, J. H., 1978, The extracellular patch clamp: A method for resolving currents through individual open channels in biological membranes, *Pfluegers Arch.* **375**:219–228.

Nelson, D. J., and Sachs, F., 1979, Single ionic channels observed in tissue-cultured muscle, *Nature* **282**:861–863.

Olek, A. J., Pudimat, P. A., and Daniels, M. P., 1983, Direct observation of the rapid aggregation of acetylcholine receptors on identified cultured myotubes after exposure to embryonic brain extract, *Cell* **34**:255–264.

Osterrieder, W., Brum, G., Hescheler, J., Trautwein, W., Flockerizi, V., and Hofmann, F., 1982, Injection of subunits of cyclic AMP-dependent protein kinase into cardiac myocytes modulates Ca^{2+} current, *Nature* **298**:576–578.

Ozawa, S., 1981, Biphasic effect of thyrotropin-releasing hormone on membrane K^+ permeability in rat clonal pituitary cells, *Brain Res.* **209**:240–244.

Ozawa, S., and Kimura, N., 1979, Membrane potential changes caused by thyrotropin-releasing hormone in the clonal GH3 cell line and their relationship to secretion of pituitary hormone, *Proc. Natl. Acad. Sci. USA* **76**:6017–6020.

Patlak, J., and Horn, R., 1982, Effect of N-bromoacetamide on single sodium channel currents in excised membrane patches, *J. Gen. Physiol.* **79**:333–351.

Podleski, T. R., Axelrod, D., Ravdin, P., Greenberg, I., Johnson, M. M., and Salpeter, M. M., 1978, Nerve extract induces increase and redistribution of acetylcholine receptors on cloned cells, *Proc. Natl. Acad. Sci. USA* **75**:2035–2039.

Putney, J. W., 1979, Stimulus–permeability coupling: Role of Ca in receptor regulation of membrane permeability, *Pharmacol. Rev.* **30**:209–245.

Quandt, F. N., and Narahashi, T., 1982, Modification of single Na$^+$ channels by batrachotoxin, *Proc. Natl. Acad. Sci. USA* **79:**6732–6736.

Reuter, H., 1967, The dependence of the slow inward current on external Ca concentration in Purkinje fibers, *J. Physiol.* **192:**479–492.

Reuter, H., 1983, Calcium channel modulation by neurotransmitters, enzymes and drugs, *Nature* **301:**569–574.

Reuter, H., and Scholz, H., 1977, The regulation of the calcium conductance of cardiac muscle by adrenaline, *J. Physiol.* **264:**49–62.

Reuter, H., Stevens, C. F., Tsien, R. W., and Yellen, G., 1982, Properties of single calcium channels in cardiac cell culture, *Nature* **297:**501–504.

Ritchie, A. K., 1983, Activation of K$^+$ permeability in the GH3 anterior pituitary cell line by thyrotropin releasing hormone, *Soc. Neurosci. Abstr.* 22.

Roberts, W. M., and Almers, W., 1984, An improved "loose patch" voltage clamp for muscle fibers and neurons, *Biophys. J.* **45:**185a.

Sachs, F., 1983, Is the acetylcholine receptor a unit-conductance channel?, in: *Single-Channel Recording* (B. Sakmann and E. Neher, eds.), Plenum Press, New York, pp. 365–376.

Sachs, F., and Lecar, H., 1973, Acetylcholine noise in tissue culture muscle cells, *Nature New Biol.* **246:**214–216.

Sakmann, B., and Neher, E., 1983, Geometric parameters of pipettes and membrane patches, in: *Single-Channel Recording* (B. Sakmann and E. Neher, eds.), Plenum Press, New York, pp. 37–51.

Sakman, B., Patlak, J. and Neher, E., 1980, Single acetylcholine-activated channels show burst-kinetics in presence of desensitizing concentrations of agonist, *Nature* **286:**71–73.

Siegelbaum, S. A., Camardo, J. S., and Kandel, E. R., 1982, Serotonin and cAMP close single K channels in *Aplysia* sensory neurones, *Nature* **299:**413–417.

Sigworth, F. J., 1982, Fluctuations in the current through open ACh-receptor channels, *Biophys. J.* **37:**309a.

Sigworth, F. J., 1983, Electronic design of the patch clamp, in: *Single-Channel Recording* (B. Sakmann and E. Neher, eds.), Plenum Press, New York, pp. 3–35.

Sigworth, F., and Neher, E., 1980, Single Na$^+$ channels in cultured rat muscle cells, *Nature* **287:**447–449.

Sine, S. M., and Steinbach, J. H., 1984, Activation of a nicotinic acetylcholine receptor, *Biophys. J.* **45:**175–185.

Smith, T. G., Jr., Futamachi, K., and Ehrenstein, G., 1982, Site of action potential generation in a giant neuron of *Aplysia californica*, *Brain Res.* **242:**184–189.

Stühmer, W., and Almers, W., 1982, Photobleaching through glass micropipettes: Sodium channels without lateral mobility in sarcolemma of frog skeletal muscle, *Proc. Natl. Acad. Sci. USA* **79:**946–950.

Stühmer, W., Roberts, W. M., and Almers, W., 1983, The loose patch clamp, in: *Single-Channel Recording* (B. Sakmann and E. Neher, eds.), Plenum Press, New York, pp. 123–134.

Tan, K. N., and Tashjian, A. H., 1984, Voltage-dependent calcium channels in pituitary cells in culture. II. Participation in thyrotropin-releasing hormone action on prolactin release. *J. Biol. Chem.* **259:**427–434.

Tillotson, D., 1979, Inactivation of Ca conductance dependent on entry of cation in molluscan neurons, *Proc. Natl. Acad. Sci. USA* **76:**1497–1500.

Tixier-Vidal, A., and Gourdji, D., 1981, Mechanism of action of synthetic hypothalamic peptides on anterior pituitary cells, *Physiol. Rev.* **61:**974–1011.

Trautwein, W., Taniguchi, J., and Noma, A., 1982, The effect of intracellular cyclic nucleotides and calcium on action potential and acetylcholine response of isolated cardiac
cells, *Pfluegers Arch.* **392:**307–314.

Tsien, R. W., 1983, Calcium channels in excitable cell membranes, *Annu. Rev. Physiol.*
45:341–358.

Unisicker, K., Griesser, G. H., Lindmar, R., Loffelholz, K., and Wolf, U., 1980, Establishment, characterization and fibre outgrowth of isolated bovine adrenal medullary
cells in long-term cultures, *Neuroscience* **5:**1445–1460.

Vandenberg, C. A., and Horn, R. A., 1984, Kinetic properties of single Na channel, *Biophys.
J.* **45:**11a.

Vassort, G., Rougier, O., Garnier, D., Sauviat, M. P., Coraboeuf, E., and Gargouil, Y.
M., 1969, Effects of adrenaline on membrane inward current during the cardiac action
potential, *Pfluegers Arch.* **309:**70–81.

Weiberg, C. B., Reinoss, C. G., and Hall, E. W., 1981, Topographical segregation of old
and new acetylcholine receptors at developing ectopic end plates in adult rat muscle,
J. Cell Biol. **88:**215–218.

Williams, J. A., 1976, Stimulation of Ca efflux from rat pituitary by luteinizing releasing
hormone and other pituitary stimulants, *J. Physiol.* **260:**105–115.

Wong, B. S., Lecar, H., and Adler, M., 1982, Single calcium-dependent potassium channels
in clonal anterior pituitary cells, *Biophys. J.* **39:**313–317.

Yamamoto, D., Yeh, J. Z., and Narahashi, T., 1984, Voltage-dependent calcium block of
normal and tetramethrin-modified single sodium channel, *Biophys. J.* **45:**337–344.

Yellen, G., 1982, Single Ca^{2+}-activated nonselective cation channels in neuroblastoma,
Nature **296:**357–359.

Young, S. H., and Poo, M.-M., 1983, Spontaneous release of transmitter from growth
cones of embryonic neurones, *Nature* **305:**634–637.

Index